# THE ROYAL COLLEGE
# OF PHYSICIANS AND SURGEONS
# OF GLASGOW

A

# THE ROYAL COLLEGE OF PHYSICIANS AND SURGEONS OF GLASGOW

*A short history based on the portraits and other memorabilia*

*by*

TOM GIBSON
*Honorary Curator of the Art Collection*

ISBN 0 86334 016 4 (Trade Edition)

ISBN 0 86334 018 0 (College Edition)

Published by Macdonald Publishers (Edinburgh),
Edgefield Road, Loanhead, Midlothian EH20 9SY



Printed in Scotland by Macdonald Printers (Edinburgh) Ltd.

# CONTENTS

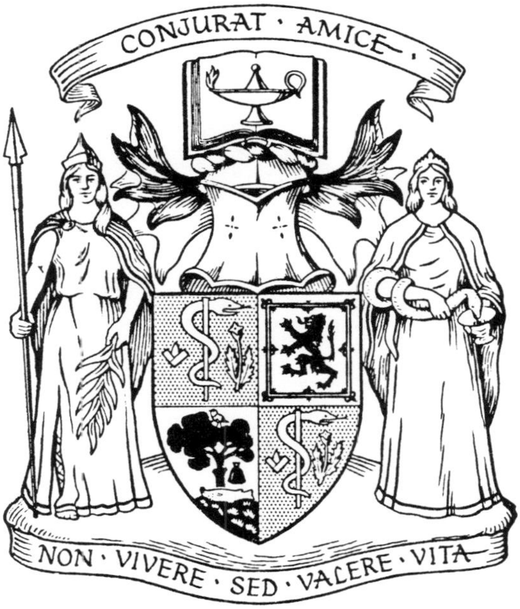
CONJURAT · AMICE ·
NON · VIVERE · SED · VALERE · VITA

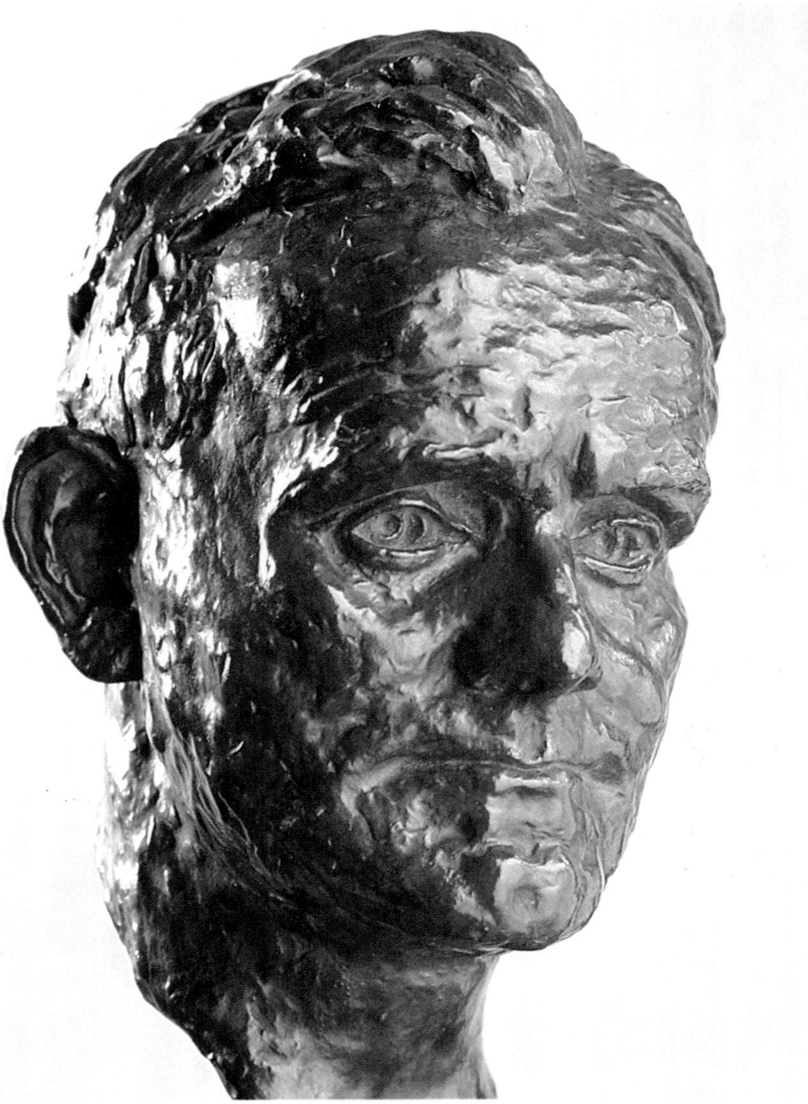

*This head of Dr T. J. Honeyman in bronze by Benno Schotz was presented to the Royal College by Dr Honeyman's family in 1971.*

*Dr Honeyman, a Fellow of the Royal Faculty, gave up medicine for art and became Director of the Glasgow Art Galleries. He continued his interest in the Faculty, however, and was the first Honorary Curator of the Art Collection.*

*During the 1960s he sorted the portraits stored in the basement and had them properly stacked. He also purchased a number of paintings for the College and is responsible for the acquisition of the portrait of James VI.*

# FOREWORD

It began as an intention. Requests for information about those whose portraits hang in the Royal College were frequent, not just from visitors but from Fellows and Members. Some years ago, Sir Robert Wright compiled some brief notes about them but these were incomplete and are now hard to acquire; something more detailed, more comprehensive and more easily available seemed desirable.

The intention became an urgent must when the portrait cellar in the basement was explored in 1979. Here, stored in a rack devised many years before by the late Dr T. J. Honeyman, which at least prevented their traumatising each other but left them exposed to the damp for which the basement is notorious, were more than a dozen portraits in oils and some framed photographs. One or two were damaged or dilapidated beyond recovery but the remainder have been cleaned, restored and mostly reframed. Some were named, some were not; even some of those named were unfamiliar or only vaguely so. With the acquisition of 234 St Vincent Street, new wall space was available; surely if these old portraits had been worthy of being hung in the past, they were not only worthy of being hung today but worthy of an adequate and permanent record.

The writing of this record began as an alphabetical list of biographical sketches. This was soon found unsatisfactory; it meant repeating basic historical background and troublesome cross-indexing; take, for example, the alphabetical separation of Lowe, Hamilton and Spang in such a list. Others could also be grouped in certain historical contexts but an overall pattern did not always emerge at once; indeed, much had been written before some of the pieces were finally placed. In the Faculty/College's history many worthies left no portrait behind, while of those whose portraits survive some are more worthy than others. Some, too, achieved fame in more than one field.

There are however sufficient portraits to span, however briefly, through the lives of their subjects, about three-quarters of our history. I have added an outline sketch of the other quarter to try to make a fairly continuous narrative although, with such a many-facetted institution, there had to be occasional secondary narratives within the main stream.

This book is in no way a definitive College history and a number of important aspects have had to be ignored. It is to be regarded as no more than what it is entitled: data about the subjects of our portraits arranged historically, rather than alphabetically, with sufficient background linkage material to add perspective. Historical writing is often dull and unattractive, because 'there are no pictures', and wherever possible illustrative material from the College collections additional to the portraits themselves has been introduced.

Every writer of history has two personal privileges: the selection of material and comment.

Selection was variably difficult. Some individuals like Lister, Macewen, Livingstone have had whole books written about their lives and data selection had to be ruthless and severe; what was chosen was that which seemed of most interest to the history of the College, medicine and Glasgow. Others with portraits had so little data about them available that even what there was, hardly made a 'sketch'. It was the same with the historical background. Little is known of the Faculty between 1682 and 1733 because the second minute book was accidentally burned. On the other hand, the litigations between the Faculty, and Universities, the Colleges and the Government in the first half of the 19th century fill volumes; to 'sketch' them adequately for a simple narrative took long, and much interesting detail had to be omitted. But the selection is mine and represents much of what I have always wished to know about the College, its portraits and its history. I hope that it may appeal in the same way to others.

To comment is a great temptation and is to be resisted in a work of this kind. Where possible I have let the characters speak for themselves. But this of course inevitably involves selection and indirectly comment. I have tried to make it neither effusive, unkind nor uncalled-for.

With an occasional exception there are neither references nor footnotes. It is not that kind of historical work; the text has been deliberately left uncluttered for easier readability. The sources are many: Duncan's *Memorials* is the standard work for the earlier material but then there are obituaries, the *Dictionary of Eminent Scotsmen*, Comrie's *History of Scottish Medicine*, Medical Directories, *Who's Who*, *Reminiscences of Old Glasgow*, and so on. All are available in the College Library but without the help of Mr A. Rodger, the Librarian, and his staff the book would never have been written. Miss Elizabeth Wilson is worthy of especial thanks: she is a mine of information about all aspects of the College History and has a knack of discovering references and documents previously unknown which have proved invaluable. Mr D. J. A. McIlroy is responsible for the illustrations and I am grateful for his ungrudging assistance.

Miss Lesley M. Cook has typed the manuscript with her usual skill, speed, and accuracy.

# INTRODUCTORY NOTES

The fact that it has had three main homes and several different titles since it was founded in 1599 can be confusing to new readers and visitors to the College; the following outline dates may ease understanding.

1599: No name given in the Charter.
1629: Facultie.
1657: Facultie of Chirurgeons and Physitians.
c 1700: The Faculty of Physicians and Surgeons of Glasgow.
1909: The Royal Faculty of Physicians and Surgeons of Glasgow.
1962: The Royal College of Physicians and Surgeons of Glasgow.

1599: Several *ad hoc* Meeting Places.
1697: First Faculty Building next to Tron Church.
1791: Second Faculty Building in St Enoch Square.
1862: Third and present Faculty Building at 242 St Vincent Street.
1900: Extension next door to 238 St Vincent Street.
1975: Again extended next door to 234 St Vincent Street.

# 1

## THE FOUNDERS AND THE CHARTER

King James VI and I (1566 to 1625)
Maister Peter Lowe (c 1550 to 1610)
Robert Hamilton (c 1565 to 1629)
William Spang (c 1545 to c 1610)

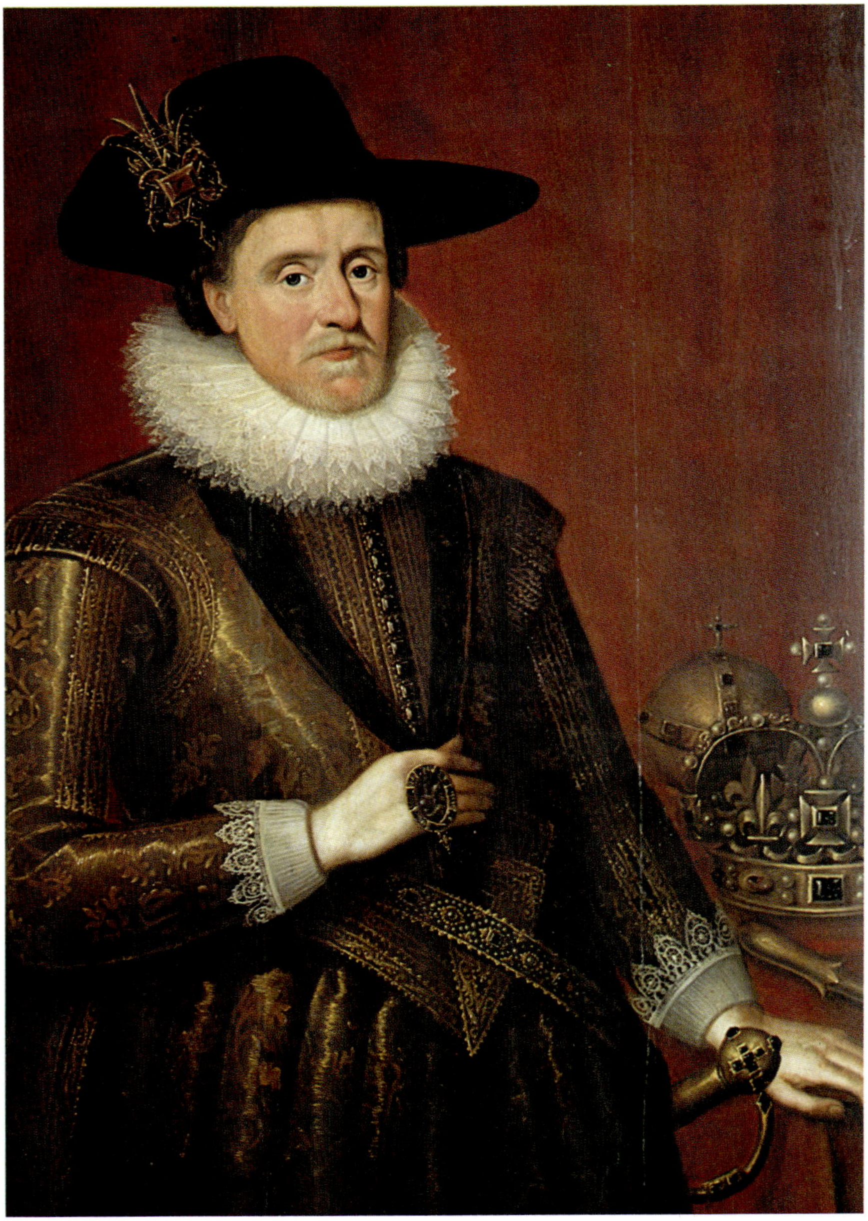

*James, the son of Mary Queen of Scots, was born in 1566, reigned as King James VI of Scotland from 1567 to 1625 and as King James I of England from 1603 to 1625. The portrait was painted by the Dutch artist Somer (or van Someren).*

# KING JAMES VI AND I

1566 to 1625

## KING JAMES VI OF SCOTLAND, 1567 to 1625
## KING JAMES I OF ENGLAND, 1603 to 1625

*The portrait, by the Dutch artist Somer or van Someren (1576-1621), is painted on wood and was discovered and obtained at auction about 1950 by the late Dr T. J. Honeyman who was then Director of the Glasgow Art Galleries. The painting was in poor condition and in three pieces but it was restored and subsequently purchased and presented to the Royal Faculty by Professor Geoffrey B. Fleming (President, 1946 to 1948) in 1952. Comparing it with other surviving portraits of the king, it appears to be an excellent likeness.*

James VI was the son of Mary, Queen of Scots, and Lord Darnley, her consort. When Mary was six months pregnant with James, she witnessed in the anteroom of her bedchamber in Holyrood Palace, the murder by multiple stab wounds of David Rizzio, her confidant and, perhaps, lover. In 1567, when James was about a year old, his father Darnley was found dead from suffocation in the garden of the house in which he had been staying and which had been blown to pieces by large quantities of gunpowder.

It is still arguable if Mary was directly concerned in her husband's murder but many believed that she was. 'Burn the whore!' cried the Edinburgh crowds as she was driven through their streets; shortly afterwards she abdicated in favour of her infant son who was crowned James VI in Stirling on 29th July 1567.

James' tutors and the Regents who governed during his childhood left him in no doubt that his mother was a murderess and this partly explains why he made no attempt to free her from the house arrest in which she was confined after she fled to England or to prevent her beheading in 1587 on the orders of her kinswoman, Elizabeth, Queen of England. Violent death was then the accepted method of acquiring and maintaining power and occurred so frequently as to be almost acceptable. James had four Regents until he began actively to reign in his twelfth year in 1578. The first two Regents were murdered; the third died 'because he loved good peace and could not have it', and the fourth, the Earl of Morton, was beheaded on a guillotine-like machine called 'The Maiden' which he himself had introduced into Scotland.

James' prime ambition was to succeed to the throne of England on the death of Elizabeth. The 'virgin' Queen had no children and James' claim through his great grandmother, Margaret Tudor, the sister of Henry VIII, was strong but not unassailable. Obviously his first priority was to stay alive and the history of his forebears was not encouraging. The James's I, II, III and IV were either murdered or slain in battle; nothing went right for James V who died broken in health and spirit in 1542 when his daughter, Mary, Queen of Scots, was less than a week old. Not only James VI but his mother Mary began their reign as children with Regents in charge of the affairs of the kingdom with all the intrigue and power politics which that entailed.

The background to much of the intrigue was the Reformation of the Christian Church. The break from the autocracy of the Pope and the Roman Catholic hierarchy was progressing rapidly in many parts of Western Europe by the middle of the 16th century although to some, particularly those in power, or desirous of power, Protestantism was often but a cloak to be worn or discarded as the occasion demanded. In Scotland the Protestant beginnings were almost defeated by Mary of Guise, the strongly Catholic mother of the girl queen Mary. She was on the point of burning a number of the more outspoken clergy when John Knox returned from exile in 1559 and so dominated and forwarded the Protestant cause that the Scottish Parliament in 1560 confirmed it as the established church of Scotland. It differed markedly from the Protestant Church in England where Henry VIII had broken with the Pope who would not allow him a divorce and a further marriage from which he might gain a male heir. He arrogated to himself all the powers of the Pope but made little change in doctrine or organisation of the Church. There was a temporary swing back to the Pope during the reign of his successor, Mary Tudor, but her successor Elizabeth returned to the ways of Henry. She was the head of state not only civil but ecclesiastical and controlled the revenues from both.

James was unhappy about the Scottish Kirk. Unlike England with its pyramid of priests, bishops, archbishops and the sovereign at the apex, there was no higher officer of the Kirk than the minister, and a series of courts, with the General Assembly as the highest, managed its affairs and controlled its discipline and its exchequer.

On the Continent of Europe there were problems too which might defeat James' purpose. France, a close ally of Scotland against England, was staunchly Roman Catholic; Henry of Navarre admittedly championed the Protestant Huguenots but after he became King of France in 1593, he reigned as a Roman Catholic. 'Paris was worth a mass', he said. Further south, Philip II of Spain was also a staunch Catholic who believed that he too had an excellent claim to the throne of England. But his great Armada sent against England in 1588 to establish his claim and re-establish Roman Catholicism was soundly defeated.

So James trod warily. He sailed to Denmark to take the Protestant Princess Anne as his bride. (Later in 1600 she was converted to Roman Catholicism). He remained on fairly friendly terms with the Pope, although, while according him high status in Christian affairs, he denied his supremacy over Kings. He preserved, too, many of the old Franco-Scottish bonds forged against the common enemy, England, and thus appeased and neutralised concerted Roman Catholic opposition to his accession to the English throne. At the same time he pleased the English Protestants by re-introducing bishops into Scotland.

And so on; the details of those years until the Union of the Crowns fill volumes. Whether regarded as double-dealing, fence-sitting, wire-walking or skilful politics, James played his part well and his accession to the English throne on the death of Elizabeth in 1603 was accomplished without a hitch and without rancour on either side.

James reigned over both Scotland and England until his death in 1625. He probably did more for Scotland than any of his sovereign predecessors, although there are those today who would see Scotland regain the independence she lost when James moved to London. He was a well educated man, witty in prose and speech, and both painting and architecture flourished during his reign. His Queen, Anne, was dull and no match for his intelligence and wit, and in his later years he made much of male favourites.

Apart from the Union of the Crowns he is generally remembered for three things:

His 'Authorised' version of the translation of the Bible of 1611, still in use today, although sadly superseded in some Kirks by more modern versions;

His 'Counterblast to Tobacco' which if heeded then would have spared much pulmonary misery;

The description attributed to Henry IV of Navarre that he was 'The wisest fool in Christendom'.

In the history of medicine, however, James holds a unique place. By his Charter of 1599 he was the first to join together surgery and medicine in a single corporation ordained to restrict medical practice over a wide area to properly qualified practitioners and with powers for controlling public health, medical jurisprudence and the control of drugs. In return the doctors had to provide a free medical service for the poor.

# THE CHARTER OF 1599

The original Charter of James VI was still extant in the first half of the 19th century, but has since been lost, probably in the course of the series of lawsuits between the Faculty and the University. A notarised copy has however been reprinted many times and is readily available. Written in Scots often picturesque and not always easy to understand, it starts by noting 'the grit abuisis quhilk hes bene comitted in time bigane, and zit daylie continuis be ignorant, unskillit and unlernit personis, quha, under the collour of Chirurgeanis, abuisis the people to their plesure, passing away but tryel or punishment, and thairby destroyis infinite number of oure subjectis'. It had jurisdiction in Glasgow, Renfrew, Dumbarton, Renfrewshire, Clydesdale, Lanark, Kyle, Carrick, Ayr, Cunningham; in effect much of the south-west of Scotland.

It gives to 'Maister Peter Low, our Chirurgiane . . . with the assistance of Mr. Robert Hamiltone, professoure of medicine'* and their successors power to examine and license all those practising surgery who are found properly trained and of good character. In addition each candidate for membership had to produce a 'testimonial of the minister and eldris, or magistratis of the parochin quhair they dwell'. Practice without such licence was punishable in a variety of ways culminating in fines and imprisonment.

Secondly, it laid upon the visitors (i.e. Low, Hamiltone, or their successors) the duty of visiting 'everie hurt, murtherit, poisonit, or onie other persoun tane awa extraordinarly and to report to the Magistrate of the fact as it is'.

Thirdly, it allowed the visitors with the advice of their brethren to 'mak statutis for the comoun weill of our subjectis anent the saidis artis'.

Fourthly, it dealt with the position of the physicians, allowing them to 'exercise' medicine if they had 'ane testimonial of ane famous universitie quhair medecine be taught or at the leave of oure and oure dearest spouse chief medicinarie'.

Fifthly, no person was to sell drugs in the area unless he had been inspected by the visitors and by William Spang the apothecary.

Sixthly, no dangerous drugs, 'retoun poison, asenick or sublemate', were to be sold except by apothecaries who had to take caution for 'coist, skaith and damage'.

Seventhly, the Faculty must convene on the first Monday of each month 'at sum convenient place, to visite and give counsell to pure disaisit folkis gratis'. The Royal College still meets on the first Monday of most months and the minutes of the previous meeting invariably end with the phrase, 'The poor were visited gratis and the College was adjourned'.

In return for all these commitments, the brethren were excused from certain civic duties such as serving on juries except as expert witnesses, paying certain taxes, and such military duties as 'wappin shawengis, raidis, oistis and beiring of armour'.

In 1672, the Faculty had the Charter ratified by the Scottish Parliament. Although certain anomalies were included, this immeasurably strengthened the powers of the original Charter and was to prove subsequently of much value in negotiations with other similar bodies and the Government.

* The presence or absence of the last 'e' of their names varies with Low(e) and Hamilton(e). In later documents Lowe and Hamilton are commonest.

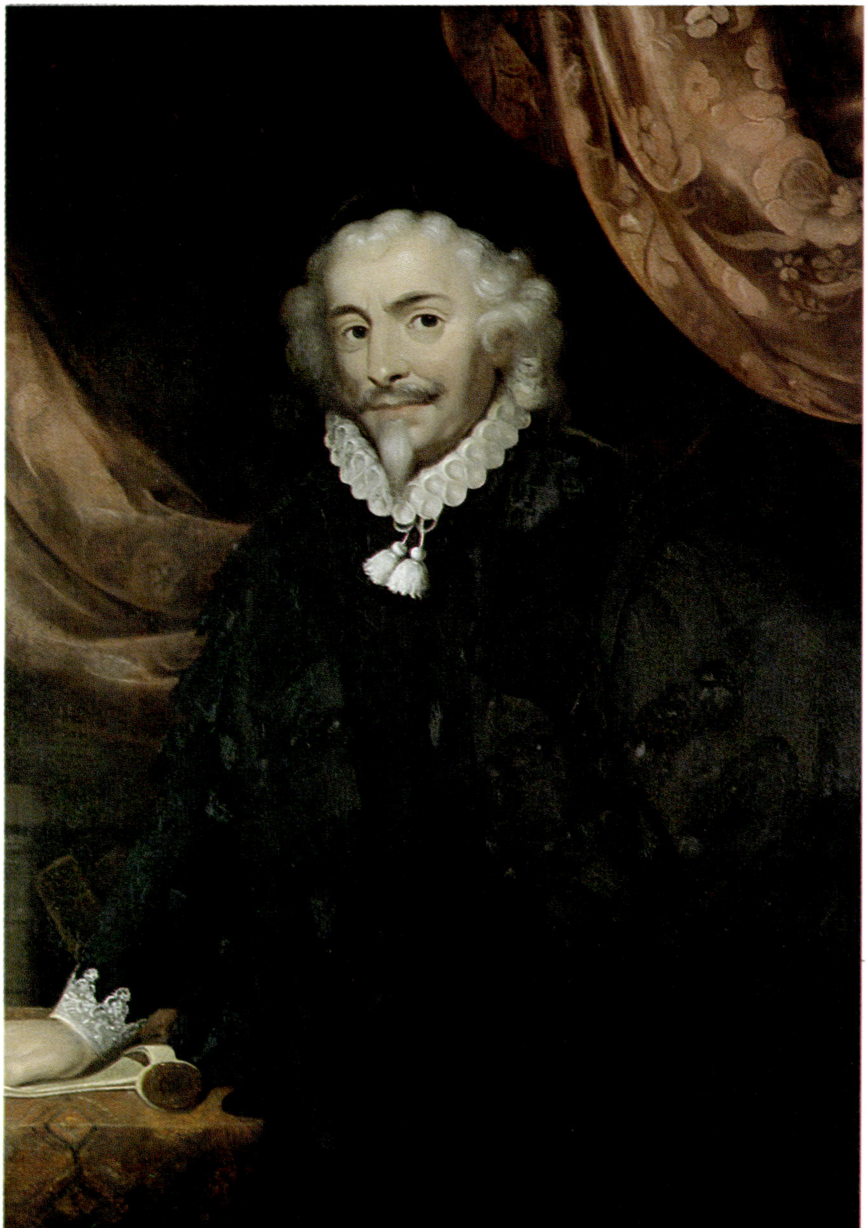

*Maister Peter Lowe (c 1550 to 1610) was described by James VI in his Charter of 1599 as 'our Chirurgiane and chief chirurgiane to oure dearest son the Prince'. The portrait is a copy made in 1822 of an ancient one which had deteriorated beyond repair.*

# MAISTER PETER LOWE

c 1550 to 1610

*The painting is a copy of an original by an unknown artist. In a minute of the Faculty of 3rd November 1795 it was noted that their 'ancient portraits were fast going into decay' and the then President, Dr Peter Wright (he was five times President of the Faculty) was asked to 'put them in a proper state but not to spend too much money upon them'. He appears to have heeded the need for economy, for the early portraits had deteriorated to such an extent by 1822 that copies were made of those of 'the three first members of Faculty, Drs. Hamilton and Low* (sic) *and Mr. Spang'. The cost of the three pictures and frames was £59.10s. They were intended as a kind of triptych with that of Lowe almost twice as big as the others. A press photograph of 1949 shows Hamilton's portrait firmly screwed to the wall on Lowe's right and Spang's was no doubt similarly fixed on his left. Today only Lowe's is fixed in the place of honour opposite the entrance.*

We know but a sketchy outline of Peter Lowe's life and some of that is tenuously based. So many of the records of the time were kept by the churches and were destroyed in the sackings and burnings of the Reformation. Peter Lowe was born about 1550 perhaps of a Catholic family who, fearful of the Calvinist ogre, packed him off to the European Continent to further his education but, equally perhaps, of a middle or upper class family of either faith who sent him, as many young Scots were sent before him, to study in the Low Countries or France, particularly if medicine were his goal. In the preface to the second edition of his *Chyrurgerie* there are a few autobiographical lines and one of them, in which he says he was 'chirurgian maior to the Spanish Regiments at Paris 2 yeeres', gives us the dates of the Siege of Paris, 1589 and 1590. He says he was before this in practice for 22 years in 'France, Flanders and elsewhere'. After the siege of Paris he was 'Chirurgian ordinary to Henry the fourth, the most Christian King of France and Navarre'. By 1596 he was back in Britain; his *Easie, certain and perfect method to cure and prevent the Spanish Sicknes* appeared in that year and in 1597 *The Whole Course of Chirurgerie*, both published in London. He was in Glasgow in 1598 and received the Charter from James VI in 1599. He had a son John by his first wife Grizell Pollart and a daughter Christine by his second wife Helen Wemyss. On his will, which has been preserved, the date of his death is given as 15th August 1610, but his tombstone in Glasgow Cathedral churchyard bears the date 1612. He was survived by his second wife and his children but the line subsequently became extinct.

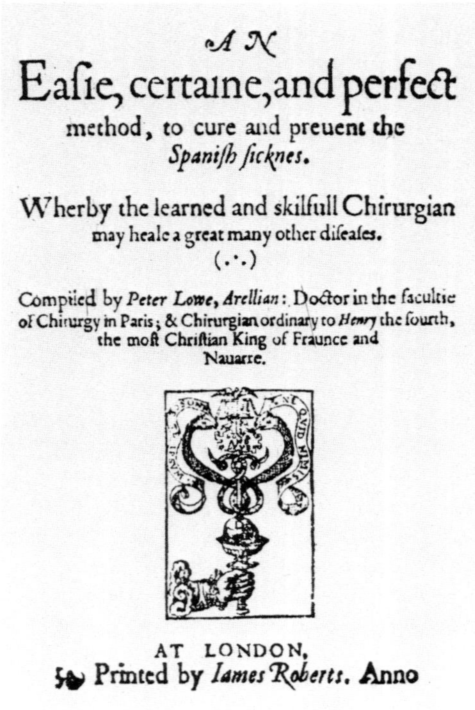

AN
Easie, certaine, and perfect
method, to cure and preuent the
*Spanish sicknes.*
Wherby the learned and skilfull Chirurgian
may heale a great many other diseases.
(.·.)
Compiled by *Peter Lowe, Arellian*: Doctor in the facultie
of Chirurgy in Paris; & Chirurgian ordinary to *Henry* the fourth,
the most Christian King of Fraunce and
Nauarre.

AT LONDON,
Printed by *Iames Roberts.* Anno

*Lowe's book on the 'Spanish Sicknes'*
*was published in 1596.*

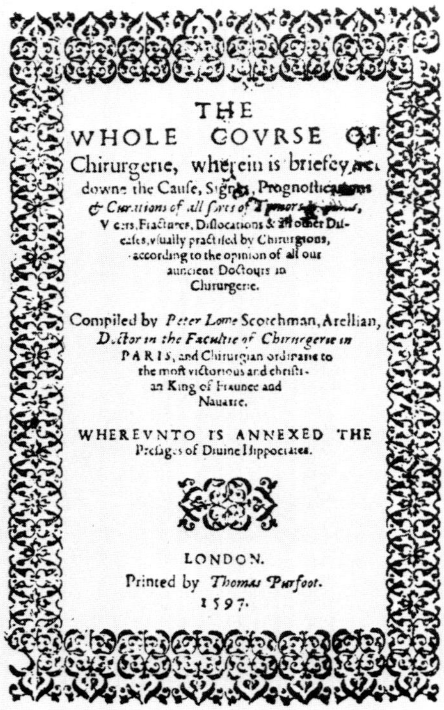

THE
WHOLE COVRSE OF
Chirurgerie, wherein is briefly set
downe the Cause, Signes, Prognostications
& *Curations of all sorts of Tumors, Wounds,*
Vlcers, Fractures, Dislocations & all other Dis-
eases, vsually practised by Chirurgions,
according to the opinion of all our
auncient Doctours in
Chirurgerie.
Compiled by *Peter Lowe* Scotchman, Arellian,
*Doctor in the Facultie of Chirurgerie in*
PARIS, and Chirurgian ordinarie to
the most victorious and christi-
an King of Fraunce and
Nauarre.
WHEREVNTO IS ANNEXED THE
Presages of Diuine Hippocrates.

LONDON.
Printed by *Thomas Purfoot.*
1597.

*The frontispiece of Lowe's second book*
The Whole Course of Chirurgerie *of 1597.*

These are the bare bones of his life and do little to explain how he, who described himself as a 'Scotchman' or 'Scottishman', could return to his homeland after more than 30 years abroad and within the space of a year or so persuade his King to grant him a charter which made him the most powerful medical man in all Scotland. But a little flesh may be added.

In the *Spanish Sicknes* he calls himself 'Peter Lowe, Arellian' and in the *Whole Course of Chirurgerie*, 'Peter Lowe, Scotchman, Arellian'. This word 'Arellian' has given rise to much unresolved speculation; one plausible explanation is that it is a form of 'Aurelian' meaning 'of Orléans' but it is equally possible that it is a latinised form of his place of birth, and Ayr, Airlie and Errol have all been suggested. He is always referred to as 'Maister' which is a corruption of *Magister*, which in turn signifies that he had graduated *Magister Artium*, perhaps at Orléans, although Paris is another possibility. He was certainly a well educated man; although he wrote his books in English, he could write excellent Latin and must have been fully fluent in French, with some German and Spanish from his practice in Flanders and his work with the Spanish Army.

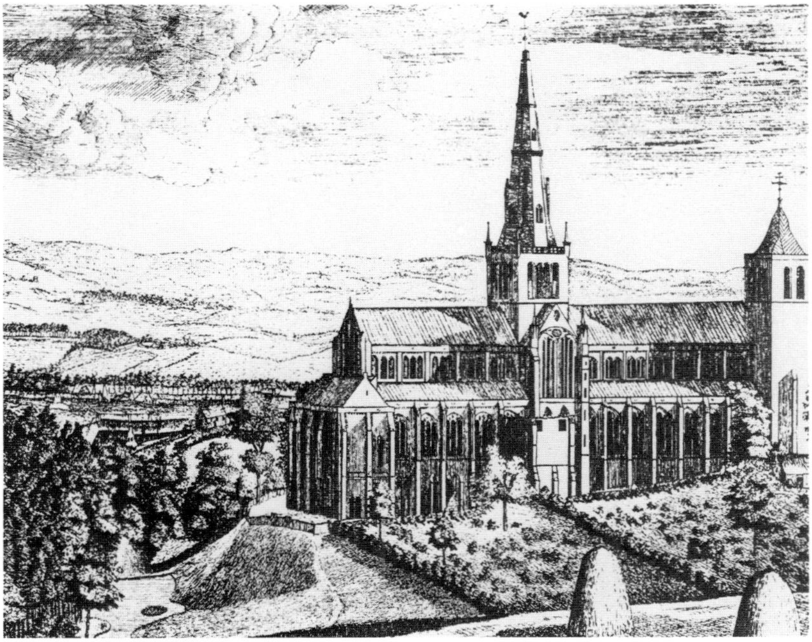

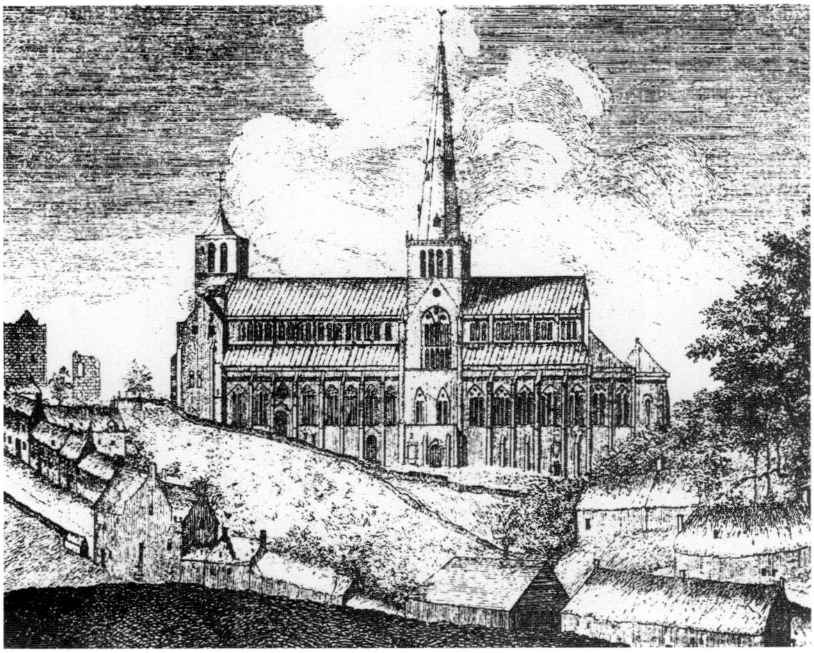

*Two views of Glasgow Cathedral made by Robert Paul about 1750. At the time of the Charter, Glasgow was a small town clustered around its Cathedral and the neighbouring College, and even 150 years later the setting is still rural. The upper view is from the north, the lower from the south.*

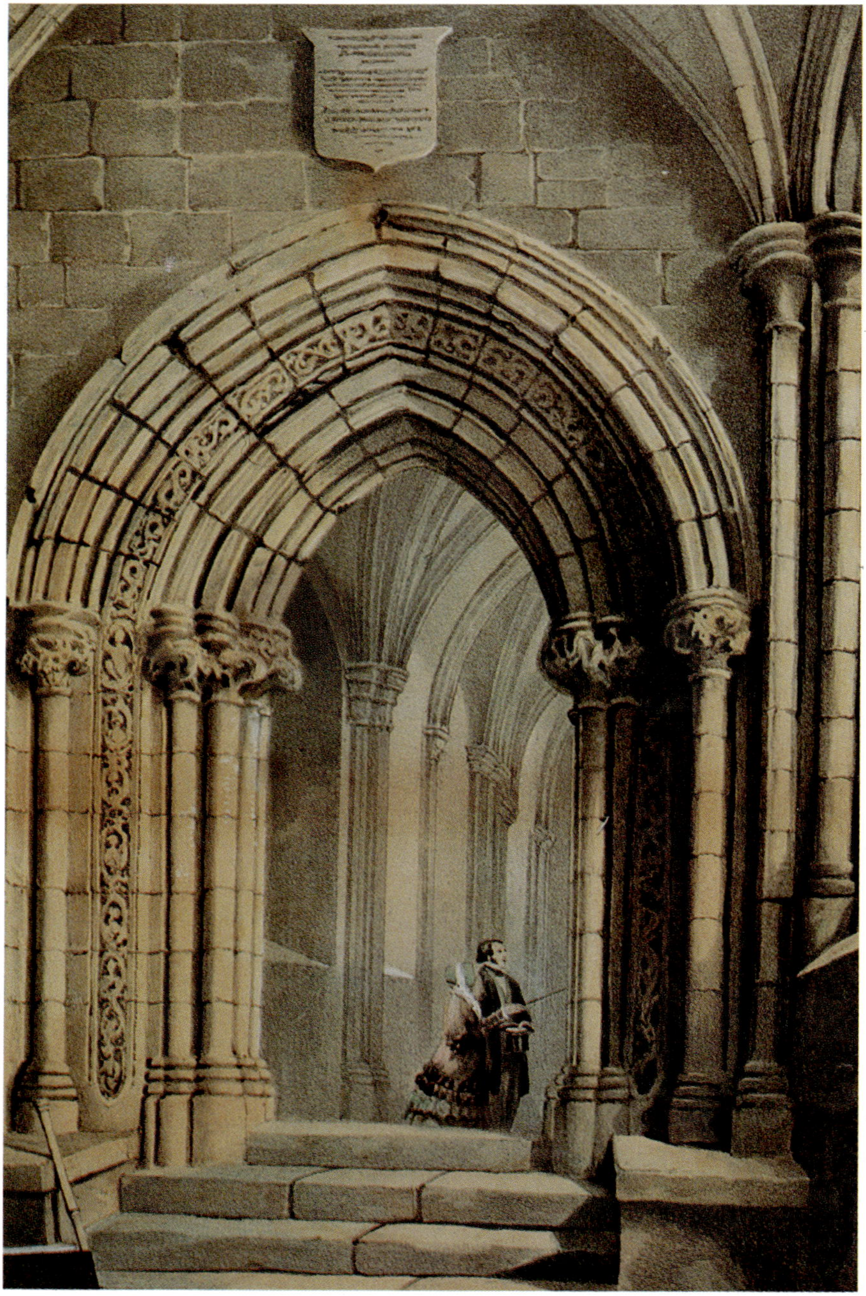

*This painting by Fairbairn (1850) shows the partly restored doorway into the Cathedral Crypt and is a good example of the richly carved and columned style of mediaeval decorated English architecture. It forms the entrance to the Crypt founded by Bishop Lauder. Peter Lowe's second wife was Helen Wemyss, the daughter of the first presbyterian minister of the Cathedral.*

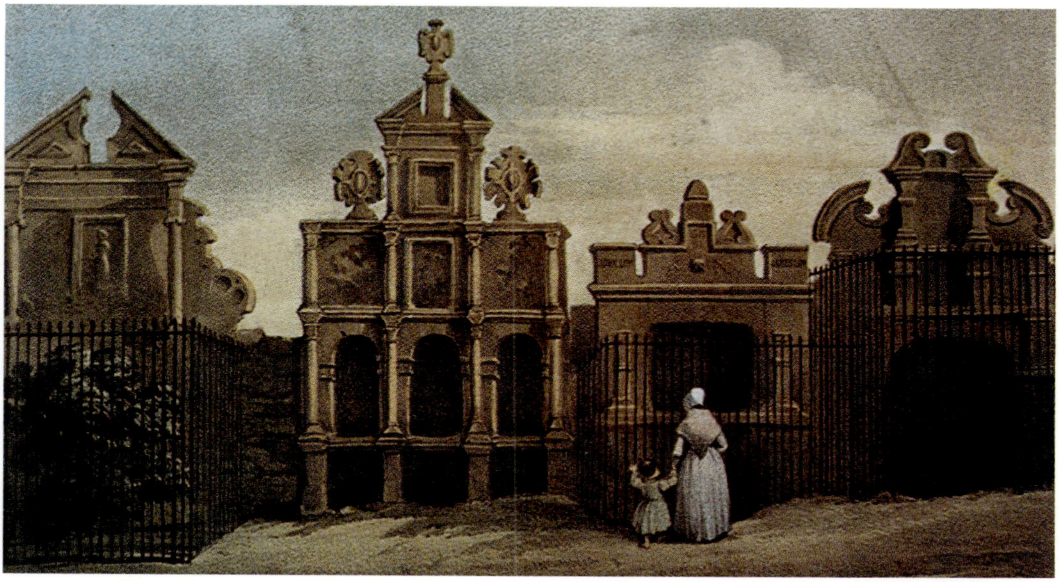

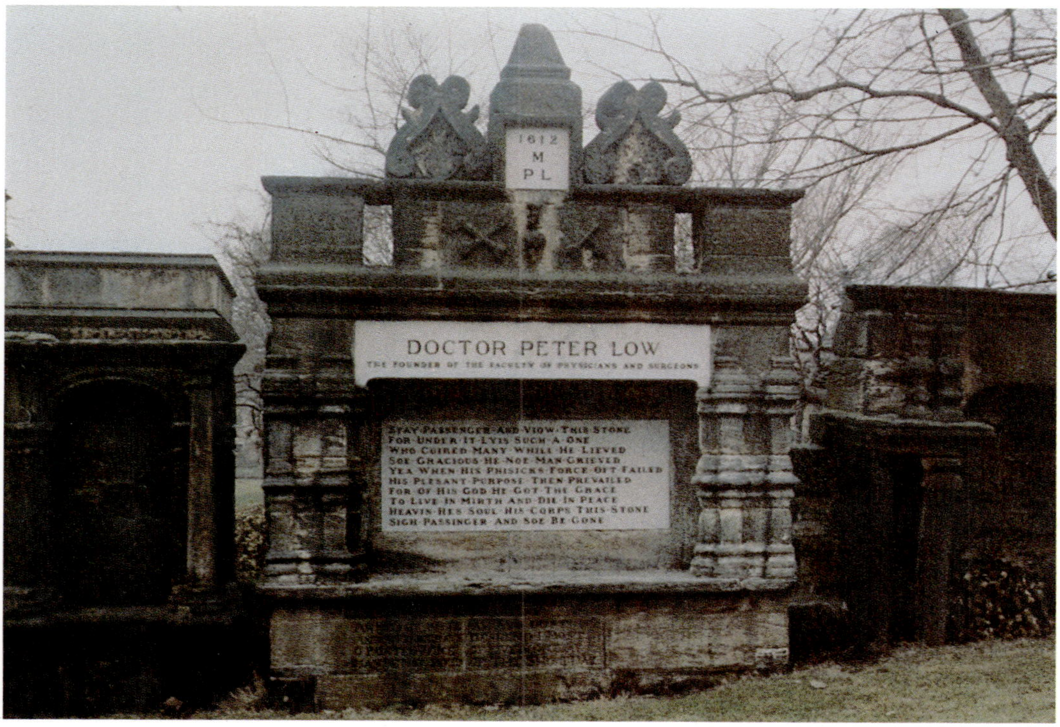
1612
M
PL
DOCTOR PETER LOW
THE FOUNDER OF THE FACULTY OF PHYSICIANS AND SURGEONS
STAY·PASSENGER·AND·VIOW·THIS·STONE
FOR·UNDER·IT·LYIS·SUCH·A·ONE
WHO·CUIRED·MANY·WHILL·HE·LIEVED
SOE·GRACIOUS·HE·NOE·MAN·GRIEVED
YEA·WHEN·HIS·PHISICKS·FORCE·OFT·FAILED
HIS·PLESANT·PURPOSE·THEN·PREVAILED
FOR·OF·HIS·GOD·HE·GOT·THE·GRACE
TO·LIVE·IN·MIRTH·AND·DIE·IN·PEACE
HEAVIN·HES·SOUL·HIS·CORPS·THIS·STONE
SIGH·PASSINGER·AND·SOE·BE·GONE

*Peter Lowe's tomb in Glasgow Cathedral cemetery. The upper picture is by Fairbairn (1850) and Lowe's tomb is second from the right. It was purchased by the Faculty in 1834; the anti-grave-robber railings have since been removed and the edifice restored and repaired on at least two occasions. Below is the appearance of the tomb today.*

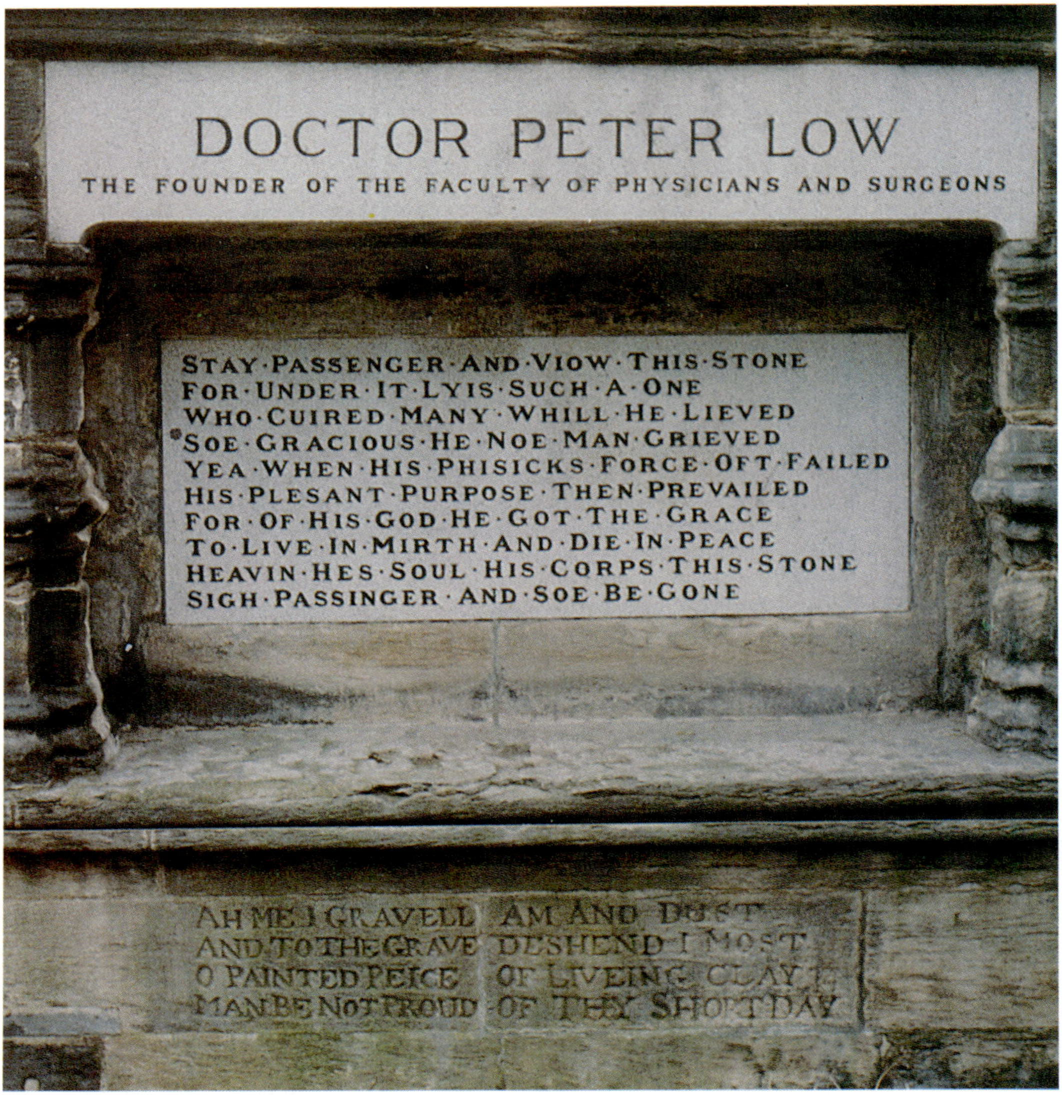


*The inscriptions on Peter Lowe's tomb. The lower, which is rather indistinct, reads:*

AH ME I GRAVELL AM AND DUST
AND TO THE GRAVE DESHEND I MOST
O PAINTED PEICE OF LIVEING CLAY
MAN BE NOT PROUD OF THY SHORT DAY

In the *Calendar of Scottish Papers* (Vol. IX) of 1588 there is to be found in a letter from a Wm. Asheby to Lord Burghley, the English Ambassador, the following: 'There is one Peter Lowe a Scotchman and a pirate; he has taken an English ship of Wells in Norfolk laden with corn for Berwick'. Lowe sailed the ship to Montrose and sold the corn, and the writer suggests sending an English man-o-war to these waters to 'encourage the King and the Protestants'. If this were our Peter Lowe he was then a Catholic pirating an English Protestant ship.

The second entry in the *Calendar of Scottish Papers* (Vol. XI) is more convincing. Dr Macartney writes to Robert Bowes on 23rd May 1595 that 'a new admittit chirurgien' to the King of France called Mr Lowe had prepared 'to perfection' a casket of documents including 'some secret devices of England, domestic and foreign, with a description of the "depis" of all the havens there' and brought it to l'Aubespin in Paris. This material he had collected a year or two previously when he had travelled in England with Alexander Dickson, the secretary to the Earl of Errol, both well known Catholics. Was Lowe acting for James or his 'master' Henry or as a go-between for both?

The last seems most likely. Like James, he favoured Catholicism or Protestantism as the situation demanded. Catholic with the Spaniards, Protestant and then Catholic with Henry of Navarre, Protestant when he returned to Glasgow and married the daughter of Wemyss, the first Protestant minister of Glasgow Cathedral. That King James and Lowe were firm friends is illustrated by the fact that James sent Lowe with the Earl of Lennox on an ambassadorial visit in 1601 to the Catholic court of Henry in Paris at a time when James' plans for the English crown were coming to fruition. The Earl of Lennox was a powerful friend of James and represented the King in Scotland after the Union. Who better than Lowe with his education, knowledge of Henry's court and his language to assist him?

James in the Charter described Lowe as 'our Chirurgiane and chief chirurgiane to oure dearest son the Prince' (Prince Henry, who died in 1612), suggesting a very close relationship between Lowe and the Royal Family. The granting of the Charter to Lowe can best be explained as an unusually lavish gift for substantial services rendered by a friend and ally, with perhaps a hint of blackmail by an astute, well-travelled intermediary at a time when favourable opinions in as many quarters as possible were essential for James' plans.

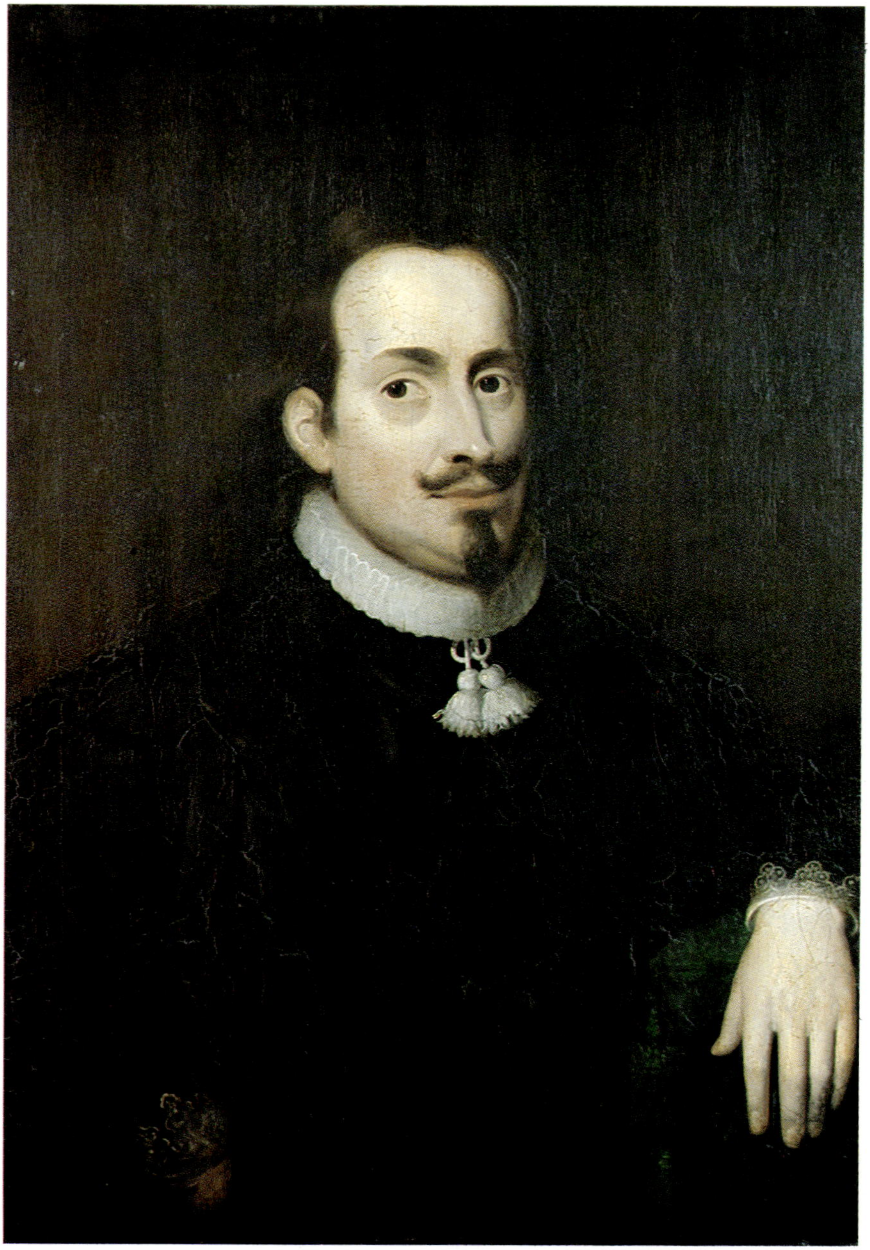

*Mr Robert Hamilton (c 1565 to 1629) was the physician assistant to Peter Lowe specified in the Charter. Like Lowe's portrait, this is an 1822 copy of an old decayed version.*

## ROBERT HAMILTON

c 1565 to 1629

*The painting has the same history as that of Lowe: a copy made in 1822 of a previous decaying portrait.*

The Hamiltons were a large family and the Dukes of Hamilton were closely related to the royal Stewarts and among the most powerful nobles in Scotland. When our particular Robert was born is unknown though he is noted in 1587 as the servant of the Commendator (i.e. the titular Bishop) of Pluscardine Priory which lies in the north-east of Scotland and was one of the last strongholds of Catholicism. He appears to have gone to the Low Countries perhaps to further his medical studies, for there is a record of his return in the *Calendar of Scottish Papers* (Vol. XI): 'July 21st, 1594. News from Scotland. On Tuesday, last week, there landed a Flemish ship at Aberdeen wherein were the Bishop of Ross, Mr. James Gordon, Jesuit, Doctor Hamilton and another servant. They went on foot to the old town of Aberdeen where many Catholics are thought to dwell. There they took horse immediately'. Where to is not recorded but presumably it was Pluscardine. Here then is Robert Hamilton, a known Catholic, arriving in Scotland when Lowe was preparing his casket of documents for France. He must have been known to both James and Lowe because he shares equal powers with Lowe in the Charter. In the Charter he is described as 'professoure of medicine', in his will as 'doctor of physic' and in the Privy Council records of 1628 as 'doctor of medicine'. But there is no record of an MD and probably those terms merely implied that he was a practising physician. He is also called 'Mr.' which suggests that he too was *Magister Artium.*

He was the senior office bearer or Visitor of the incorporation during most of its first 20 years. His will is still extant and shows that he died in October 1629. Curiously, although he had been left lands in Ireland by a kinsman, Sir Claude Hamilton of Shawfield, and was a successful physician for many years, the total value of his estate was only 84 pounds Scots or about £7 sterling. Of the character of the man we know nothing.

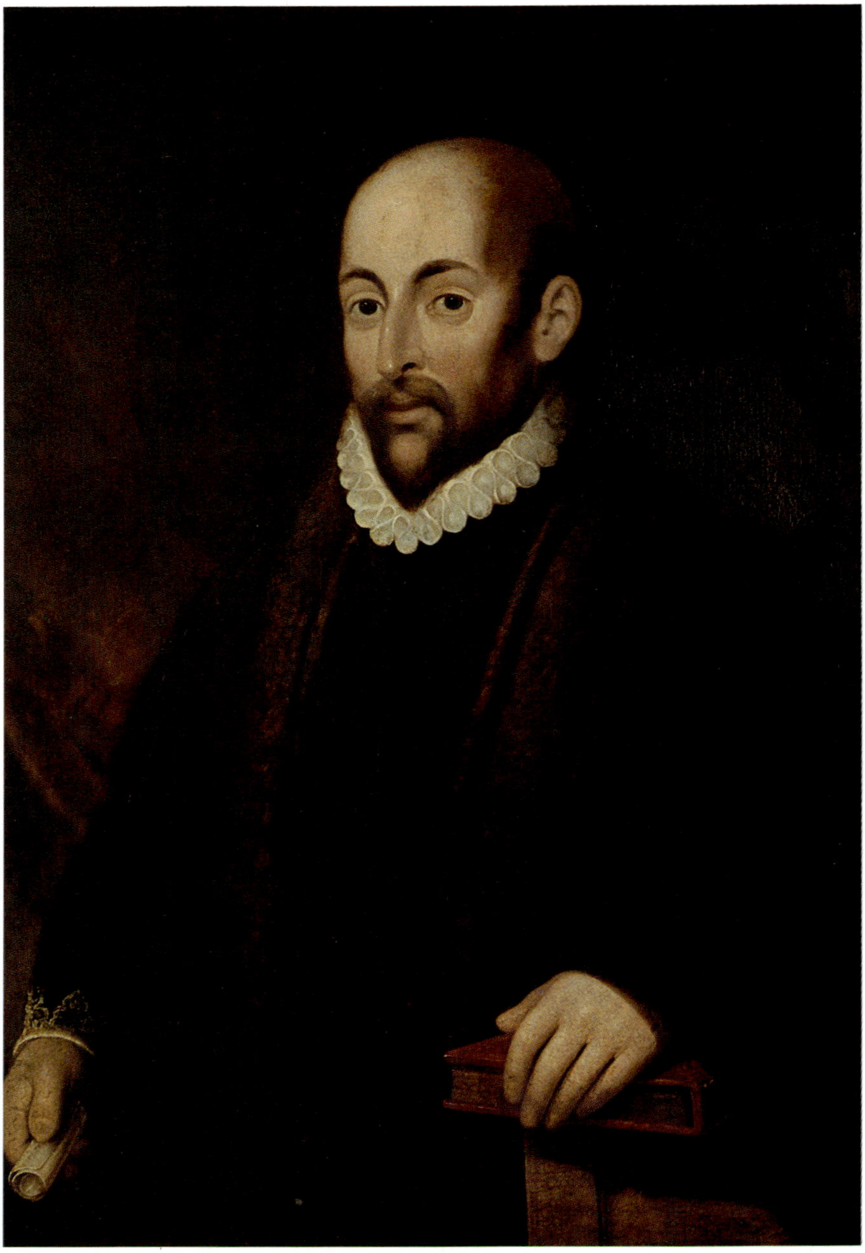

*William Spang (?1545 to ?1610) was an apothecary specified in the Charter as the inspector of any shops selling drugs. This painting, too, is an 1822 copy.*

# WILLIAM SPANG

c 1545 to c 1610

*Like those of Lowe and Hamilton the portrait is a copy of an earlier one and the painter is unknown.*

Little is recorded about Spang. He is noted as being in practice as a pharmacist in 1574. He was appointed a Burgess and Freeman of the City of Glasgow 'for his support to hald his booth in MEDISENE DROGIS for serving of the town and UTHERIS' on 21st August 1576. He was thus an older man than either Lowe or Hamilton, as is obvious from his portrait, and was sufficiently well respected to be named in the Charter as inspector of drugs. He was appointed 'Visitor' (i.e. President) of the incorporation in 1606. He had a son, also William, who became a member in 1602.

And that is all we know of him.

# 2

# IN THE BEGINNING: SURGEONS AND BARBER SURGEONS

In the beginning they had no name and no home. They were just the 'Visitors', Mr Peter Lowe and Mr Robert Hamilton, and they held their first meeting on the 3rd of June 1602, in Blackfriars Kirk where they first presented their Charter to the Provost of the Burgh of Glasgow and three of his Baillies and then proceeded to admit five new members. At the same time they relinquished their personal powers under the Charter and invested these in the newly formed body. One of the new members was William Spang, the apothecary mentioned in the Charter; of the others, only one bore the title 'Mr.' and we know nothing of any.

Two other new members were admitted shortly afterwards and these nine individuals probably included all the reputable practitioners of the healing art in the Burgh. For Glasgow was a small community of only 7,000 or so inhabitants, and even by the end of the 17th century the population was only around 11,000. Seaborne trade from Spain, France, the Low Countries and Scandinavia came up the east coast into Edinburgh; so did much of the traffic from London to Scotland. It was not until the next century that the balance of trade shifted from East to West as the transatlantic trade with the American colonies increased, and Glasgow and the West of Scotland, importing raw materials like tobacco and sugar, and developing such industries as coal mining, textiles and shipping, became the major industrial centre of Scotland. But, in the 17th century, Glasgow was but a cathedral town with its University next its Cathedral on the banks of the Molendinar burn which joined the river Clyde half a mile away in a large pool where salmon fishing was still a thriving industry.

With the exception of Mr Robert Hamilton, it is unlikely that any of the early members were physicians. Two grades were permitted to practise medicine by the Charter: holders of a medical degree from a known university where medicine was taught, and those approved by the royal physician. No Scottish university then taught medicine and MD's of foreign universities were rare, and when James moved south in 1603 his personal physicians took little thought thereafter for any possible colleagues in the south-west of Scotland. In addition, the practice of a physician was purely consultative and only lucrative in larger centres where he was already well known and respected.

So nearly all of the group were surgeons and some at least must have risen from the ranks of the barber surgeons as did the great Ambroise Paré half a century earlier. The barbers were the obvious choice for such minor operations as venesectomy or abscess incision for they had the skill of imparting the keenest edge to small knives: the sharper the blade, the quicker the cut, the less the pain. But having tasted blood, some ventured too far; the Faculté de Chirurgie in Paris, of which Lowe claimed a doctorate, railed against them as did Lowe himself: 'usurping the name of Chirurgien, they have scarce the skill to cut a beard'.

But they were there and they could not be ignored; so six weeks after the first meeting in 1602 they were accepted as a 'pendecle', an appendage of surgery, and could be admitted on payment of a fee, but had few corporate privileges and had to promise 'not to meddle with anything further belonging to surgery'. Usually when a barber was noted in the minutes as having been admitted he was cited as a 'simple barber surgeon to meddle only with simple wounds', after which was a list of operations with which he must not 'meddle' on pain of a fine or expulsion.

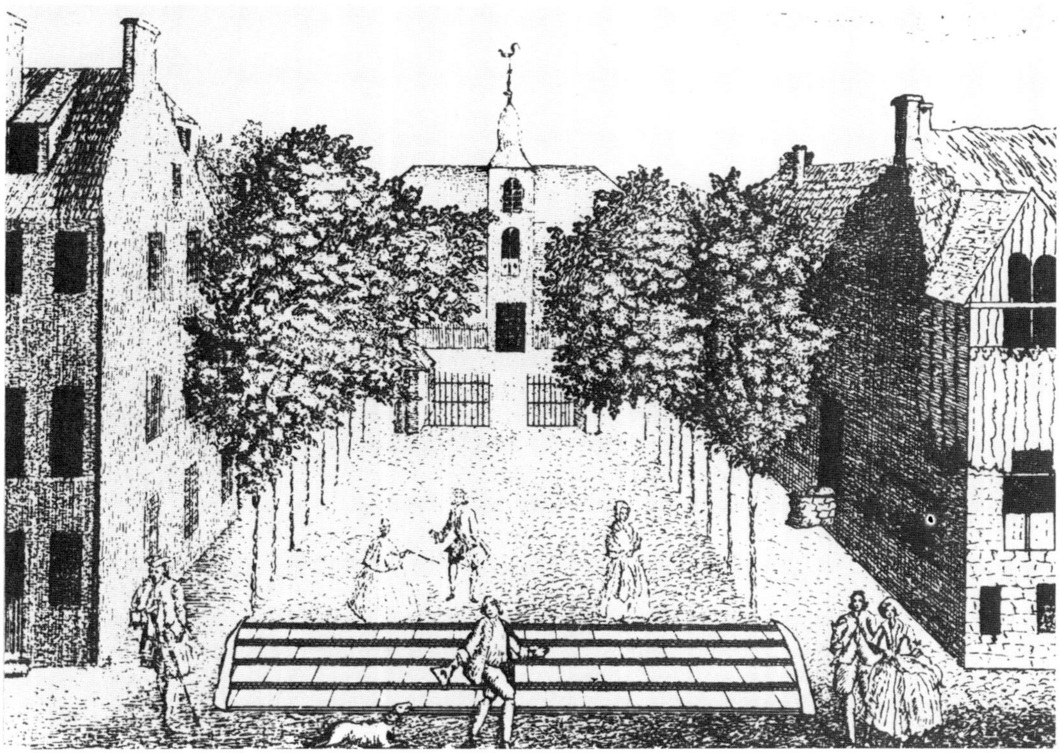

'A prospect of the entry into the Blackfriars Church, Glasgow,
March 1st, 1736.
R. Paul Sculp.'

*The first meeting under the Charter was held in this Kirk on 3rd June 1602 and it was an occasional meeting place until the first Faculty Hall next to the Tron Kirk was built in 1697.*

It was an unhappy relationship; the best of the barber surgeons was probably as efficient at surgery as some of the admitted surgeons but had no say in the running of the corporation, no vote in the election of the Visitor (President) and thus no elected representative in the Trades House. There seems to have been goodwill and sympathy on both sides, however, and the Surgeons and the Barbers, in 1656, applied to and received from the Town Council a 'Seal of Cause' or 'Letter of Deaconry', in effect a Municipal Charter which formed them jointly (but not with the physicians) into a Craft or Trade with equal representation in the Trades House. But they still had unequal privileges; the Barbers had no say in the election of the Visitor and appear to have been systematically excluded from all offices. The minutes of all meetings from 1682 to 1733 were destroyed in a fire but from Town Council minutes it appears that the few barber members accepted their lot until after the turn of the century when the Town Council was increasingly pestered with complaints from the Surgeons against the Barbers and from the Barbers against the Surgeons. In 1707 the Town Council granted the Barbers virtually equal

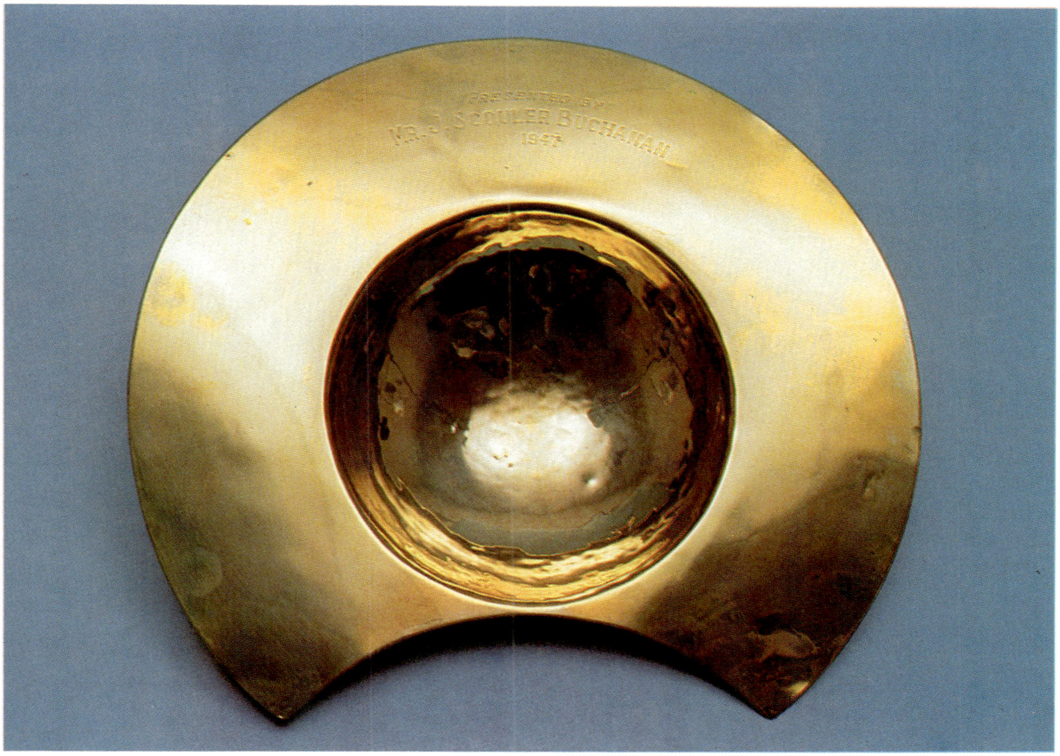


*A bleeding bowl of the kind used by the barber surgeons. The concavity was fitted into the flexed elbow before one of the anticubital veins was lanced.*

privileges to those of the Surgeons and this was followed by the admission of so many barbers that they outnumbered the surgeons.

But the days of barber surgeons were numbered. The Barbers separated from the Surgeons in Edinburgh in 1719 and in London in 1745, and in Glasgow talk and plans for separation continued from 1708 until the divorce was finally made absolute in 1720. The Letter of Deaconry was renounced, the Barbers received one-fifth of the value of the joint assets and formed their own Craft. The two sides parted amicably and to this day the Incorporation of Barbers sends an annual donation to the College Library.

Although they had no name in the beginning and referred to themselves as the 'Brethren of Chirurgerie' or the 'Craft of Chirurgerie', the term 'Facultie', probably based on the Parisian *Facultés*, appears in the minutes in 1629. Although nearly all members were surgeons, they did not want to lose the physicians and from 1654 they called themselves the 'Facultie of Chirurgeons and Physitians' but, as will now be told, the physicians gradually took over from the surgeons in the second half of the 17th century and by 1700 the title was 'The Faculty of Physicians and Surgeons of Glasgow'. It remained thus until, in 1909, King Edward VII graciously permitted the use of the adjective 'Royal'. Finally, in 1962, because of the changes in meaning of the word 'faculty' and to bring the institution into line with other similar bodies, it became, by Act of Parliament, 'The Royal College of Physicians and Surgeons of Glasgow'.

# 3

## THE 'PURE' PHYSICIANS IN CHARGE
1672 to 1820

John Moore (1729 to 1802)
Peter Wright (c 1740 to 1819)
Robert Cleghorn (c 1760 to 1821)

In the first half of the 17th century only two physicians were admitted to the Faculty; both had university degrees and, in accordance with the Charter, no examination was required of them. Although the number of physicians in the area was not large, it was certainly more than this. Most of them appear to have stood aloof from an organisation they regarded as little more than a craft with members who were tradesmen. This was one ill effect of the increasing liaison between the surgeons and the barbers and the Municipal Charter they had negotiated.

But there was also an increasing desire on both sides for a much closer association. On the one hand the physicians were in need of a professional body; on the other, the surgeons saw their status declining and the ideal of a joint corporation of surgeons and physicians, as envisaged in their Charter, almost vanished. In 1656 Oliver Cromwell tried to set up in Edinburgh a College of Physicians for Scotland. The Edinburgh College of Surgeons rebelled at the scheme and wrote to the Glasgow Faculty who reacted in the same way and the matter was dropped. In Edinburgh a separate College of Physicians was instituted in 1681; in Glasgow the physicians took over the Faculty and retained and strengthened its joint medical and surgical status.

Matters came to a head in 1671 when Dr John Colquhoun and two other physicians, all university graduates in medicine and resident in Glasgow, requested admission as a right under the Charter of James VI. The Faculty declared by a majority vote that the mere fact of possession of a medical degree did *not* carry with it the right of admission. The wording of the Charter is undoubtedly vague but such a decision was contrary to previous rulings and tradition. The unease which the Faculty must have felt about it gave rise to a second vote at the same meeting when they agreed to admit the three physicians while in no way conceding their right of entry as medical graduates.

The physicians would have none of it; they saw their status being determined by lesser mortals and held out for the principle of the right of admission when holding a university degree in medicine.

The next overture came from the Faculty who were empowered to offer Dr Colquhoun virtually every advantage he wished for the physicians, the exceptions being that the surgeons would not separate from the barbers and in no circumstances would they concede the right of unexamined entry of university qualified physicians.

The physicians, shrewdly led by Colquhoun, stepped down from their demand for absolute privilege and thereby gained virtual control of the Faculty. In all matters the physicians were to take precedence over the surgeons and the physicians were given the veto of any resolution passed by the Faculty which they considered 'derogatory to their degree'. Even their concession that they had no absolute right of admission without examination was so wrapped round with provisos that never again would their admission depend on the 'bare call of the Chirurgianes'. There were to be two 'Visitors', a Physician-Visitor and a Surgeon-Visitor, and when matters were finally adjusted, Dr John Colquhoun 'did condescend and immediately thereafter did accept in and upon himself the office of Physician-Visitor'.

The first act of Dr Colquhoun and his Surgeon-Visitor colleague was to select those surgeons with whom the physicians would deign to associate. It had become customary with some of the barber surgeons to give them leave to practice a few listed operations; all such, however, and all barbers with the general non-meddling clause were weeded out.

There were now in effect two separate corporations: the Faculty of Physicians and Surgeons (in that order!) and the Incorporation of Surgeons and Barbers. The physicians would have no truck with the latter and their disdain and disapproval must have played a major part in its final dissolution.

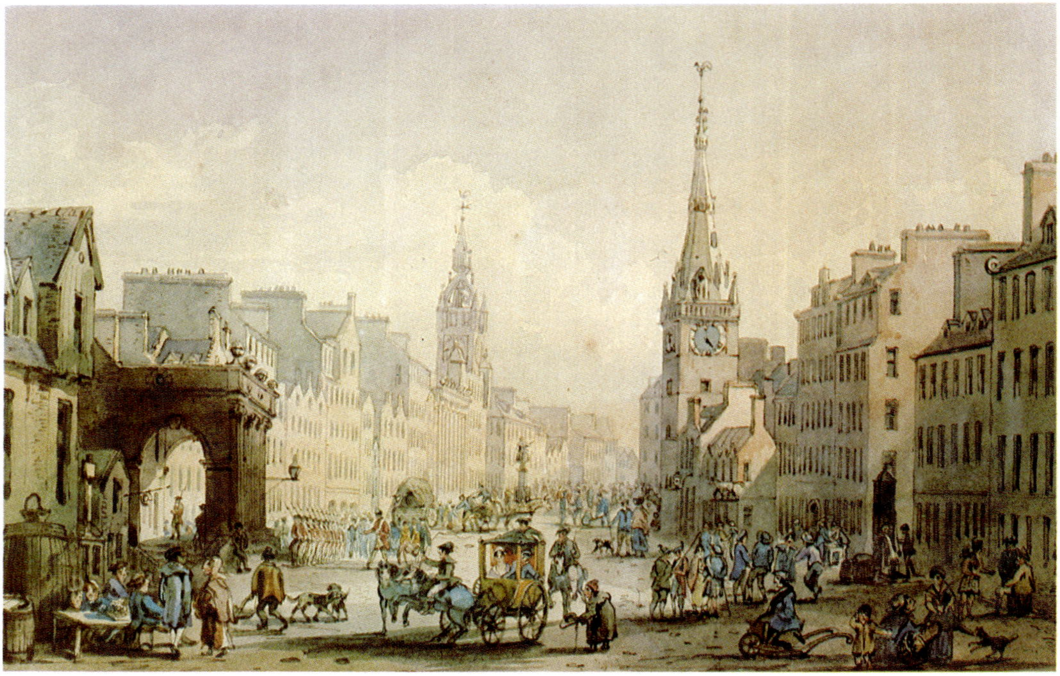

*The Trongate looking east during the mid 18th century. The Tron Kirk is on the right and the first Faculty Hall was built on this side of it and opened in 1698.*

The missing minutes of the meetings from 1682 to 1733 must have contained much of interest of the early relationship between physicians and surgeons. There is no doubt that the Faculty had become a much more active body. In 1697 they acquired, next to and on the west side of the Tron Church, a property which they knocked down and on the site erected the first Faculty Hall which opened in 1698. At the same time they began there the Faculty Library with donations of books from 60 different donors: some surgeon and some physician members and a number of outside bodies.

Although the holders of the posts of Physician-Visitor and Surgeon-Visitor had equal powers so far as convening and chairing meetings were concerned, there was a gradual change in emphasis and by the time of the first surviving minute of the 18th century, of the meeting on 8th November 1733, it was already established that the Physician-Visitor was the Praeses or President and the Surgeon-Visitor simply the Visitor or Vice-President; so it remained until 1820 when the supply of pure physicians dried up and others became eligible for the office of President. All the Presidents of whom we have records from 1672 till 1820 were MD's of a variety of universities, some in Britain including Glasgow, some in Europe. They were 'pure' physicians in so far as they did no general practice or surgery, although they might combine their consulting medical practice with lecture- or professor-ships. This 'purity' was jealously guarded. If a physician strayed and undertook surgical or general practice the Faculty treated him as a surgeon and he had to sit the examination. In 1745 a Mr Andrew Morris who was a graduate of the University of Rheims wanted admission to the Faculty as a graduate physician but also insisted on opening a surgery in Glasgow and practising as a general practitioner. The Faculty challenged his right to do so; he in turn challenged the Faculty's right to proscribe him until, some years of litigation later, he gave in, took the examination and was admitted as a surgeon.

The practice of the established 'pure' physician was undoubtedly lucrative; few of the well-off citizens would die without adding guineas to his coffers. But to become established and respected took time and it was common for the practitioner to be admitted first as a surgeon and embark in general practice, and later take an MD and become a physician. The subject of our next portrait illustrates this sequence.

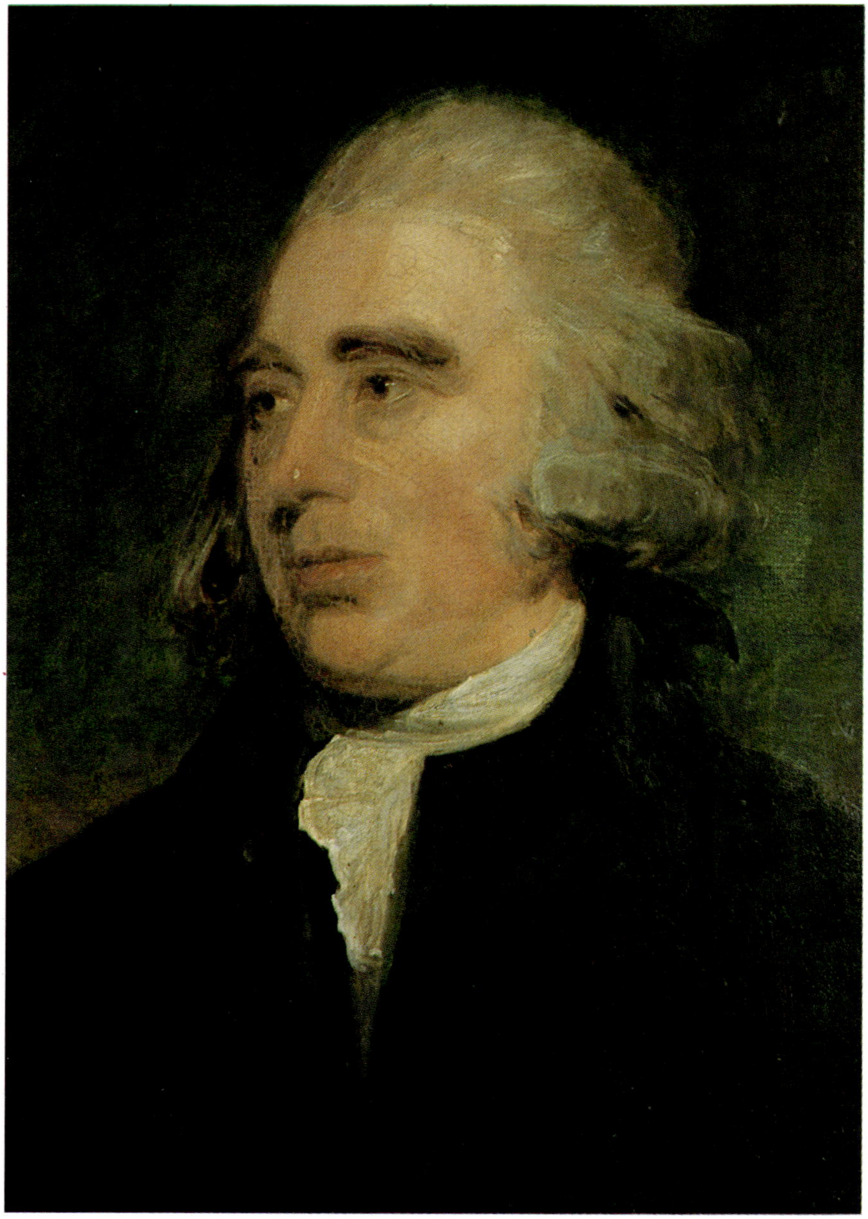

*John Moore (1729 to 1802) was first a surgeon, later a physician, a man of letters and the father of Sir John Moore of Corunna whose statue stands in George Square. The portrait is a copy by James Barr of the original by Sir Thomas Lawrence.*

# JOHN MOORE

1729 to 1802

*The portrait is a copy made by James Barr of an original by Sir Thomas Lawrence which belonged to Moore's grandson, John Carrick Moore of Corsewall, Wigtownshire. The copy was commissioned and presented to the Faculty in 1865 by the President, Dr John Gibson Fleming.*

John Moore was the son of the Reverend Charles Moore, a minister in Stirling, and was educated in Glasgow Grammar School and Glasgow University where he attended courses in medicine, literature, history and philosophy. He was at this time an apprentice to a very well known surgical partnership, that of Mr William Stirling and John Gordon. Some years before, the partners had another never-to-be-forgotten apprentice, Tobias Smollett, who, like Moore, is more remembered for his literary works than his doctoring.

When he had completed his apprenticeship in 1747, Moore served in the Low Countries as surgeon's mate with the 54th Regiment under Colonel Campbell, later the 5th Duke of Argyll. He worked first in Maestricht with the wounded from the Battle of Laffeldt and his competence earned him a recommendation to the Earl of Albemarle, who was then Colonel of the Coldstream Guards, and he next became assistant to the surgeon of that regiment. After peace was made at the Treaty of Aix-la-Chapelle in 1749, Moore returned to London where he attended the lectures of William Hunter. To pursue further his medical studies he then went to Paris, widely acknowledged at that time to be *the* centre for medical training, and spent two years there. He was greatly aided by the sponsorship of the Earl of Albemarle who was now the British Ambassador in Paris and appointed Moore surgeon to his household.

His erstwhile master, John Gordon, invited him back to Glasgow and to a partnership in 1751. This Moore was happy to accept, but on his way back to Glasgow he paused in London to attend more of William Hunter's lectures and also those of William Smellie, the great obstetrician and another Scot from Lanarkshire. He 'entered' the Faculty as a general practitioner/surgeon after he reached Glasgow.

Moore spent almost 20 years successfully in practice in Glasgow until in 1770, and now 41 years old, he graduated MD at Glasgow University and turned physician. But this phase of his career only lasted two years. In 1769 the Duchess of Hamilton had asked Moore and William Cullen to see her ailing son James, the 7th Duke of Hamilton, but in spite of their care and after a long illness, probably tuberculosis, he died in his 15th year. He was succeeded by his younger brother Douglas whom the Duchess placed under Moore's care so completely that, in 1772, Moore gave up his practice and he and the young 8th Duke of Hamilton set out on a grand tour of Europe which was to last until 1778. When he then returned to London, Moore set up there in practice as a physician but more and more of his time was taken up in writing. First he put together the notes he had made on the Grand Tour; in 1779 he published in two volumes *A View of Society and Manners in France, Switzerland and Germany*, and in 1781 two more volumes on *A View of Society and Manners in Italy*. These met with much success and Moore gained a high reputation in literary circles. After some undistinguished *Medical Sketches*, he published his best known work, a novel called *Zeluco*, in 1786. It is a tale of vice and villainy and ends with the death of Zeluco, a Sicilian nobleman, in a duel. His two later novels, *Edward* and *Mordaunt*, deal more with virtue rewarded and have long been forgotten.

Robert Burns and John Moore had a mutual friend in Mrs Dunlop and she sent Moore in 1786 a copy of the Kilmarnock edition of Burns' poems. A correspondence followed; Moore sent Burns copies of the *View of Society and Manners* and *Zeluco*, and Burns on 2nd August 1787 sent Moore the most famous of all his letters. 'To divert myself a little in this miserable fog of Ennui, I have taken a whim to give you a history of MYSELF'. Then follows the 5,000 word autobiography which has been the basis for all biographies of Burns.

There is no doubt that Burns had an extremely high opinion of Moore's literary ability but their correspondence ceased with some ill feeling in 1794. Moore had gone to Paris in 1792 and witnessed there the destruction of the monarchy and the massacres which followed. He wrote of these experiences in *A Journal during a Residence in France* deploring the savagery and bloodshed he had seen. Burns' comment to Mrs Dunlop was neither forgiven nor forgotten. 'I cannot approve of the honest Doctor's whining over the deserved fate of a certain pair of Personages. What is there in the delivering over a perjured Blockhead, and an unprincipled Prostitute to the hands of the hangman that it should arrest for a moment, attention in an eventful hour'.

When Moore died in 1802 he left five sons, the eldest of whom, General Sir John Moore, was to die in 1809 at Corunna after winning this battle in the Peninsular War. He is perhaps more memorable than his father because of Charles Wolfe's poem—'Not a drum was heard, not a funeral note, / As his corse to the rampart we hurried . . .'. But the father is to be remembered in the annals of the College not only as a successful Glasgow surgeon, general practitioner and physician, but for his honoured place in British literature.

The pure physicians therefore often became such in the evening of their professional life and many were probably weary and unwilling to take on a new burden such as the Presidency of the Faculty. Certainly we find many Presidents being elected for a second or third term of office. The record was held by the following who was President for no less than five terms.

*Note: The Works of John Moore, MD with Memoirs of his Life and Writings* by Robert Anderson MD in 7 volumes, Edinburgh, 1820, is in the College Library.

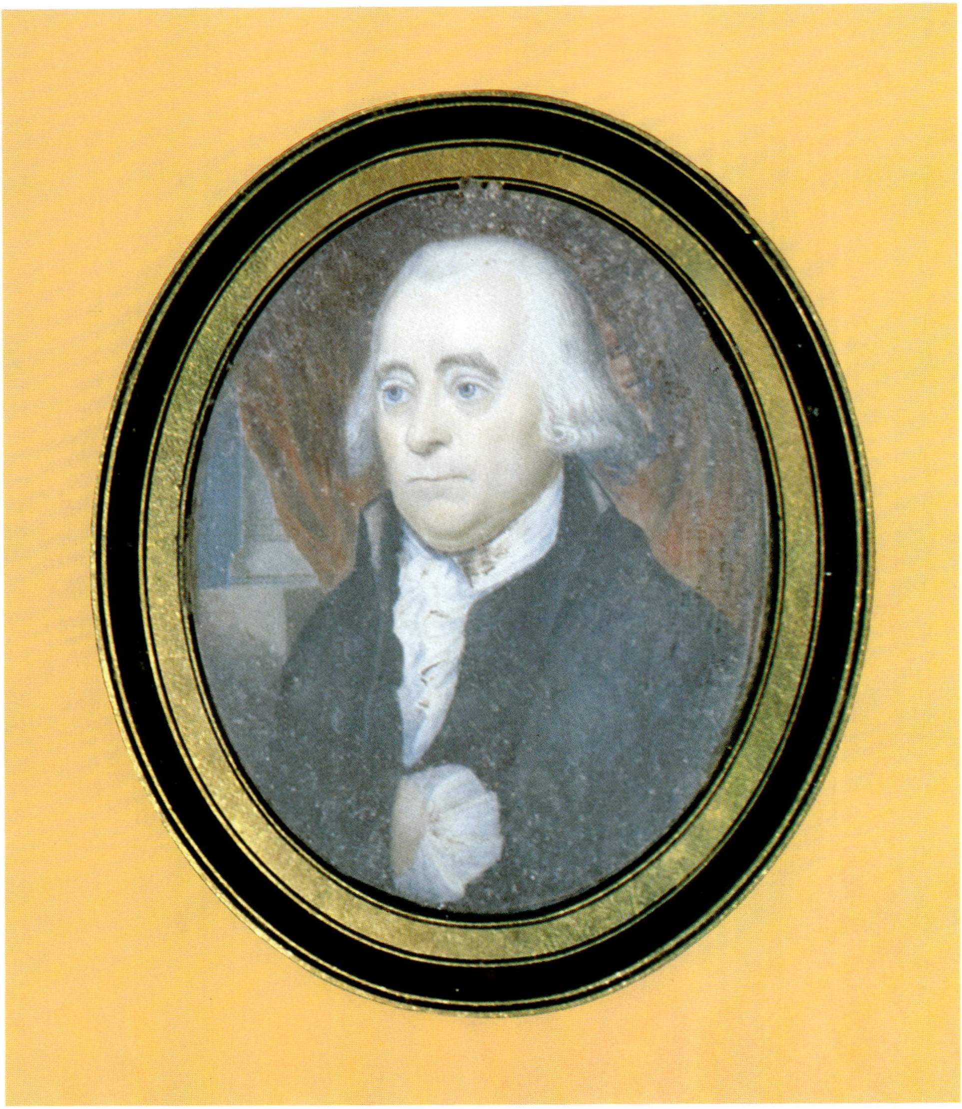

*Peter Wright (c 1740 to 1819) holds the record for having been President of the Faculty no less than five times. The name of the artist of the miniature portrait is unknown.*

*President, 1771 to 1773; 1777 to 1779; 1785 to 1787; 1795 to 1797; 1804 to 1806.*

# PETER WRIGHT

c 1740 to 1819

*The portrait is only a miniature and the artist is unknown.*

Peter Wright took an MD at St Andrews University in 1765. At that time St Andrews was not teaching medicine and it seems likely that Wright learned his doctoring elsewhere, perhaps as an apprentice in a practice, perhaps by classes at Glasgow or Edinburgh. His training and his MD, however, were good enough for the Faculty to admit him in 1766 and to make him President for the first of five terms in 1771. The approximate date of his birth, 1740, given above, is a guess based on these dates; it might well have been earlier.

It has been previously noted how, in 1795, during one of his Presidencies, Wright was asked to do something about the Faculty's ancient portraits which were decaying badly but not too much money was to be spent on them. The result is that they have all gone, although enough seems to have remained of the lineaments of Lowe, Hamilton and Spang for the present copies to be made in 1822.

Anderson's University was founded in Glasgow in 1796 and according to the will of its founder, Dr John Anderson, Peter Wright was made its first President and was also named in Anderson's will as the Professor of the Theory of Medicine. Since Anderson left only £1,000 to endow his university, it is doubtful, however, if Wright ever taught in it.

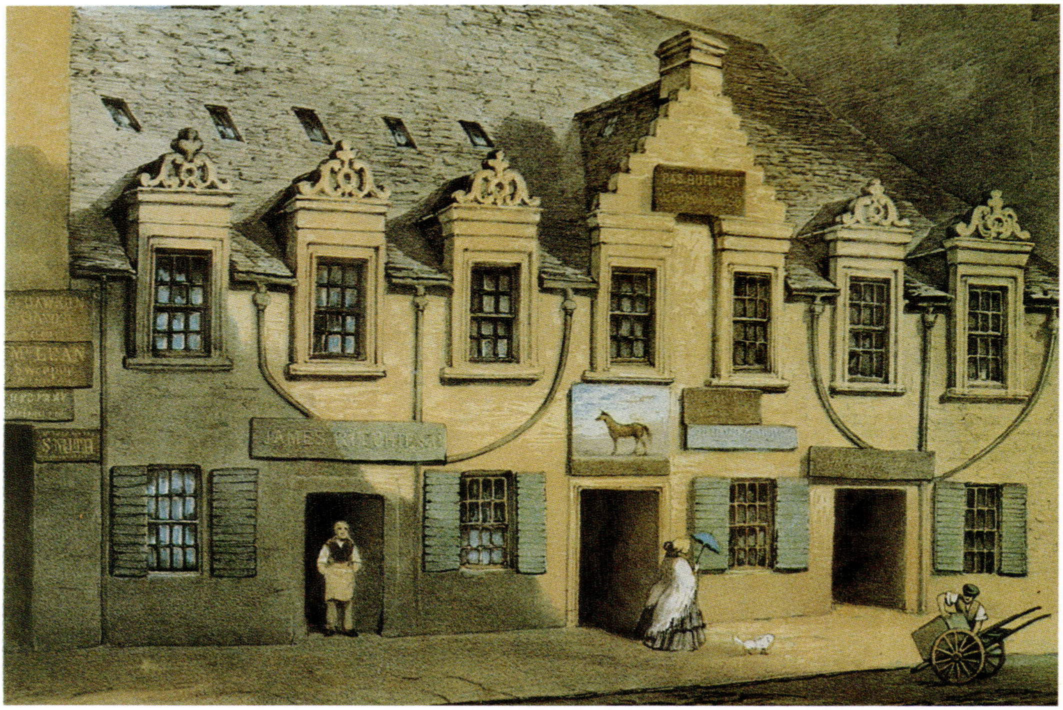


OLD HOUSE IN STOCKWELL STREET (*Fairbairn*, 1850)

*This is described as 'one of the finest specimens extant of the dwelling-houses which the Glasgow citizens of the 17th century delighted to rear for the accommodation of themselves and families'. Built about 1668, it had originally a walled garden and summerhouse at the back and belonged in turn to several of 'the mercantile aristocracy of the time'. Mr Ritchie paid £1,800 for it in 1827 but it had by then ceased to be a dwelling-house.*

*It was the type of house and the situation in which Peter Wright probably lived.*

*Another aspect of the houses of the well-to-do in Peter Wright's time is shown in this Fairbairn (1850) print, 'Court of an old Mansion House, Main Street, Gorbals'.*

*The earliest part of the building dates from 1687 and was a most desirable dwelling-house until about 1800 when the front portion became a public house. 'The tenants are to this day (i.e. 1850) humbly respectable, but they do not, of course, occupy the position in society which their predecessors did'.*

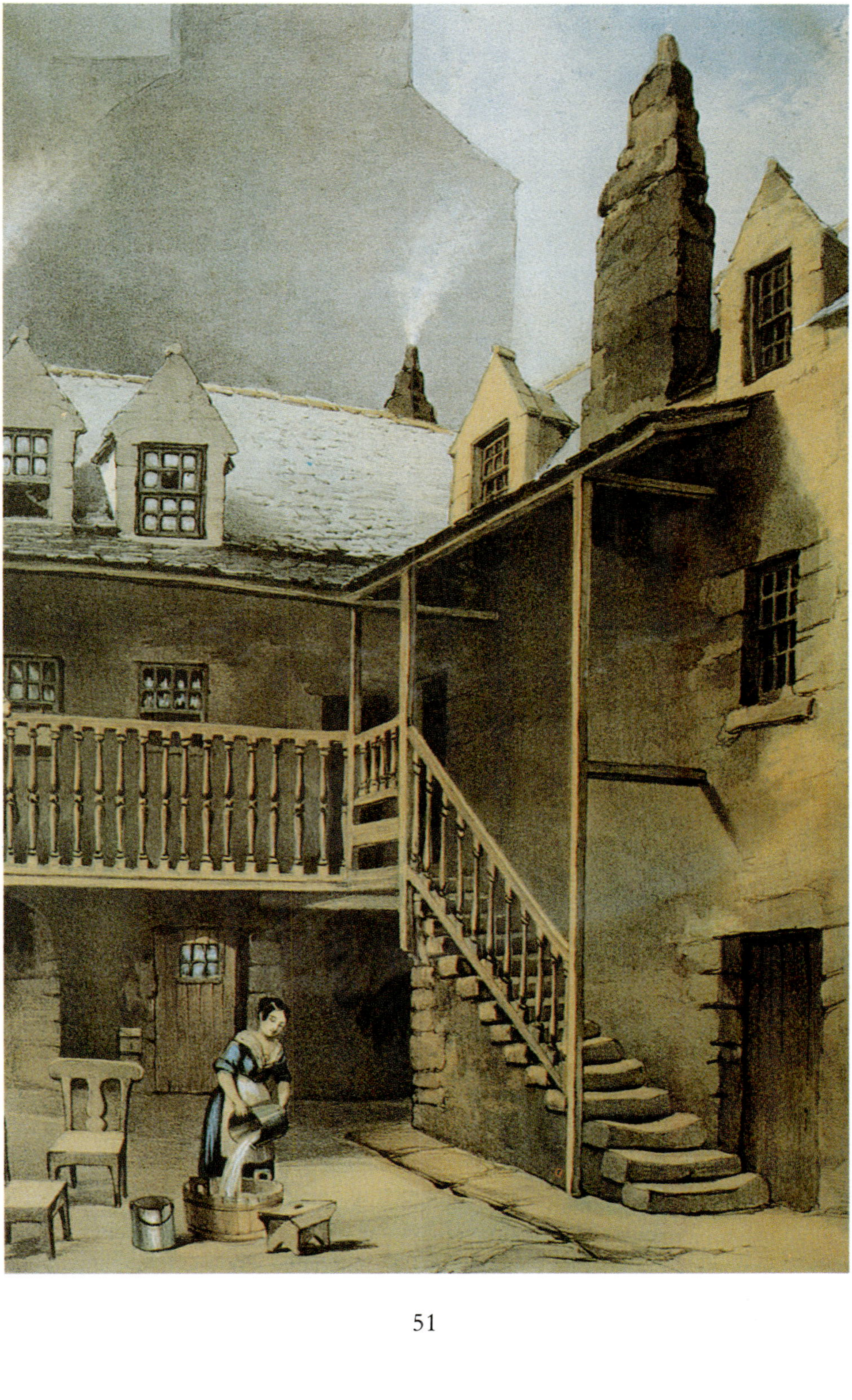

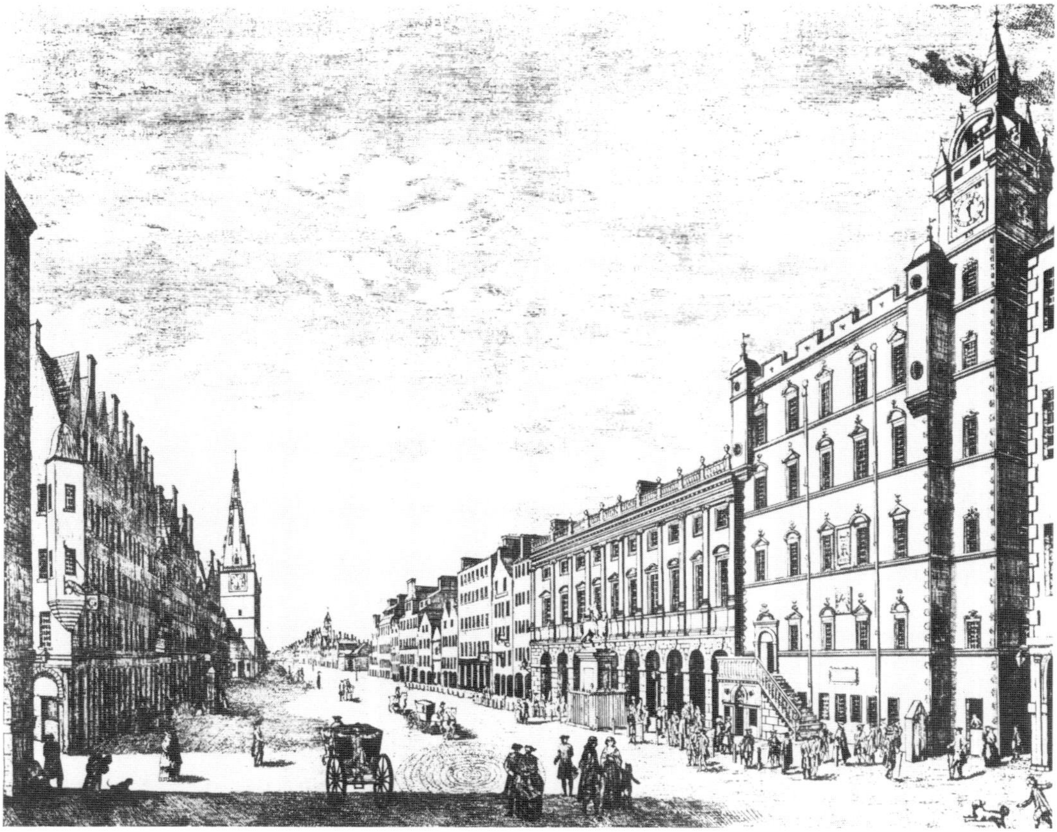

'A View of the Trongate of Glasgow from the East.
R. Paul incepit. Gul Buchananus perfecit.'
(c 1750)

*The Tolbooth is on the right, the Tron Kirk on the left. Beyond the Tolbooth are the arches of the Piazza where were the 'plainstanes'. In front of the Piazza is the statue of King William III which was later removed because of the riots which occurred around it.*

In the published reminiscences of these times, Peter Wright is a kenspeckle figure. We read:

how he attended, at the end of the 18th century, the lying-in of the Duchess of Montrose, wearing a cocked hat and a sword;

how his bag-wig danced and shook with his laughter at a meeting of My Lord Ross's Club;

how he strutted about the 'Plainstanes' in peacock magnificence in his scarlet cloak with a gold-headed cane and a cocked hat perched on powdered hair or wig.

The 'Plainstanes' were the only part of Glasgow then paved with flagstones and lay in front of the Piazzas at Glasgow Cross. It was only the upper classes, those in professions, the tobacco, sugar and cloth barons, and some *literati* who strolled on them with clean shoes. Lower classes and all females had to walk in the dirt of the roadway. Peter Wright was said to be the last person to walk the Plainstanes, 'but his scarlet cloak was then getting rather threadbare'.

He was President of the Faculty of Physicians and Surgeons of Glasgow from 1771 to 1773 and subsequently was re-elected from 1777 to 1779, 1785 to 1787, 1795 to 1797 and 1804 to 1806.

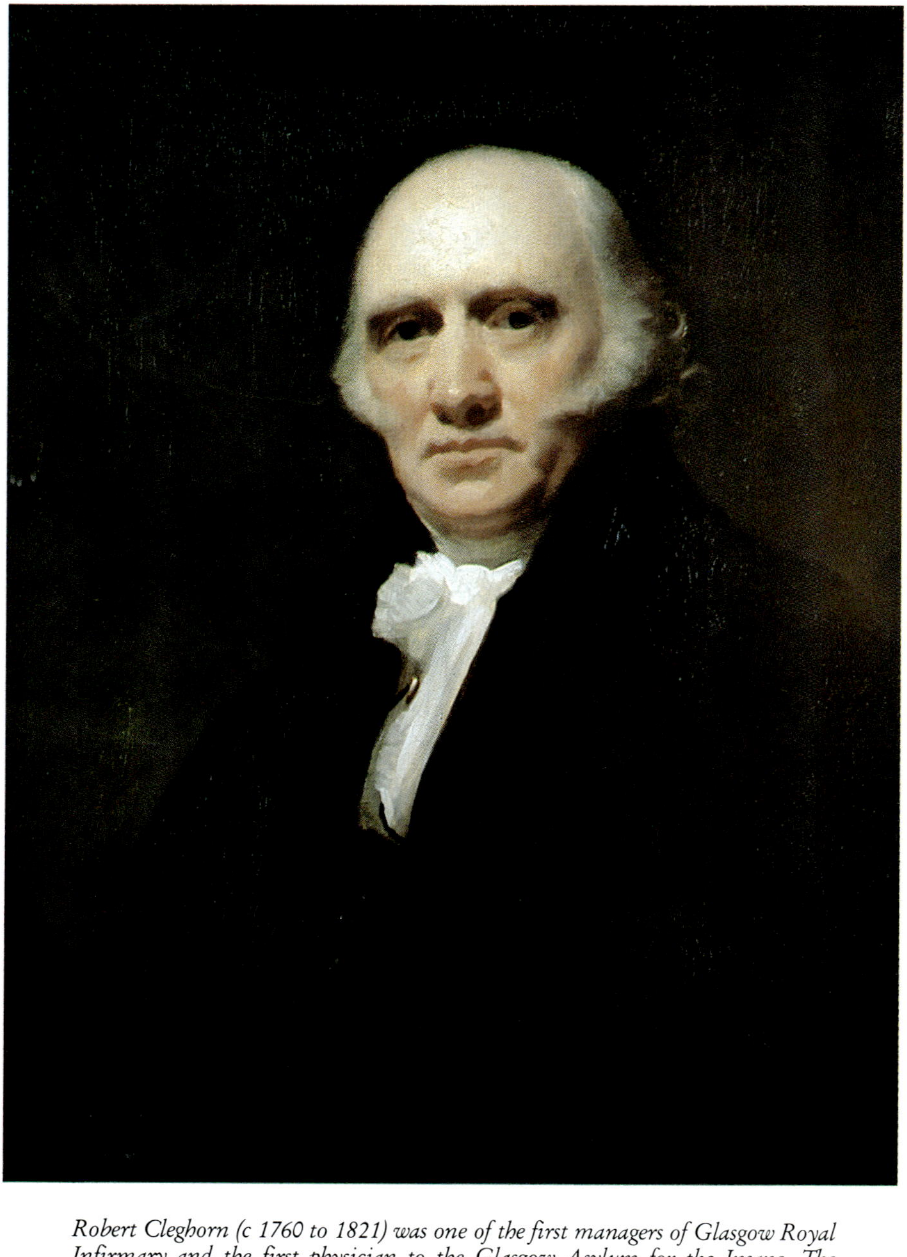

*Robert Cleghorn (c 1760 to 1821) was one of the first managers of Glasgow Royal Infirmary and the first physician to the Glasgow Asylum for the Insane. The portrait is by Sir Henry Raeburn.*
*President, 1788 to 1791.*

# ROBERT CLEGHORN

c 1760 to 1821

*The portrait is by Sir Henry Raeburn and is on extended loan from Gartnavel Royal Hospital.*

Robert Cleghorn studied at, and took his MD in, Edinburgh in 1783. Three years later he was admitted to the Faculty as a physician. In 1788 he was appointed Lecturer in Materia Medica in Glasgow University and in 1791 Lecturer in Chemistry.

A little information about Cleghorn as a lecturer and Cleghorn as a practising physician is available from Thomas Lyle's *University Reminiscences*. He was a popular lecturer and 'his oratory was certainly of the first order and so musical . . . that the student found himself in danger of being sung asleep'. Like others before and since he seems to have delivered the same lectures with the same jokes and comments year after year, but they attracted students. Lyle estimated that his fees from his students each session amounted to 600 guineas.

There have always been wide variations in medical fees, but Cleghorn's seem inordinate even in his upper class practice at that time. One disputed bill for treating the Earl of Eglinton was for £2,000, and he never treated even a member of a tradesman's family for less than a guinea while others would charge a shilling or so. Cleghorn even collected from Jamie, his porter, janitor and jack-of-all-trades, the tips which students gave him for small services, much to the disgust of the students.

These were the days of the 'resurrectionists' and the 'sack-em-up-men' who plundered the graves of the recently dead to provide bodies for dissection. Doctors were hated and feared as well as respected. Comrie tells the story of a hostile crowd gathering one night outside Robert Cleghorn's house in College Street with angry mutterings for vengeance. When the cook went to the door to find the cause, she was immediately accused of being in the act of 'roasting a bairn for the doctor's supper'! Some of the mob had to be taken inside before they could be convinced that it was only a suckling pig that was revolving on the spit. Cleghorn seems to have lived well.

It was however with hospital development in the City that he is particularly remembered. In the early days of the Faculty, Glasgow had no institutions for the

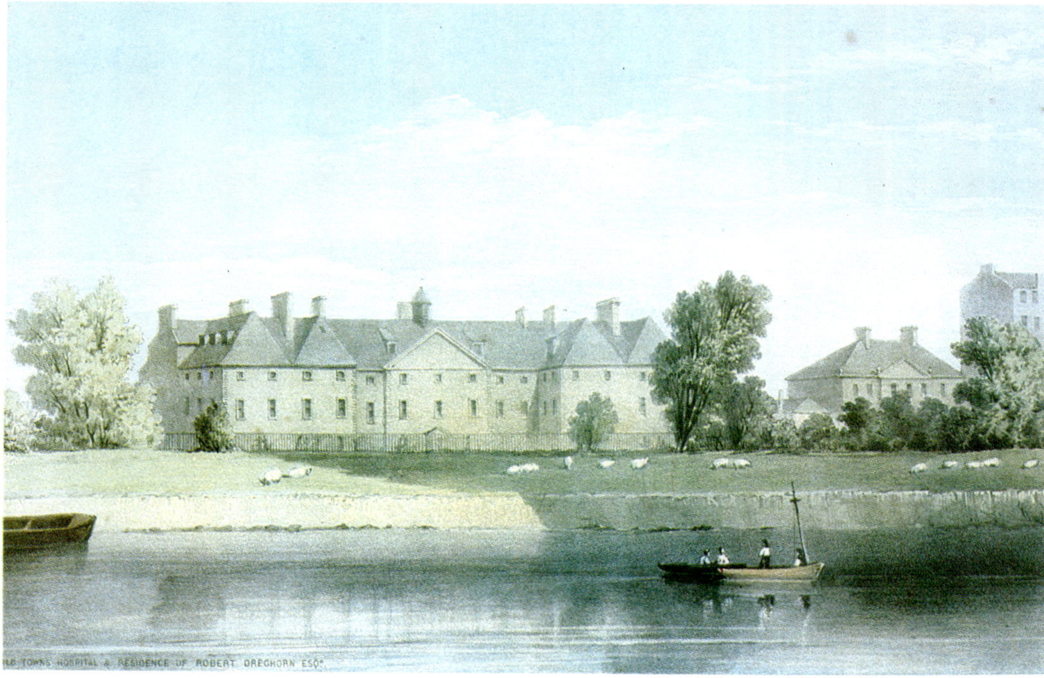


THE OLD TOWN'S HOSPITAL (*Fairbairn*, 1850)

*This was Glasgow's first major hospital and was built near what is now Clyde Street, and opened in 1733. After Glasgow Royal Infirmary opened in 1797 it remained as a poor's-house until 1844 when the inmates were moved to the old Lunatic Asylum in Parliamentary Road whose patients had been transferred to the new asylum at Gartnavel. It was used as a temporary hospital in the great cholera epidemic of 1848 and 1849 but thereafter became a warehouse and was finally demolished.*

treatment of the sick poor and the local authority seems to have relied on the Faculty's once-a-month outpatient sessions and subsidies paid to the occasional physician or surgeon, and even to a 'stonecutter'. The Town's Hospital, the first in Glasgow, was built by public subscription and opened in 1733. It fulfilled a need but the growth of the medical school in the second half of the century required something better for clinical teaching. It is said that Cleghorn taught in the Town's Hospital but it is doubtful if it was ever used much for this purpose; it was probably quite unsuitable.

The movement to build a general hospital suitable for teaching was initiated by the University, but the Faculty was keenly interested and contributed £100 on three separate occasions to the building fund. They were hard-up at the time, having been building their new hall which opened in 1791 in St Enoch Square, and their Widows' Fund had drained much of their assets; otherwise they might have given more. The Royal Infirmary took shape on its present site and was opened for patients in December 1794. Three members of the Faculty and the President *ex officio* were on the Board of Management, as were the University Professors of Anatomy and of Medicine. Since both the latter and all the senior members of the Infirmary staff were also members of

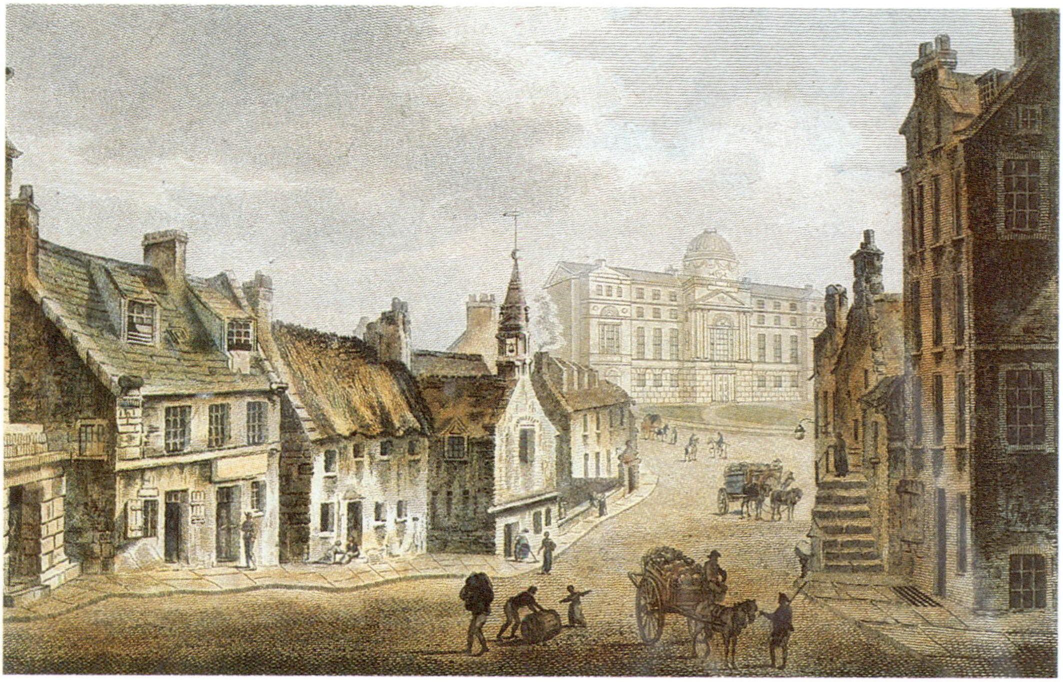

*Glasgow Royal Infirmary in 1801, seven years after it opened, seen from along Kirk Street, the upper end of High Street. The engraving is by W. Miller, Old Bond Street, London.*

the Faculty, it was understandable that the Faculty, in the beginning, took over the organisation of the Hospital much to the wrath of the Managers, and there were many early squabbles. Cleghorn was not only one of the first Managers and one of the first two physicians appointed to the Hospital, but also one of those who successfully supported the Managers in their right to make their own arrangements for running the Hospital without dictation from the Faculty.

But Cleghorn is best remembered today as the first physician to the Glasgow Asylum for the Insane, now Gartnavel Royal Hospital. In the Town's Hospital there were a few 'cells' set aside for the insane poor; for the insane well-to-do there was no accommodation whatever. The condition of the 'cells' was appalling even to the Hospital's directors who in 1805 approached the Lord Provost about building an asylum. He in turn approached the Faculty who set up a committee and contributed £100. The Asylum was built between 1810 and 1814 north of Cathedral Street in what was then green fields but became Parliamentary Road. This in turn has recently been bulldozed out of existence and a certain amount of greenery has reappeared.

The original building became too small and the present hospital was begun at Gartnavel in 1842.

In 1817 Cleghorn retired from his Lectureship in Chemistry apparently on the understanding that he would be appointed Professor; but the Chair went to another, and thereafter, according to Lyle, 'the Doctor's spirits seldom rallied above zero'. He moved to his country house on the banks of the Clyde near Rutherglen and as his health declined feared more and more that he would die in poverty and pled with his old colleagues that when his money was gone and they had to remove him to the Town's Hospital they would grant him a small room to himself. He left in fact an immense fortune which went to his only child, a daughter with club feet.

Robert Cleghorn was President of the Faculty of Physicians and Surgeons of Glasgow from 1788 to 1791.

# 4

## THE END OF THE 'PURE' PHYSICIANS
1820 to 1830

John Balmanno (c 1775 to 1840)
Alexander Dunlop Anderson (1794 to 1871)

Because of the shortage of suitable candidates for the office of President among the few pure physicians in practice, the Faculty discussed in 1812 a resolution to open the office to a surgeon equally as to a physician provided he had an MD, but this was rejected. Paradoxically, there was then almost a surfeit of young MD's. The number of students attending the University School of Medicine had increased markedly because of the demands of the Napoleonic Wars and many went on and took their MD. But they couldn't survive economically as pure physicians and many MD's practised as surgeons or general practitioners. Indeed, with the growth of the University Medical Schools more and more surgeons were graduates and the old style apprenticeship training was dying out. The whole spectrum of medical practice was changing and when the resolution was again put before the Faculty in 1820, it was passed with only one member dissenting. From then onwards the offices of President and Visitor could be held by either a surgeon or a physician, and the office of Visitor eventually became not just that of Vice-President but that of President-Elect.

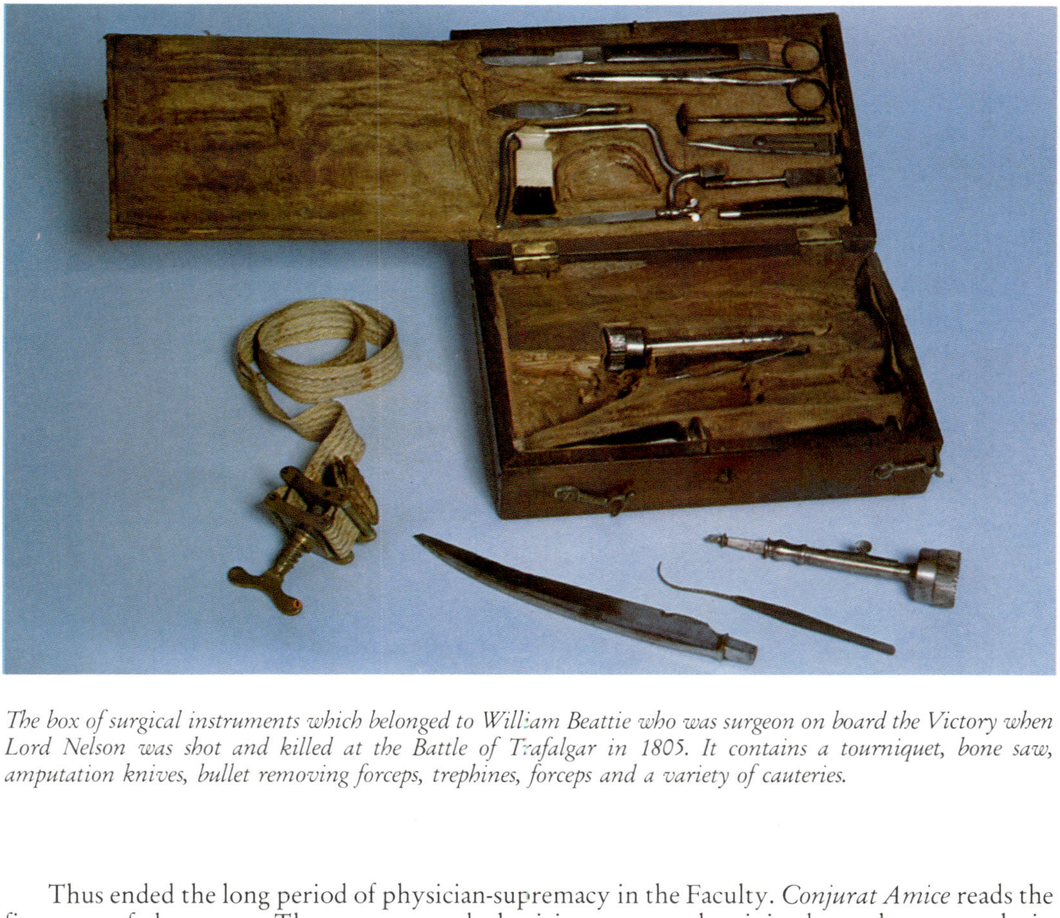

*The box of surgical instruments which belonged to William Beattie who was surgeon on board the Victory when Lord Nelson was shot and killed at the Battle of Trafalgar in 1805. It contains a tourniquet, bone saw, amputation knives, bullet removing forceps, trephines, forceps and a variety of cauteries.*

Thus ended the long period of physician-supremacy in the Faculty. *Conjurat Amice* reads the first part of the motto. The surgeons and physicians were at last joined together not only in friendship but on a basis of equality.

One of the last of the 'pure' physician Presidents was the next subject, John Balmanno. His story also illustrates the similar change in the staffing of Glasgow Royal Infirmary where at first only the 'pure' were allowed to hold staff appointments as physicians.

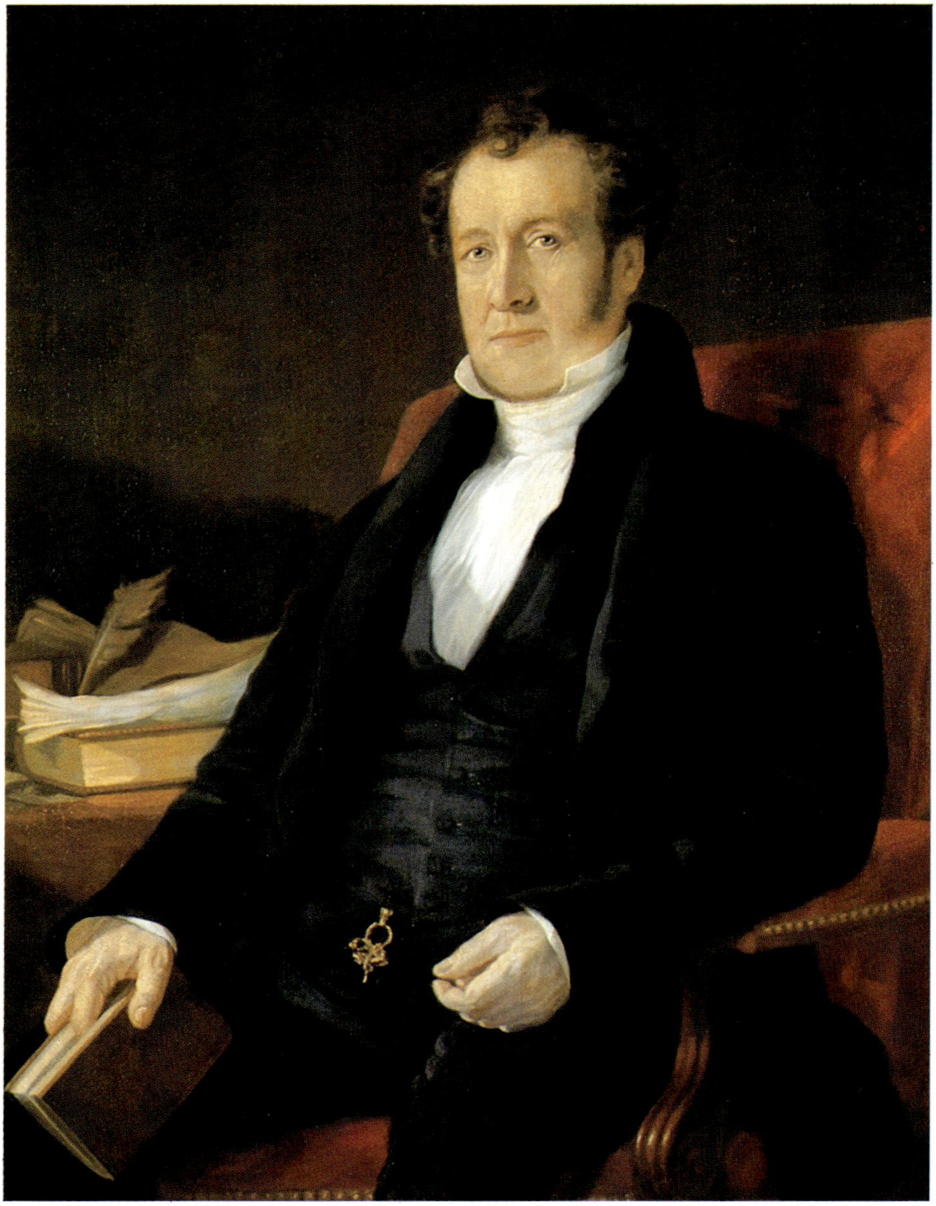

*John Balmanno (c 1775 to 1840) was one of the last of the 'pure' physicians and succeeded Robert Cleghorn as physician to the Glasgow Asylum for the Insane. The portrait, according to Duncan, is by Sir Henry Raeburn, but some modern artists have been uncertain about this.*

*President, 1800 to 1802; 1806 to 1808; 1818 to 1820; 1826 to 1828.*

# JOHN BALMANNO

c 1775 to 1840

*The portrait by Sir Henry Raeburn was housed in Gartnavel Royal Hospital until 1980 when it was loaned to the Royal College. It was cleaned, repaired and reframed at that time.*

John Balmanno was virtually the last of the 'pure' physicians in the West of Scotland and his fame was matched if not actually surpassed by that of his mother. Mrs Balmanno in the latter part of the 18th century kept a druggist's or apothecary's shop at the sign of the 'Golden Galen's Head' in the centre of Glasgow which was very well known and popular. The lady was both diagnostician and therapeutist and had her own 'physic garden' in which she grew many of the ingredients of her pills, powders and potions. This garden lay on the north side of George Street west of High Street and was later passed by Balmanno Street which ran up to Rottenrow ending in the steep Balmanno Brae. The Balmanno building at the junction of Balmanno Street and Rottenrow was originally constructed after John Balmanno's death as an 'Asylum for Indigent Old Men'. It is now much altered and is now a Hall of Residence of Strathclyde University, the original building having been demolished. It is clear that the names commemorate both the physician and his mother.

John Balmanno studied medicine in Edinburgh and graduated MD in 1798 with a thesis entitled 'De debilium palpitatione' and was admitted to the Faculty in 1801 as a physician on presentation of his Diploma. Under the will of John Anderson he was designated to the Chair of Materia Medica in Anderson's University, but it is unlikely that he ever taught there.

He was appointed to Glasgow Royal Infirmary in 1804. The appointments then were for a set period which varied from time to time, followed by a period of ineligibility and then usually reappointment. There were two physician posts to be filled in the Royal Infirmary; the regulations stated that they must be 'pure' physicians, but there were very few such remaining. By 1830 there were only two: Drs John Balmanno and Richard Millar. The Faculty's difficulties in finding 'pure' physicians for its Presidents is illustrated by the fact that Balmanno had been President twice and Millar no less than four times: 1800 to 1802; 1806 to 1808; 1818 to 1820 and 1826 to 1828.

The 'pure' physician had become an anachronism and the days of the gold-headed cane, the powdered wig, and the flowing red cloak were over. Dr Millar fought hard to retain the old system but no one supported him and the Managers of the Royal Infirmary finally agreed that 'any gentleman who shall have been 15 years in general

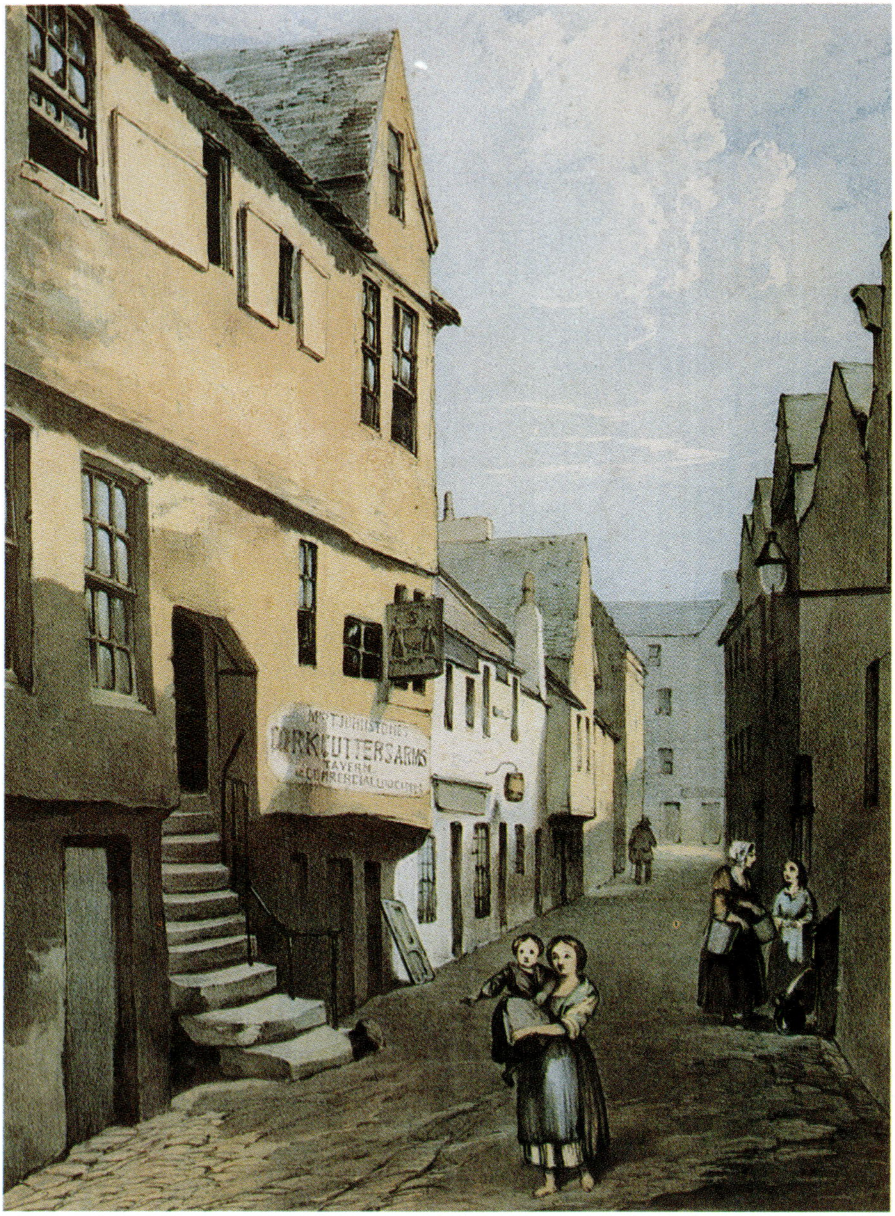


LAIGH-KIRK CLOSS (*Fairbairn*, 1850)

*A 'Closs' or 'Close' at that time meant a lane and not, as today, the common entrance to a tenement. The view looks into the Closs from the Trongate and the house on the left which also had a front on the Trongate was where Margaret Tarbet had her shop selling paints, perfumery and drugs. She married one of her shopmen called Balmanno and their son Dr John kept on the shop and lived for some time in the adjoining timber house after his mother's death.*

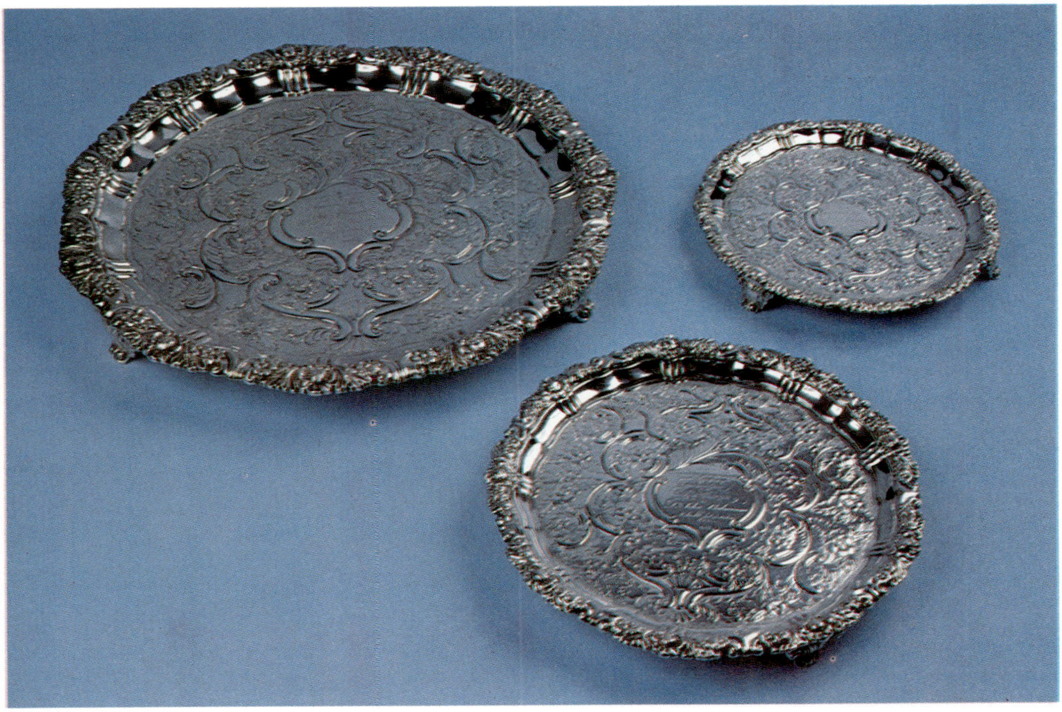

*Set of Silver Salvers presented in 1818 to John Balmanno by the Committee of Subscribers for the Suppression of Contagious Fevers. The inscription is in the text.*

practice and who shall have obtained the degree of Doctor of Medicine . . . shall be eligible to be Physician in the Infirmary'.

In Balmanno's lifetime plagues and pestilences were never far away. The ever-increasing influx of labour from Ireland and the Highlands led to such unbelievable overcrowding and insanitation that it is almost miraculous that the whole population was not wiped out. One of the most terrible epidemics occurred in 1818 and both Balmanno and Millar acquitted themselves well not only in tending the sick but in impressing the local authority on the need for action. One of the most prized possessions of the Royal College is a set of three silver salvers each of which bears the following inscription:

*Committee of Subscribers for the*
*Suppression of Contagious Fevers*
*in the City of Glasgow*
*to*
*Dr. John Balmanno*
*for valuable and gratuitous services*
*1818.*



E

The story of how these came into the College's possession is worth retelling.

Mrs Balmanno, the druggist, had a sister who was married to a William Fleming. Mr Fleming, in 1751, leased a plot of land from the Town Council beside the Molendinar burn near where the stream runs into the Clyde. There he built a sawmill which he drove with water from a dam he built on the burn. He prospered, for he was the first to use Scotch fir for making boxes, laths and other simple wooden articles previously made from imported timber. But there were complaints; his dam and its release was causing flooding in the Clyde; effluvia were damaging the fish. There may well have been an element of jealousy too, for one day in 1764, without telling Mr Fleming, the Council sent along twelve men who demolished the whole mill and threw the debris into the Molendinar. Mr Fleming, much angered, sued the Council and was awarded damages of £610 with which he purchased some farm land on the North of the city and which, in a final gesture of retribution, he called Sawmillfield. Quite by accident, apparently, this laid the foundations of the Fleming family fortunes for generations. A year after he bought the land in 1767 the Forth and Clyde Canal began to be dug and was planned to pass right through Sawmillfield. The Flemings at first protested at the inconvenience of

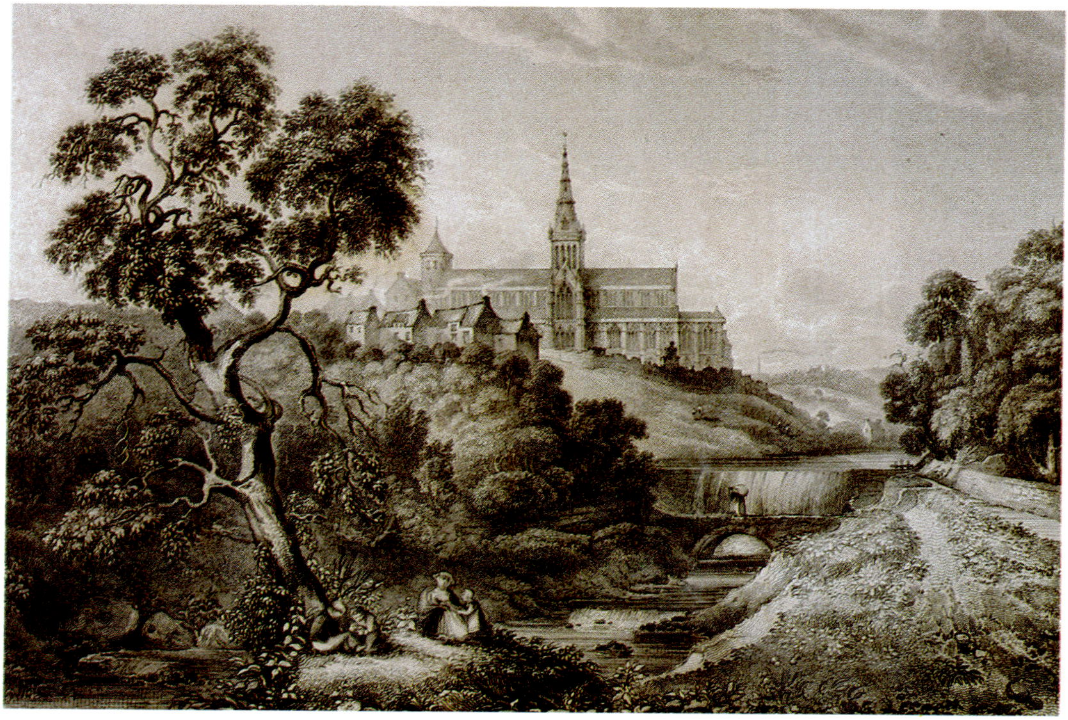

*The Cathedral and the College were both built on the banks of the Molendinar burn which supplied them with water and drainage, at least in the beginning. This undated engraving by Wm. Brown shows the Cathedral from the south and the burn running down its eastern flank.*

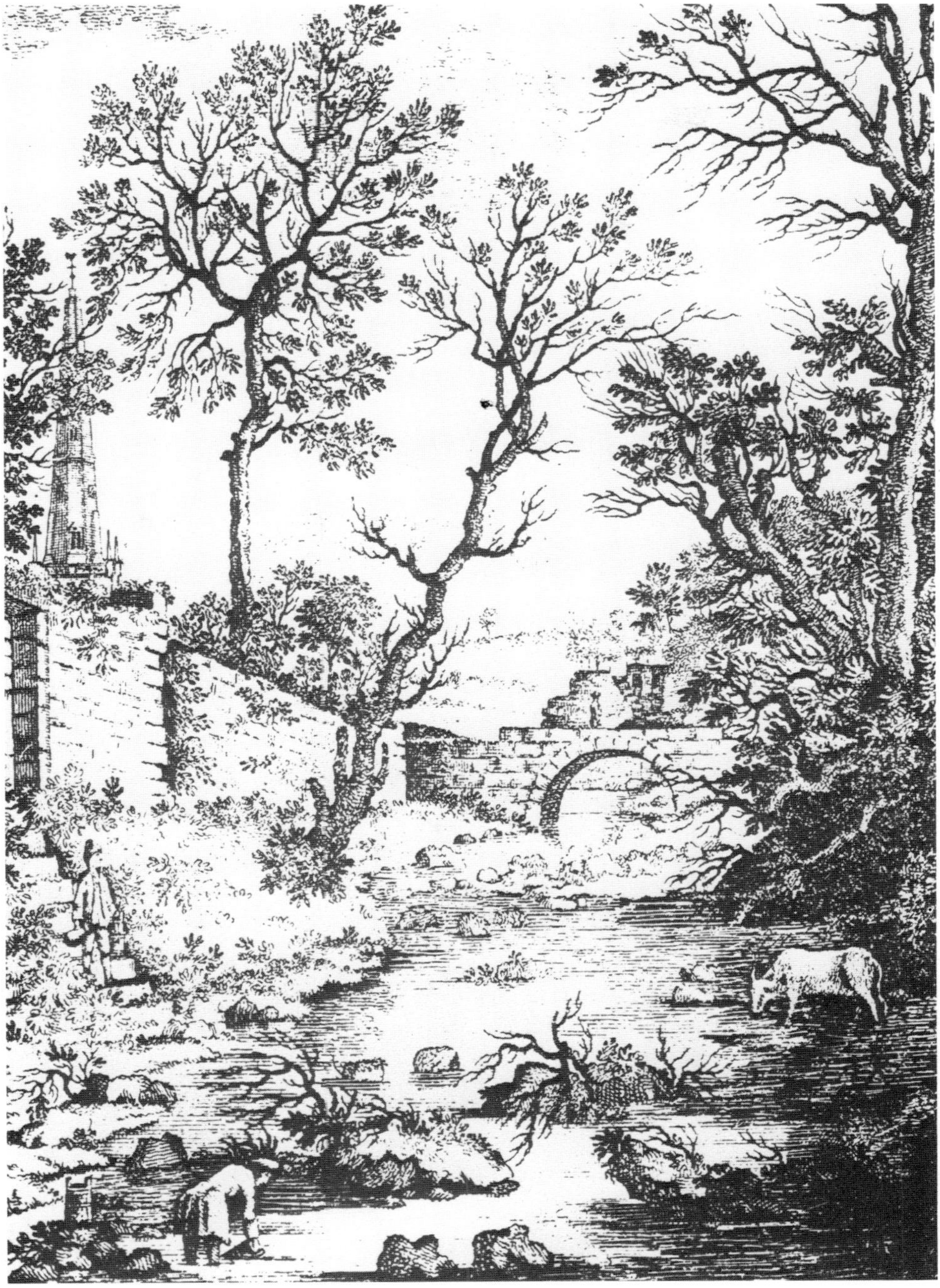

*Another view of the Molendinar, probably by Robert Paul about 1750. The Cathedral spire is on the left. The Molendinar today is the outflow from Hogganfield Loch and is completely tunnelled underground as far as the Clyde.*

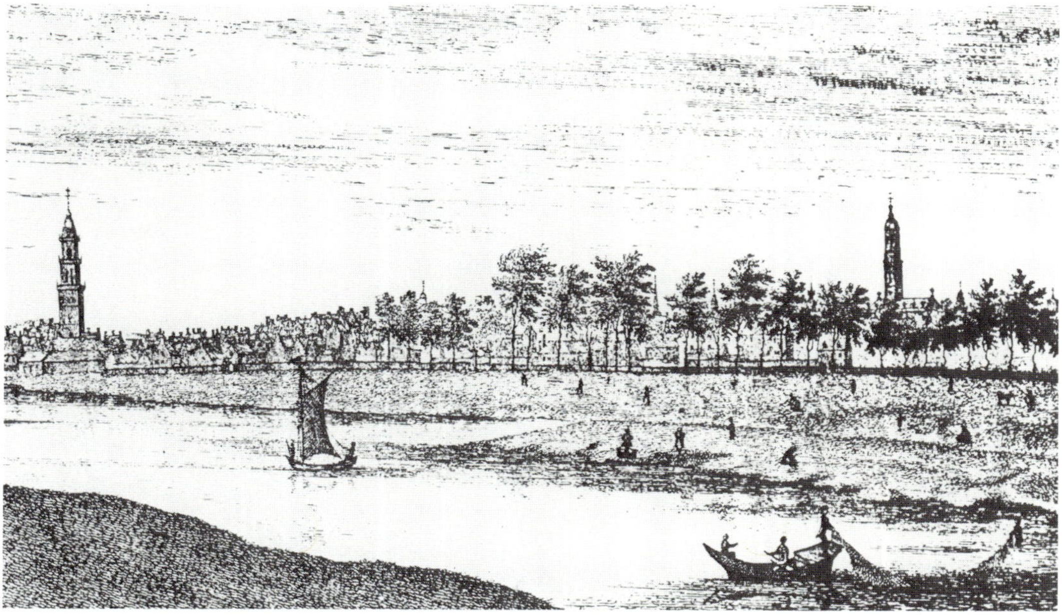

*Salmon fishing in the Clyde from an engraving by Robert Paul about 1760.*

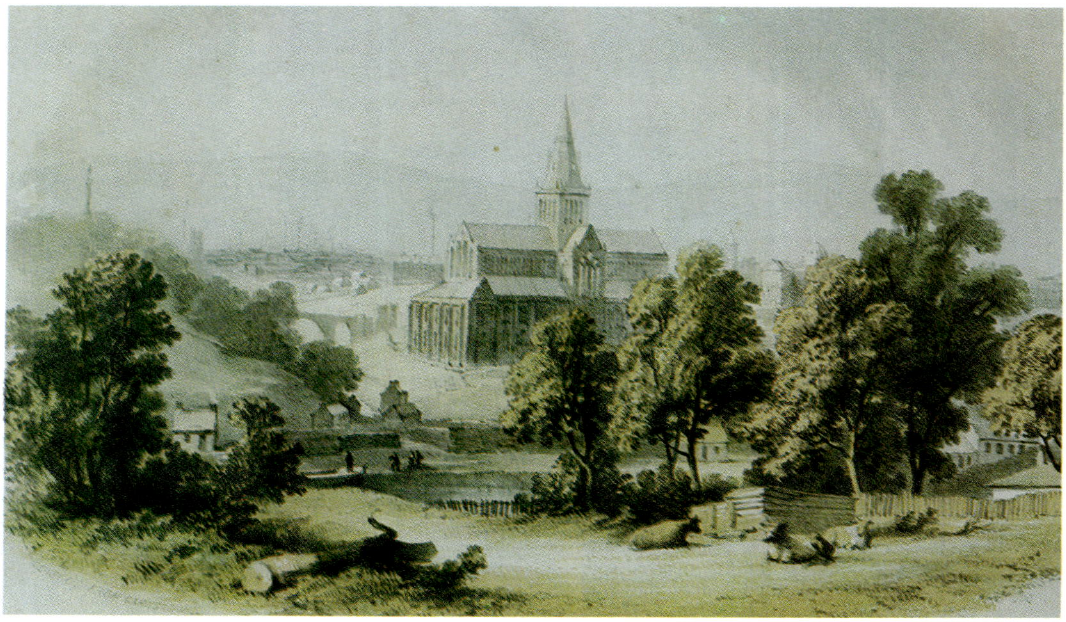

'VIEW FROM GARNGAD HILL' (*Fairbairn*, 1850)

*The Forth and Clyde Canal is in the middle foreground and the area is near the site of Fleming's 'Sawmillfield'. Today it is completely built over.*

having to ferry cattle back and forth, but soon realised that the land was now worth many times its purchase price.

William Fleming had a grandson, John Gibson Fleming (*q.v.*) and he in turn had a grandson Geoffrey Balmanno Fleming who was President of the Royal Faculty from 1946 to 1948. Geoffrey B. Fleming was Professor of Child Health in Glasgow University and appears to have inherited much of the Balmanno/Fleming wealth. A bachelor like Balmanno, he made a number of gifts to the Faculty including the Portrait of King James VI and after his death in 1952 the largest of the three salvers was bequeathed to the Faculty. The executors of his estate later donated the two smaller pieces to keep the set intact.

A student of Glasgow Royal Infirmary, writing many years later, remembered John Balmanno as 'a big-boned, somewhat ungainly looking person with features . . . for the most part austere but expressive of power. He had a ringing voice which resounded through the ward and compelled attention'. He was a popular clinical teacher who still used Latin in giving instructions to his juniors, one favourite phrase being '*Descendat in balneam tepidam, hora somni*'. A warm bath before going to sleep was both cleansing and relaxing, and, ordered in Latin, had probably more therapeutic effect; at least it complied with the basic principles of all treatment: *nihil nocere*, 'do no harm'.

John Balmanno succeeded Robert Cleghorn as Visiting Physician to Glasgow Royal Asylum on the death of the latter in 1821. In his later years the Asylum work increased to such an extent that it took up nearly all of his time and when he died in 1840 the post of resident physician superintendent was created.

John Balmanno was President of the Faculty of Physicians and Surgeons of Glasgow on two occasions: 1802 to 1804 and 1812 to 1814.

The next subject is one of those who started their hospital appointments as surgeons because they were not sufficiently 'pure' to be physicians, but later when the rules changed were appointed physicians.

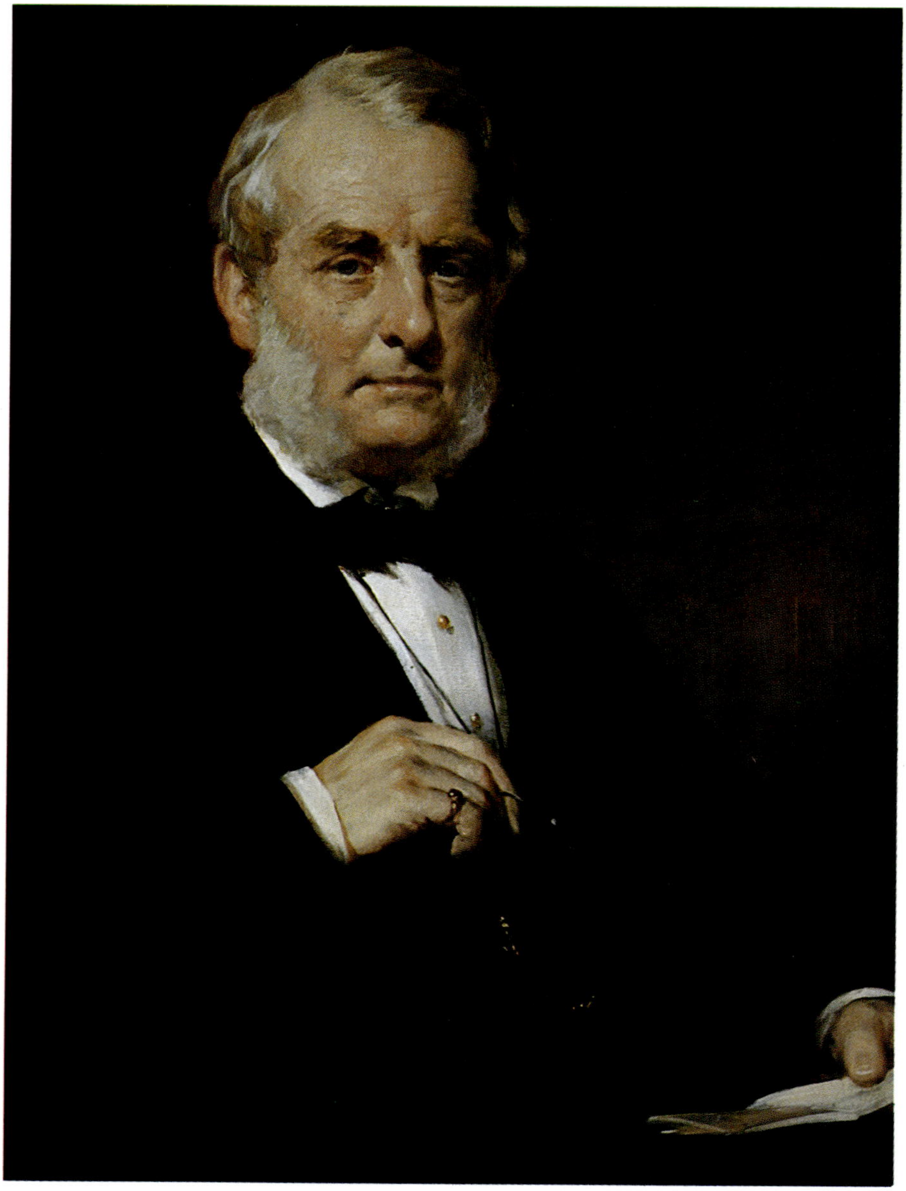

*Alexander Dunlop Anderson (1794 to 1871) was first a surgeon in Glasgow Royal Infirmary and then, after the rules about 'purity' of physicians changed in 1830, he became a physician. He was the father of Sir Thomas McCall Anderson, Regius Professor of Medicine in the early 1900s. The portrait is a delightful example of the work of Sir Daniel Macnee.*

*President, 1852 to 1855.*

# ALEXANDER DUNLOP ANDERSON

1794 to 1871

*The portrait is by Sir Daniel Macnee. It was commissioned by the Faculty in 1869 'as a mark of great respect and esteem the Fellows entertain for his high character as a Physician and private friend and their appreciation of the interest and attention he has always taken in the affairs of the Faculty and the many important services he has rendered to the Corporation during a period of nearly fifty years'. A special meeting was held in the Faculty Hall for the portrait's unveiling in 1870.*

Alexander Dunlop Anderson was born in Greenock to Andrew Anderson, a merchant in the town. John Anderson, who founded Anderson's University, was a brother of Andrew and thus the uncle of our Alexander. Alexander was in due course the father of Sir Thomas McCall Anderson who became Regius Professor of Medicine in Glasgow in 1900 and achieved international fame as a dermatologist. Alexander was also the uncle of another Andrew Anderson who was Professor of the Practice of Medicine in Anderson's College, an ophthalmologist of note, and President of the Faculty of Physicians and Surgeons of Glasgow from 1868 to 1870.

But that is enough of Anderson genealogy! The ramifications of this famous academic and medical family need a treatise to themselves.

The family was obviously well-to-do and Alexander was able to study medicine in Glasgow, Edinburgh and London. He became a member of the London College of Surgeons in 1816. The system there was somewhat similar to the present MRCP/FRCP and Anderson was elected a Fellow in 1844. Some of his studies appear to have been carried out after he had joined the Medical Service of the Army at the age of nineteen. He served as assistant surgeon for six years, i.e. until 1819, with the 49th Regiment and spent some time with them in Canada.

He graduated MD in Edinburgh in 1819, settled in practice in Glasgow in 1820 and the following year joined the Faculty of Physicians and Surgeons of Glasgow.

In the end he became a physician and it may be that in spite of, or because of, his Army experience, he always had leanings towards medicine rather than surgery.

However, the rule about 'pure' physicians in the Glasgow Royal Infirmary still prevailed and in the 1820s he filled a series of surgical appointments:

1823—Junior Surgeon 1st Year
1824—Junior Surgeon 2nd Year
1827—Senior Surgeon 1st Year
1828—Senior Surgeon 2nd Year

After the rules had been changed in 1830, Anderson applied for a vacancy and was appointed Physician to the Infirmary in 1838. He was also for a time Physician to the Institution for the Deaf and Dumb.

He wrote a few short papers, mostly case reports, but one on the treatment of burns with cotton wool in the *Glasgow Medical Journal* of 1828, while he was still a surgeon, is memorable. He noted that the scalds which a small child had received from hot porridge and which had been wrapped in cotton wool which the mother was carding at the time, were completely healed when he removed the wool some days later. He describes 14 cases of burns treated with freshly carded cotton; some patients died, some lesions were deep, others just blisters, and, while he claims relief from pain and other symptoms, the paper resembles a host of others on burns in being little more than anecdotal. His final advice, however, is sound for many burns dressings: having applied the cotton wool, leave it be. Only remove it for very pressing reasons and certainly not because of the offensive smell or because the patient thinks that nothing is being done for him.

The Western Medical Club which still flourishes today was formed in 1845. It began when a group of the most eminent Glasgow physicians and surgeons had dinner together at Bell's Inn at Bowling Bay, a mile or two down the north bank of the Clyde. The evening 'was spent with great hilarity and it was agreed to institute a club with the object of providing friendly and social intercourse among the members of the medical profession in Glasgow and the West of Scotland'. Three subjects of our portraits were the office bearers. A. D. Anderson was appointed chairman, Robert Perry was vice-chairman, and John Gibson Fleming, whose words are quoted above, was secretary.

When A. D. Anderson died on 5th June 1871 the President, Dr John Gibson Fleming, called a special meeting of the Council which resolved to request his family to allow the funeral to take place from the Faculty Hall 'as a recognition of his long and valuable services to the Faculty and of the esteem in which he was held as a professional brother'. The family agreed.

Alexander Dunlop Anderson was President of the Faculty of Physicians and Surgeons of Glasgow from 1852 to 1855.

# 5

## THE FACULTY AND THE UNIVERSITY, I: WILLIAM CULLEN AND HIS PUPILS

William Cullen (1710 to 1790)
Joseph Black (1728 to 1799)
William Hunter (1718 to 1783)

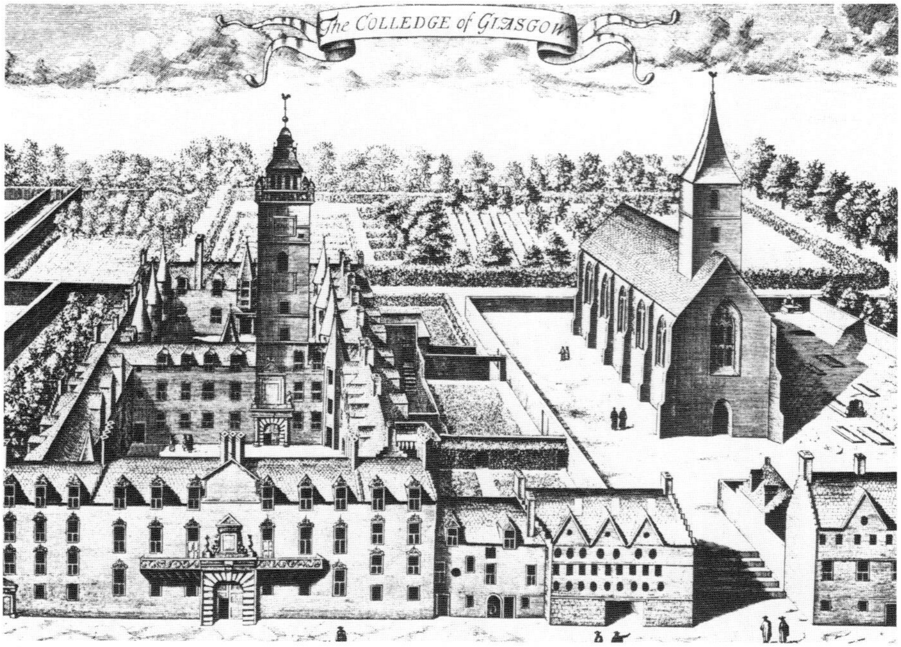


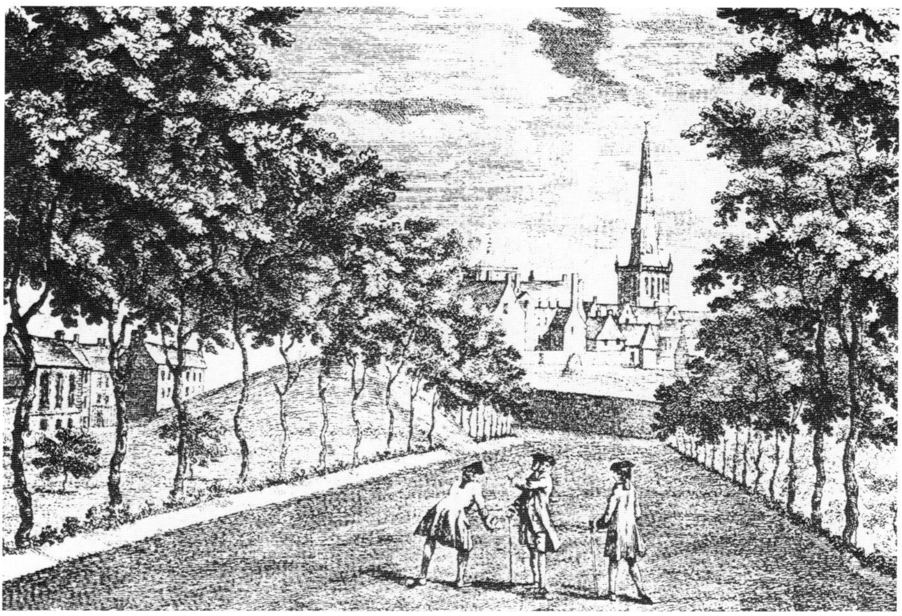

*The College of Glasgow, as the University was originally called, was founded in 1451 and built south of the Cathedral on the west bank of the Molendinar. The grounds and gardens were spacious, as may be seen from the lower engraving: 'A View of the Middle Walk in the College Garden'. It is by Robert Paul and dated 1762. The upper engraving is undated but is probably by the same hand and about the same date.*

The papal bull of Nicholas V which founded Glasgow University in 1451 empowered the granting of degrees in theology, canon and civil law, and '*quavis alia licita facultate*', in any other recognised discipline. The University had therefore every right if it had so wished to have a medical faculty and grant testimonials. There is indeed a record of one early '*doctor in medicinis*', Mr Andreas de Garleis, admitted as such to the University in 1469, but this was an isolated instance. The first Professor of Medicine was Dr Robert Mayne who was appointed in 1637 'to teach a public lecture of Medicine . . . once or twice every week except in vacation times'. There is some evidence that he did so but none that it had any impact on medical training. When he died in 1646 the professorship lapsed. The University made another attempt to set up a medical school in the early years of the 18th century. Dr John Johnstoune was appointed to the chair of Medicine in 1714 and Dr William Brisbane to that of Anatomy and Botany in 1720. But the professorships were largely titular and a contemporary wrote in 1745 that neither gave lectures. They did, however, fill the chairs to the exclusion of others for many years. Brisbane died in 1742 and was succeeded by Dr Robert Hamilton, a brother of the Thomas Hamilton who was John Moore's partner. With only a handful of students and the current impossibility of legally obtaining subjects for dissection, Hamilton at least made a start and paved the way for the real beginning of Glasgow University Medical School when William Cullen was appointed in 1751 to succeed Dr Johnstoune who had held on to his sinecure of a chair for 30 years before resigning in 1750.

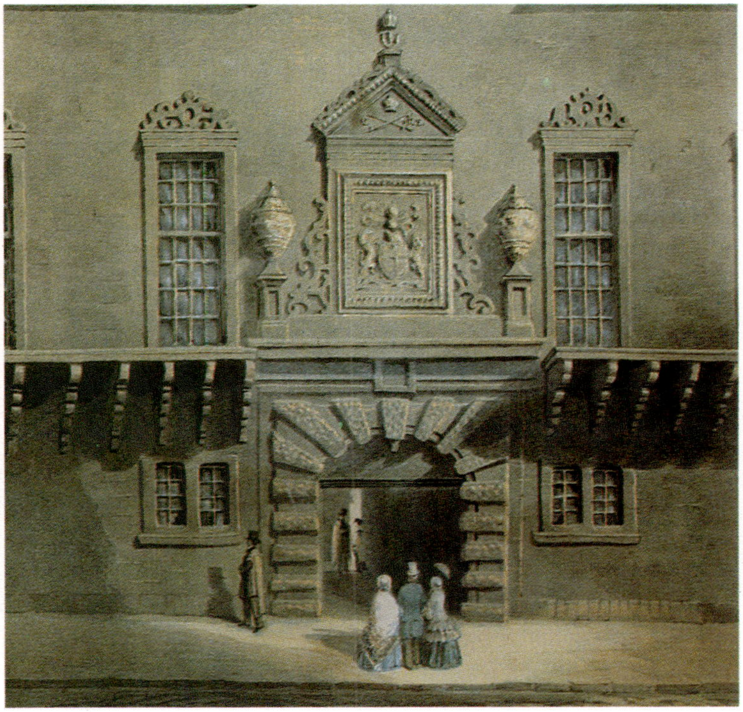

THE FRONT GATE OF THE COLLEGE (*Fairbairn*, 1850)

*Much of this gateway with the Royal Arms and the initials of Charles II above it was removed from the old University in College Street and built into the north-east entrance to the new University on Gilmorehill in 1870 where it remains.*

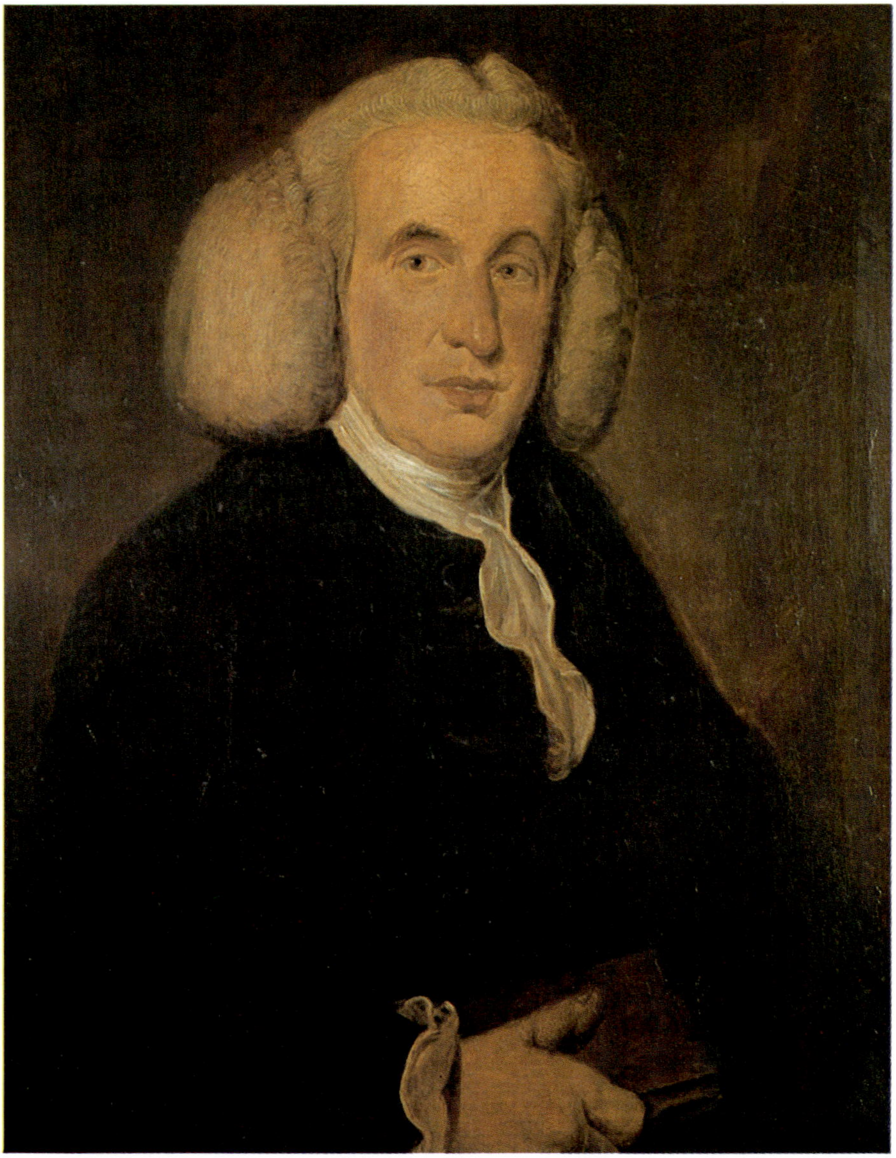

*William Cullen (1710 to 1790) was the real founder of the Glasgow University Medical School, although he later left it for Edinburgh. At first a general practitioner/surgeon he attained international fame as a physician and his research in chemistry was the inspiration of Joseph Black. The portrait is a copy of that by W. Cochrane in Glasgow University.*

*President, 1747 to 1749.*

# WILLIAM CULLEN

1710 to 1790

*The portrait is a replica of that by W. Cochrane in the Hunterian Museum at Glasgow University. It was presented to the Faculty in 1869 by Dr Tannahill.*

Cullen was born in 1710 in Hamilton, a small country town about 10 miles from Glasgow. His early schooling was at the local grammar school and when aged about fifteen he was apprenticed to John Paisley who had an extensive general practice in Glasgow. Paisley was also the librarian to the Faculty and possessed a worthwhile medical library of his own which he later made available to Cullen's students. During his apprenticeship Cullen attended some of the Arts classes at Glasgow University. In 1729 he went to London where he obtained a surgeon's post on a merchant ship sailing between London and the West Indies. His experience on ship-board and in the Islands greatly extended his medical knowledge. Captain Cleland, the master of the ship, liked and respected the lad and two or three years later invited him to stay on his estate and look after his ailing son. It so happened that this estate was at Shotts, not far from Hamilton, and so Cullen was able to look after his family affairs which had devolved on him and at the same time start up a general practice in a district which housed some of the most respected and powerful families in Scotland. He might well have settled there comfortably but after two years, avid for more knowledge, and helped by a small legacy, he spent two years in Edinburgh studying at the University Medical School which had made an excellent start with, among others, Munro *primus* as Professor of Anatomy. Now 26 years old, Cullen set up in practice in Hamilton where he was employed by the Duke of Hamilton and the other landed gentry in the neighbourhood. One of his apprentices from 1737 to 1740 was William Hunter (*q.v.*). He graduated MD at Glasgow University in 1740 and moved from Hamilton to Glasgow in 1744.

There is no doubt that this move was intended to give him the opportunity to teach medicine to others, in the way he had seen it taught in Edinburgh. In his first year, he

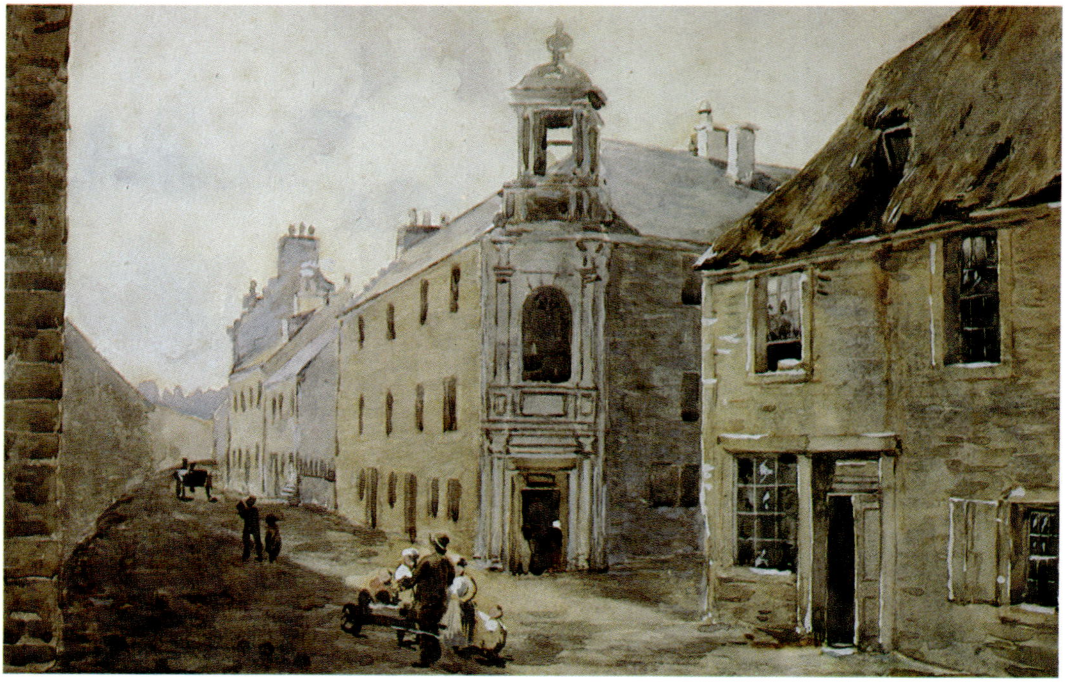

*William Cullen's House in Castle Street, Hamilton. The picture was presented to the Royal Faculty by Dr Freeland Fergus, but neither artist's name nor date is recorded.*

gave a course of lectures outside the University. The Professor of Medicine, Dr Johnstoune, appears to have been sympathetic, however, and in 1746 Cullen gave his lectures on medicine under the aegis of the University. But to try to start a medical school like that of Edinburgh he found that he would have to do everything himself with the exception of anatomy, with which Hamilton was coping admirably. He started teaching chemistry in 1747 after the University had fitted out a laboratory for him, and in 1748 added materia medica and botany. Johnstoune resigned in 1750 and Cullen was appointed Professor of Medicine in 1751.

Cullen broke with tradition in his lectures; he did not read them but merely used notes, and he delivered them in English while most of his university colleagues were still declaiming in Latin. But his lectures were only part of his work; he had a busy practice as a physician and he carried out experimental work in 'pure' chemistry, i.e. not just that with pharmaceutical applications. In this he was the stimulus for Black's (*q.v.*) enthusiasm and accomplishments in this field; indeed Cullen may have already laid the groundwork of some of Black's discoveries.

But Cullen was restless and ambitious and saw in Edinburgh better opportunities for his teaching methods and research, and so in 1755 he accepted the post of Professor of Chemistry in that University. He must have been a superb lecturer; his first class in chemistry had only 17 students, the next 59, and later the number rose to 145. He began to give clinical lectures in Edinburgh Royal Infirmary and these, too, became widely popular. The Chair of the Practice of Physic became vacant in 1766 and Cullen was very disappointed when Dr John Gregory and not he was appointed. But the Chair of the Institutes of Physic became vacant shortly afterwards and Cullen was appointed. He and Gregory seemed to get on well and they lectured year about on the theory and practice of medicine. When Gregory died in 1773 Cullen succeeded him and held the chair until 1789. He was then 79 years old, frail in body and mind, and died shortly afterwards.

His writings were many and varied from medicine to physiology to agriculture; translations appeared in Latin, French, German and Italian, and Cullen was undoubtedly one of the most read and respected European physicians of the second half of the 18th century. His merit was widely recognised: President of the Edinburgh College of Physicians, 1773 to 1775; Foreign Associate of The Royal Society of Medicine in Paris, 1776; Fellow of the Royal Society of London, 1777.

William Cullen was President of the Faculty of Physicians and Surgeons of Glasgow from 1747 to 1749.

*Note:* A full biography of William Cullen and his work is available in *Account of the life, lectures and writings of William Cullen*, Vol. 1, published in 1832, now reissued; Vol. 2, commenced by John and William Thomson and concluded by David Craigie (edited by Allen Thomson), 2 vols., 8vo, Edinburgh 1859.

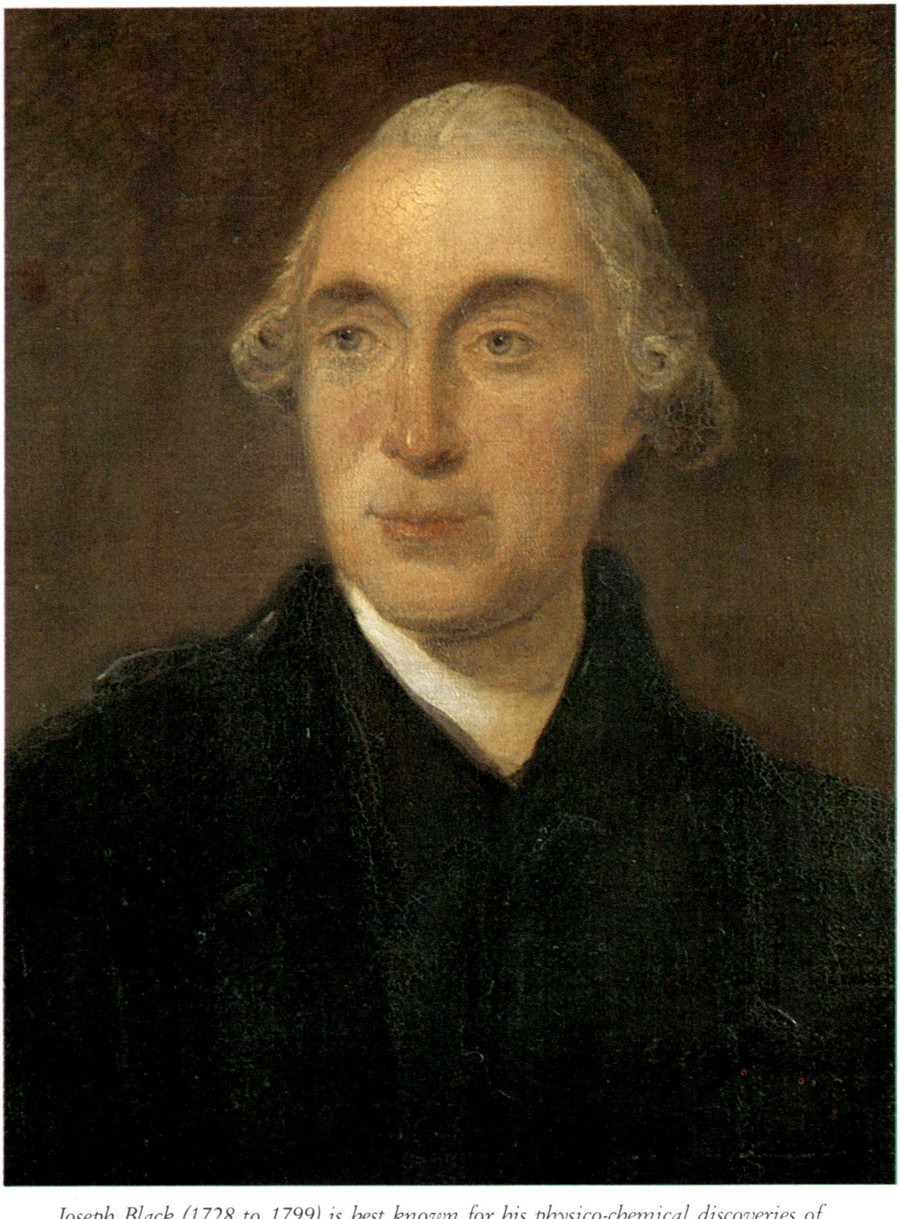

*Joseph Black (1728 to 1799) is best known for his physico-chemical discoveries of carbon dioxide and latent heat. The portrait is a copy by James Barr of the original by David Martin.*

*President, 1759 to 1761 and 1765 to 1766.*

# JOSEPH BLACK

1728 to 1799

*His portrait, of which that in the College is a copy, was painted by David Martin of whom Raeburn was a pupil. It was in the possession of the Royal Medical Society in Edinburgh when the copy was made by James Barr for the College in 1865.*

Joseph Black was born in Bordeaux. His father, a wine merchant, although from a Scottish family, had been born in Belfast and came to reside in Bordeaux where he married the daughter of another Scottish wine merchant. Young Joseph was first sent to school in Belfast and when eighteen years old came to Glasgow University to study medicine. Cullen was already lecturing in medicine and when he began teaching chemistry in his new laboratory in 1747, Black became his assistant there. The friendship between the two lasted throughout their lives and was of great benefit to both. In 1751 Black went to Edinburgh for further study in medicine and qualified MD in 1754. The subject of his graduation thesis which was later expanded for publication as *Experiments upon Magnesia alba, Quicklime and some other Alkaline Substances* was one of the major discoveries of inorganic chemistry. In essence, he discovered carbon dioxide; but this is almost as great an over-simplification as that in the *Dictionary of Eminent Scotsmen* which says that he discovered 'that a cubic inch of marble consisted of half its weight of pure lime and a quantity of air equal to six gallons measure'.

His basic innovation was exact measurement. That, and his care and accuracy in experiments and the urge to learn more, led to the inescapable conclusions that some forms of matter were compounds of other forms and that at least one gas other than air existed.

His experiments were many and most exist today only in the notes taken by students. It is still a simplification but so far as carbon dioxide is concerned, the experiments showed essentially:

if a given mass of chalk is roasted, half that mass of quicklime remains;

if an acid such as oil of vitriol is added to chalk and quicklime, the same amount of acid will dissolve twice as much chalk as quicklime *but* during the process the chalk will effervesce while the quicklime will not;

the gas effervescing from the chalk, when collected, will snuff out a candle and will not support life.

Black called the gas 'fixed' or 'mephitic' air. The fact that it differed from the air which he knew, was complicated by the fact that quicklime will absorb carbon dioxide from the air to reform chalk, but one of the foundations of organic chemistry had been established.

When Cullen left the Chair of Medicine in Glasgow and went to Edinburgh in 1755, Robert Hamilton succeeded him. This left the Chair of Anatomy and Botany in Glasgow vacant and to this Black was appointed in 1756. Next year, Hamilton died and Black became Professor of Medicine. While in Glasgow he made his second great discovery: that of latent heat.

It arose from observation and deduction of simple everyday events. In a cool room objects of wood and metal will feel cool to the touch but if contact is maintained will soon lose their coolness; a piece of ice in the same room will stay cool until all the ice has melted. The experiments which followed had to wait till the depth of winter when ice could be obtained; then he showed that the amount of heat required just to melt a quantity of ice would raise the temperature of the same quantity of water by many degrees. The same phenomenon occurs when water is boiled into steam and Black himself coined the phrase 'latent heat' which is still used.

Either of his two discoveries was enough to ensure immortality for his name, but Black did not seek fame. He wrote little and most of his researches are known only from his lectures which did much to make chemistry acceptable as a discipline of its own. He went back to Edinburgh in 1766 to take up the Chair of Chemistry which had fallen vacant when Cullen moved to that of the Institutes of Physic, and he held this post until 1799 when one day his manservant found him dead, seated at table with some bread and a few prunes before him and a bowl of milk unspilled on his knees. He was frugal in his habits, of delicate health and to some degree indolent, but he was a popular practitioner and counted among his friends many important contemporaries such as

Adam Smith, the Glasgow Professor of Moral Philosophy who later wrote the *Wealth of Nations*, David Hume the Scottish philosopher and James Hutton, the Edinburgh doctor who founded the theory of modern geology.

Joseph Black was twice President of the Faculty of Physicians and Surgeons of Glasgow, from 1759 to 1761 and from 1765 to 1766.

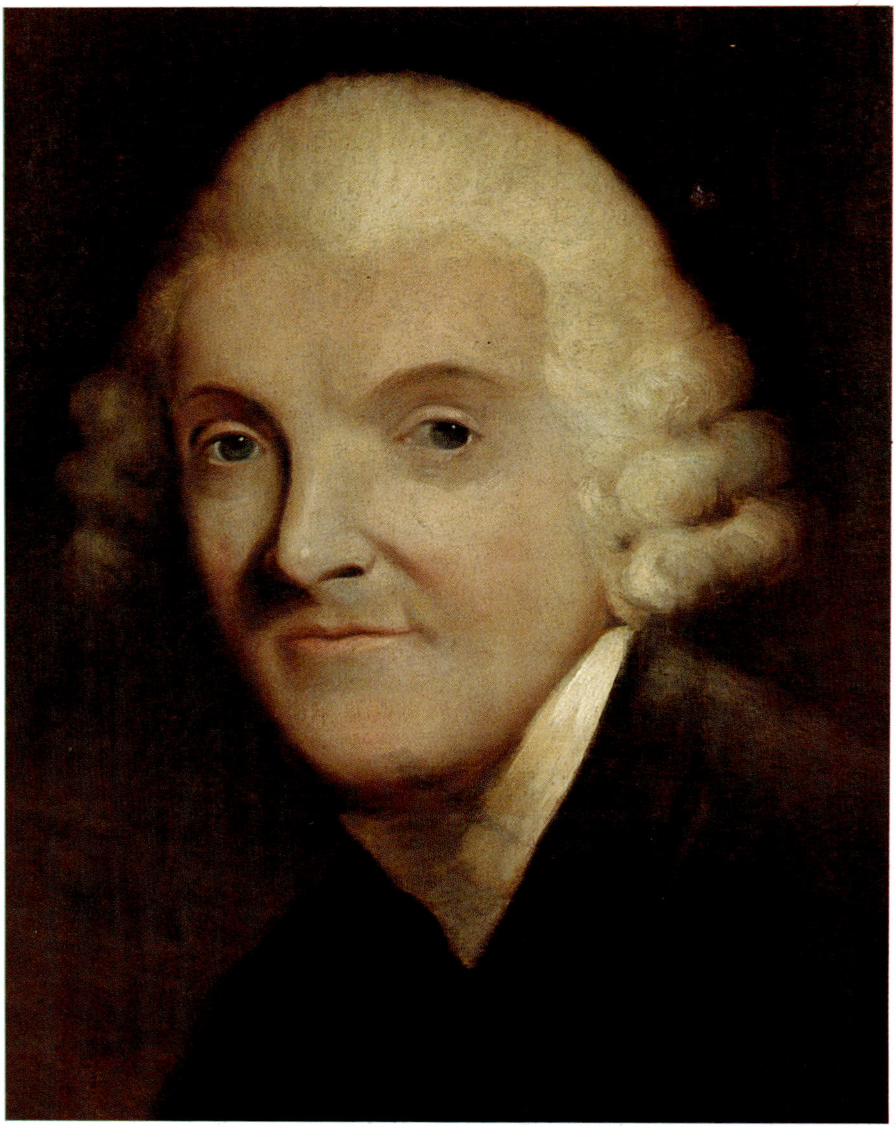

*William Hunter (1718 to 1783) was the elder of the famous Hunter brothers, a pupil of William Cullen, who spent most of his life in London where he prospered greatly as physician and obstetrician. His priceless collections of books, coins, pathological specimens and other historical material are now housed by Glasgow University. The portrait is a copy of part of the original by Sir Joshua Reynolds in the Hunterian Museum there.*

*William Hunter was the second individual to become an Honorary Fellow of the Faculty.*

William Hunter has been included in this section because he was a pupil of Cullen. Although he had nothing to do with Glasgow University Medical School, he and Cullen had great respect and liking for each other throughout their lives and there is a tantalising might-have-been. To Cullen in Edinburgh in 1765, Hunter wrote suggesting that Cullen and Black should join with him to found a 'School of Physic upon a noble plan in Glasgow. I would propose to give all my Museum and Library and build a Theatre at my own expense and I should ask nothing for teaching but the credit of doing it with reputation. You and Black with those we would choose, I think could not fail of making our neighbours stare. We should at once draw all the English, and I presume most of the Scotch students'.

But Glasgow's exported talent rarely returns and it was not to be.

## WILLIAM HUNTER

1718 to 1783

*The portrait is a copy of the head and shoulders of a three-quarter length portrait by Sir Joshua Reynolds in the Hunterian Museum in Glasgow University.*

William Hunter was the seventh child of a family of ten, of whom his equally famous brother John was the last. The family home was Long Calderwood, a small farm then on the outskirts of the village of East Kilbride. It is preserved today as a museum for the Hunter brothers, but the surroundings are mostly built over by the East Kilbride Development Corporation.

After local schooling he went to Glasgow University at the age of fourteen where he appears to have impressed his teachers with his ability and diligence. At first designed for the Church, he became acquainted with William Cullen who was then established in practice in the neighbouring town of Hamilton; thereafter medicine became his overriding ambition. He was apprenticed to Cullen in 1737 and stayed in the Cullen home for nearly three years during which he and Cullen became lifelong friends. A partnership was agreed upon in which Hunter would take over the surgical part of the practice (Cullen disliked surgery) on the understanding that Hunter would go and study further at Edinburgh and London before settling in Hamilton.

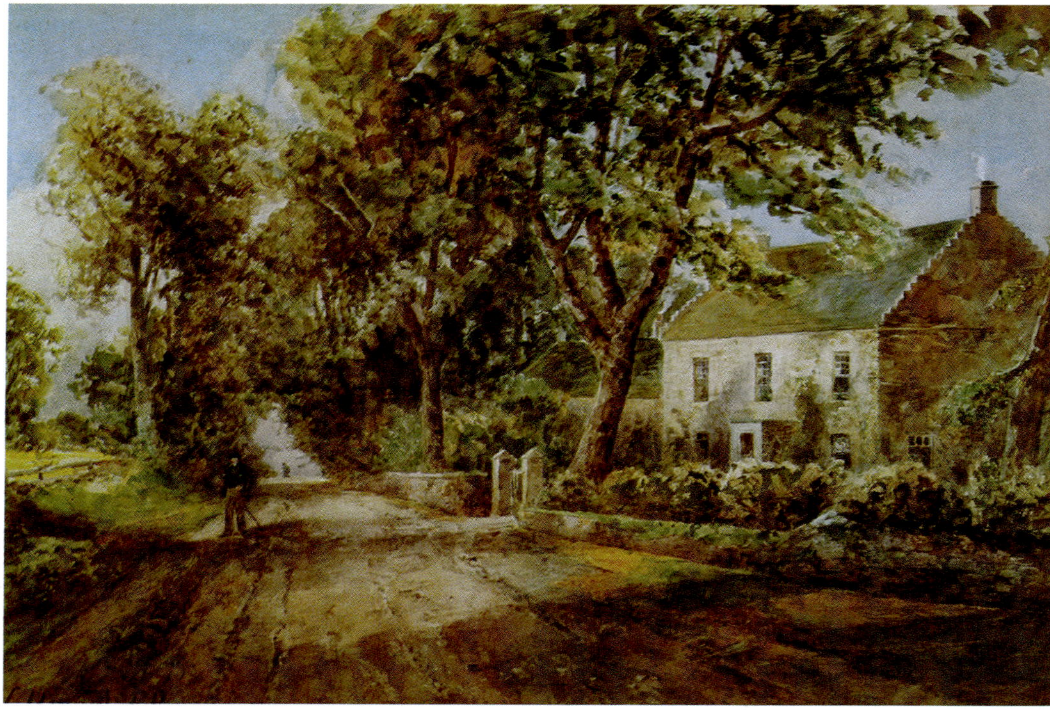

*The farm of Long Calderwood at East Kilbride where William and John Hunter were born. The Faculty minutes of June 1894 record that the picture 'had recently been painted and was now presented to the Faculty by Dr. Charles Blatherwick RSW—Helensburgh'. The house is maintained today as a small museum by the Hunter Trust, but the rural setting has disappeared with the expansion of East Kilbride as an industrial and residential centre.*

He spent six months or so in Edinburgh attending the medical lectures at the University, including those of Munro *primus*, and then went to London. Expatriate Scots in London looked after their own; at first William Smellie, who a short time previously had gone south from his practice in Lanark and who was to become a great obstetrician, took him in; then a letter from Foulis the Glasgow printer to James Douglas the anatomist gained him not only an assistantship but also accommodation in the Douglas home where he tutored the son. Although Douglas died in the following year Hunter remained with the family as before.

Cullen, seeing his pupil well set on a London based career, readily cancelled their agreement. In any case Cullen was shortly to leave the practice in Hamilton for a more academic career in Glasgow.

Douglas had been not just an anatomist but also a successful surgeon and obstetrician and Hunter took over much of his practice. Apart from Smellie, whose manners were coarse and unprepossessing, there were only two obstetricians of note in London at that time and the death of one and the retirement of the other left the field open to Hunter. His endeavours in man-midwifery led eventually to his great work on the *Anatomy of the Gravid Uterus*.

He obtained an MD from Glasgow University in 1750 and in 1751 revisited his homeland and was then honoured by the Faculty who created him an Honorary Member, only the second individual to be so distinguished.

This was one of his last contacts with Glasgow and the Faculty. Several biographies have been written about him and his brother John and the remainder of his life need not be detailed here. His success in practice, his personal charm, his integrity, his capacity for hard work and his frugality, all led to the accumulation of great wealth which he spent on the collections of books, coins, pathological specimens and curiosa and memorabilia of many kinds and which he willed to Glasgow University on his death. The pathological specimens were recently restored and remounted by the late Professor Burton and are housed in the Pathology Department at Glasgow Royal Infirmary; the other Hunterian collections are in Glasgow University.

*Note:* A succinct readable biography of William Hunter is that by Sir Charles Illingworth published by Livingstone in 1967.

# 6

# THE FACULTY AND THE UNIVERSITY, II: CONTENTION AND LITIGATION c 1800 to c 1860

The period around the turn of the 18th/19th centuries was one of continual expansion and change in every field, industrial, academic, medical and social. The Faculty was changing too after being relatively static for two centuries.

In 1792 it began its Widows' Fund, an insurance for the widows of deceased members. This had the immediate effect of greatly increasing the admission fees. Then, as now, widows greatly outnumbered widowers, and the constant drain on the Fund made continuing increases necessary until by 1816 the entry fee had reached £150. Although, in 1850, the Widows' Fund contribution became no longer compulsory on entry, it is still noteworthy that in spite of a hundred and fifty years' inflation, the entry fee in 1960 was still only £150.

The monthly out-patient sessions when advice was given to the sick poor were no longer fulfilling a useful role in the expanding city. Admittedly two of the members in turn looked after the patients in the Town's Hospital, but with the opening of the Glasgow Royal Infirmary in 1794 with its own physicians, this was no longer a heavy commitment. In 1798 Jenner introduced vaccination and the Faculty, seeing how successful this was in preventing the ravages of smallpox, set up, in their Hall in St Enoch's Square, a Vaccination Centre in 1801. Each month two members were delegated for this duty and the Centre was open every Monday; in its first five years, 10,000 persons were vaccinated free of charge and the Centre continued until almost the end of the 19th century.

There were thus disadvantages both financial and time-consuming in joining the Faculty. 'So why join?' said the young doctors clutching their University Diploma in Medicine. Some practised only as physicians, and this was just tolerable to the Faculty, but others engaged in surgical and general practice. 'You can't do that', said the Faculty, 'unless you submit yourself to our examination and pass it and pay the fees', but many young MD's ignored them and continued practising; for the powers of the Faculty to deal with them were sadly weakened. £40 Scots, the statutory fine, had become virtually worthless and no punishment, while the cost of litigation to secure conviction was greatly in excess of any return.

In desperation, in 1815, the Faculty sued four MD's: one each of the Universities of Glasgow, Edinburgh, St Andrews and Aberdeen. In each case this was to forbid them practising surgery, but in the case of St Andrews and Aberdeen, it was also to prevent them practising at all since both Universities were notorious for selling MD's without providing any courses or examinations. The Faculty won its case with regard to the practice of surgery, but the learned judge refused to commit himself on the failings of St Andrews and Aberdeen Universities.

Glasgow University was only indirectly involved in this litigation but, to try to circumvent further suits, it introduced a degree in surgery, the CM, *Chirurgiae Magister*, in 1816. Any holder of such a degree could, it claimed, practise surgery without interference from the Faculty.

The members of the Faculty were at a loss how now to preserve their ancient rights and privileges. They were well aware that the powers granted by James VI had become totally inadequate. A new royal charter might be the answer but they were informed that the monarchy, two centuries after James, had much depleted powers in this respect and only an Act of Parliament could confer the authority which they wished. So, in 1817, they presented a petition to the House of Commons in which, *inter alia*, the name of the Faculty was to be changed to that of 'The Royal College of Physicians and Surgeons of Glasgow'. Glasgow University, however, lodged a *caveat* and the project was later abandoned. A century and a half had to pass before the new title was finally granted by Parliament.

For ten years the Faculty nursed its wrath and took no action. The CM was not a particularly popular degree but the numbers of those so qualified slowly increased and by 1826 there were 23 CM's practising in the West of Scotland. The Faculty could stand it no longer and raised an action of suspension and interdict against all of them, asking that they be prohibited from practice until they had been examined by the Faculty.

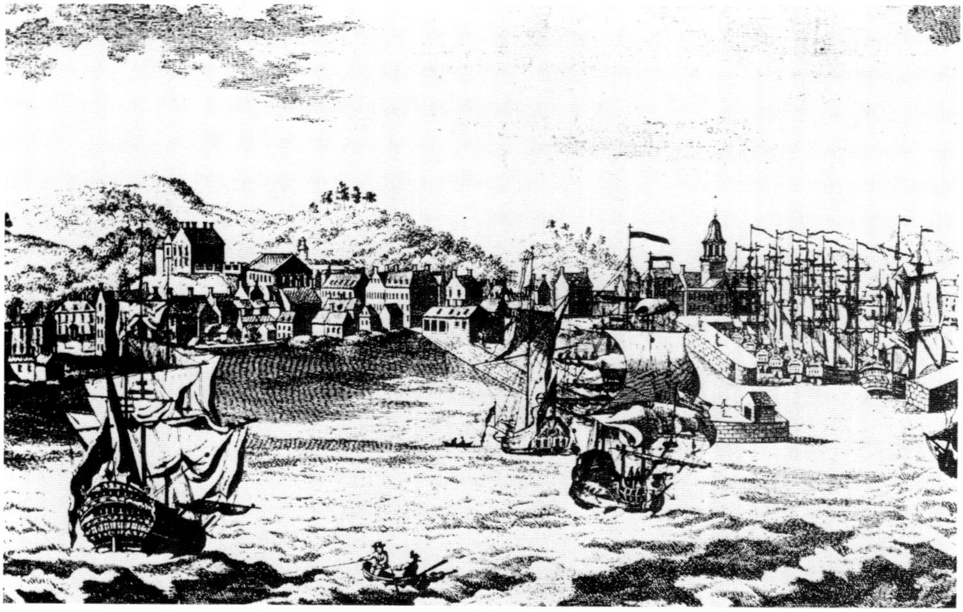

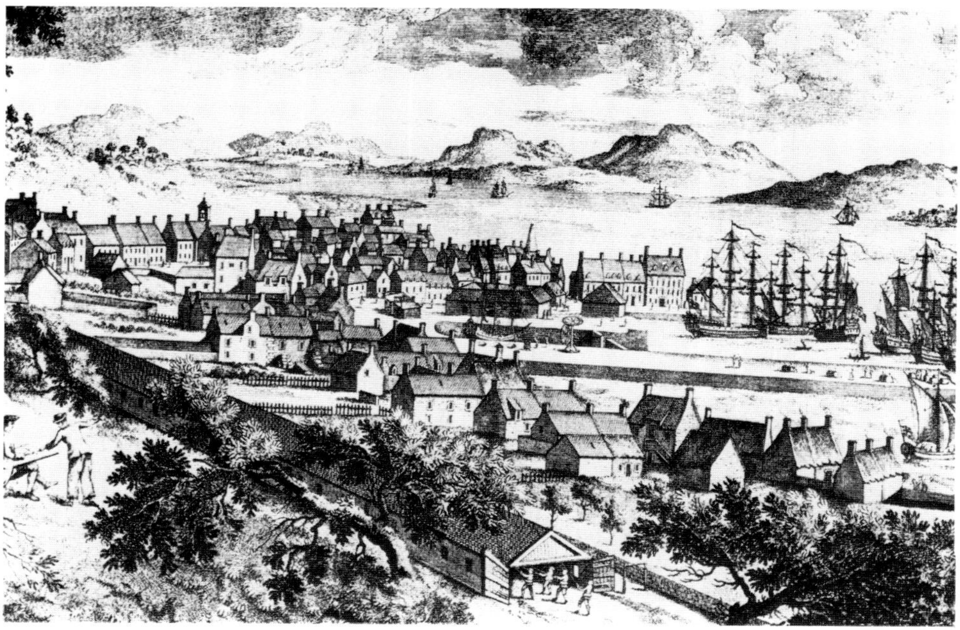

*Views of Greenock (above) and Port Glasgow (below) from which ships sailed to and from the Americas. The increasing transatlantic trade from the Clyde was a major factor in the growth of Glasgow as an industrial and commercial city.*

*The engravings were made by Robert Paul in 1768. The outline of the distant hills in the Port Glasgow view repeats the contours of Ben Lomond, as seen from the south, at least four times, and casts doubt on the accuracy of Paul's work.*

The case dragged on for 14 years. It went first to the Lord Ordinary who referred it to the Second Division of the Court of Session. At this stage Glasgow University entered the arena asking that the Court find the opposite, i.e. that holders of their CM could practise surgery freely within the Faculty's bounds. The case was then laid before the Lords of the First Division and the Lords Ordinary who in the end found in favour of the Faculty and awarded it costs against the University and the CM's.

The University appealed to the House of Lords. Not for the first or last time, there was confusion in London about the differences between Scottish and English Law. The Lord Chancellor was particularly scathing about this 'letter in which King James VI assumed to himself the power which I never heard any king had before of making his Surgeon and a Doctor of Physic a Corporation; . . . and it gives them large and extensive powers extending over about half Scotland . . .' and so on. He sent it back for advice to the Court of Session in Edinburgh who assured him that the Charter was in fact a legal and binding document, and the University's appeal was finally dismissed in 1840.

The Faculty had won, but much had been lost on both sides, particularly money and good will. Relations between the Faculty and the University were strained for many years and University professors were excluded from offices of the Faculty.

The case illustrated widespread contemporary problems: who trained doctors, who examined doctors, who licensed doctors to practise? Quacks and unqualified practitioners of all kinds were numerous and the public required not only protection from such but also some means of recognising a properly trained, examined and licensed practitioner. Long discussions which are discussed below took place for almost 20 years between parliamentary committees, the Universities, the Colleges and the Faculty before the Medical Act of 1858 became law. Both the Faculty and the University could now confer the right to practise and the way was open to a much closer cooperation between them than ever before.

# 7

# THE FACULTY, THE COLLEGES AND THE LAW: THE FIGHT FOR SURVIVAL

James Watson (1787 to 1871)

During the first half of the 19th century the Faculty was not only in contention with the University but fighting for its very existence against the Colleges and those parliamentarians whose projected Acts excluded it from all powers of licensing and accreditation in the United Kingdom. Improved communications were opening up the country. At the turn of the century a stage-coach from Glasgow could reach London in about 60 hours, and now, new roads were being constructed and Macadamised, and soon the railway network was being laid. No longer could the Faculty operate snugly and unassailed within the bounds of the Charter of James VI; it had to be recognised nationally as a licensing body with similar privileges and powers to other comparable corporations, or it would perish. The main antagonist was the Royal College of Surgeons of Edinburgh, sometimes acting on its own, sometimes in concert with the other Colleges in London and Dublin. The Royal College of Physicians of Edinburgh at this time had no licensing powers and was but little involved except in so far as it desired such powers.

Take for example the fuss over the 'Passage Vessels Regulating Bill' in 1822. One clause in this Bill, which proposed regulations for ships carrying passengers, specified the various bodies whose certificates of competence would be acceptable for surgeons employed in such vessels. The Faculty and its diplomas were nowhere mentioned in the Bill although the licences of all the Colleges of Surgeons were approved. As if to enhance the slight to the Faculty, Glasgow University's CM was to be acceptable.

One of the Faculty's members, James Corkindale, who later became President in 1834, was sent to London presumably by stage-coach to present the Faculty's case and have its name included in the Bill. He traced the problem to the Lord Advocate who had apparently acted in good faith since he had been led to believe that 'The Royal College of Surgeons of Edinburgh had a paramount control in medical affairs in the whole of Scotland'. Dr Corkindale seems to have convinced him of the real state of affairs and the Bill was withdrawn.

Sometimes the Royal College of Surgeons of Edinburgh acted with the Faculty, as in the case of the Bills to amend the English Apothecaries' Act of 1815. There were several of these drafted between 1825 and 1833, and the wording was such that they would have prevented those who possessed only Scottish diplomas from practising in England and Wales, and indeed would have confined such practice to diplomates of the London Apothecaries' Company. There was much activity, to- and fro-ing and the writing of memoranda which apparently established the Faculty's case but had no immediate effect since the final draft of 1833 was not proceeded with.

It had become apparent, however, that what was required was not so much Acts to rationalise the powers of individual corporations but an all-embracing Bill to govern the practice of medicine throughout the United Kingdom. This was reinforced by the lengthy discussions which occurred between the Colleges and Parliament over the Irish Medical Charities Bill in 1838. This Bill laid down the qualifications necessary for an applicant for any post connected with the medical care of the sick poor in Ireland. The Faculty's name was not mentioned in the Bill although all the other licensing bodies were included. The Colleges had already been deeply involved in the drafting of the Bill before the Faculty even heard of it and their insistence on having the Faculty's name inserted in the Bill led to much fruitful discussion about the various methods of medical teaching and examination. Although this Bill was also withdrawn, the Faculty appear again to have made their case. That they were at this time involved in the terminal stages of their battle with the University hindered some of the arguments, but also further underlined the need for a Medical Act which would give fair weight to the conflicting claims of the parties involved.

It took 20 years before such an Act, agreeable to all, was finally passed. Bill after bill was drafted, presented, objected to and withdrawn. Sometimes the Faculty found itself merely ignored; at others it was positively excluded. There was only one College of Surgeons in England, only one in Ireland; there should therefore only be one in Scotland! There is no doubt that the Royal College of Surgeons of Edinburgh strongly wished to become that of Scotland and succeeded in having the change written into the draft of some of the Bills.

The contest continued year after year with the Faculty fighting for its existence, paying legal expenses from coffers already depleted by the litigation with the University, and repeatedly sending delegates to London by stage-coach or perhaps by ship from Leith.

The fortunes of the Faculty waxed and waned. By 1843 it was proposed that they should have a new Charter in which they were to be constituted 'The Royal College of Physicians and Surgeons of Glasgow'. But this was later dropped and by 1848 the Faculty's name had disappeared from the then proposed Bill and the Edinburgh College was to get a new Charter entitling it to be called 'The Royal College of Surgeons of Scotland'.

Fortunately that Bill was also withdrawn and in 1850 the Faculty was finally recognised legally as having equivalent status to that of any other similar 'Corporation or Royal College in Scotland'. It was largely due to the President, Dr James Watson, even then known as 'The Father of the Faculty', that such favourable terms were obtained for the Faculty.

The *Act for better regulating the Privileges of the Faculty of Physicians and Surgeons of Glasgow and amending their Charter of Incorporation* was passed on 10th June, 1850. In addition to confirming the privileges and powers of the Faculty as an examining and licensing body, it allowed all members of the Faculty to be called Fellows as in the Colleges and it also removed the need for any contribution to the Widows' Fund in the entrance fee.

Although the standing of the Faculty was now defined by statute, long discussions were still required between the Colleges, the Universities, the Apothecaries' Company and the Faculty, each trying to maintain every traditional privilege but obviously having to compromise if any lasting agreement was to be reached. The final solution was the formation of the General Medical Council which would supervise the training, examination and licensing of properly qualified doctors by the various bodies represented on the Council. The Faculty was to have one representative on the Council, the same as each College, and this parity throughout the U.K. was finally established in the Medical Act of 1858.

There are two clauses in this Act which illustrate just what a close fight it must have been:

> Clause XLIX allows the Royal College of Physicians of Edinburgh to obtain a new Charter from Queen Victoria in order to change its name to 'The Royal College of Physicians of Scotland';
>
> Clause L makes it lawful for Her Majesty to grant to the Faculty of Physicians and Surgeons of Glasgow and the Royal College of Surgeons of Edinburgh, if they so agree, a Charter to amalgamate them into 'one united Corporation under the name of "The Royal College of Surgeons of Scotland".'

Neither of these possible changes has come to pass although there are still those who believe that a single Scottish College (or Academy) of Medicine and Surgery would be a more powerful and influential body than any of the present three Colleges.

James Watson, the subject of the next portrait, was the Faculty member most concerned with the discussions which led up to the Medical Act of 1858 and was the first Faculty representative on the General Medical Council.

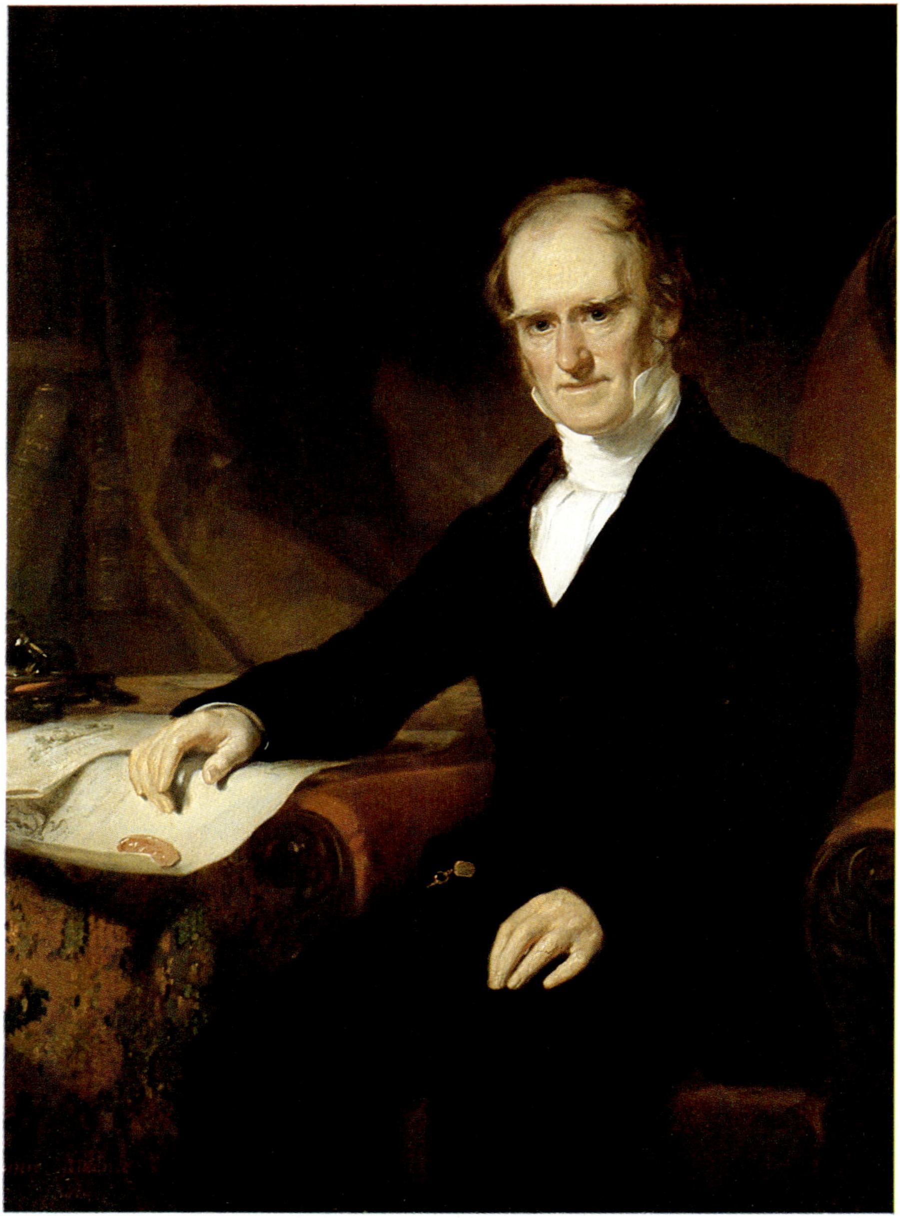

*James Watson (1787 to 1871) was known as 'The Father of the Faculty' and was largely responsible for ensuring that the Faculty had the same rights in medical licensing and education as any of the Royal Colleges. The portrait by Daniel Macnee was commissioned by the Faculty.*

*President, 1838 to 1841; 1849 to 1852; 1857 to 1860.*

# JAMES WATSON

1787 to 1871

*The portrait was painted in 1850/51 by Daniel Macnee, a Glasgow artist who was later knighted and became the President of the Royal Scottish Academy. The portrait was commissioned by the Faculty, which also paid for a similar portrait by the same artist to be presented to Dr Watson and his family.*

James Watson was born in Glasgow and educated at the Grammar School before proceeding to Glasgow University where he took the full curriculum of the arts course, having intended to study for the Church. But, although he remained a staunch Christian, and was an elder of the Scottish Kirk for many years, he later entered the medical faculty and became a member of the Faculty of Physicians and Surgeons of Glasgow in 1810. He pursued at first the usual course of general practitioner/surgeon and was appointed Surgeon to Glasgow Royal Infirmary in 1813. But he veered more and more towards medicine, graduated MD at Glasgow University in 1828 and became a Physician in the Royal Infirmary in 1842. He was also physician to the Fever Hospital in Clyde Street.

He wrote only a few short articles for the Scottish medical press but is remembered by his contemporaries as a man of many talents, a highly esteemed medical teacher and an excellent physician. His outstanding contribution, however, is the indefatigable work he carried out for the Faculty in its long struggles with the University, the Colleges and the Government which have been described briefly above. It is no coincidence that he was President of the Faculty on the three occasions on which the Faculty had succeeded in maintaining its rights and privileges against long odds:

from 1838 to 1841, during which the University lost its appeal in the House of Lords;

from 1849 to 1852, during which the Medical Act of 1850 confirming the Faculty's equivalent powers to the Scottish Colleges was passed;

from 1857 to 1860, during which there was passed the Medical Act of 1858 giving the Faculty equal privileges with the other Colleges nationwide.

Already by 1850 he was called the 'Father of the Faculty', and the Faculty were so impressed with his good work towards the 1850 Act that they not only commissioned his portrait but set up the Watson Prize Fund which survives to this day. But his

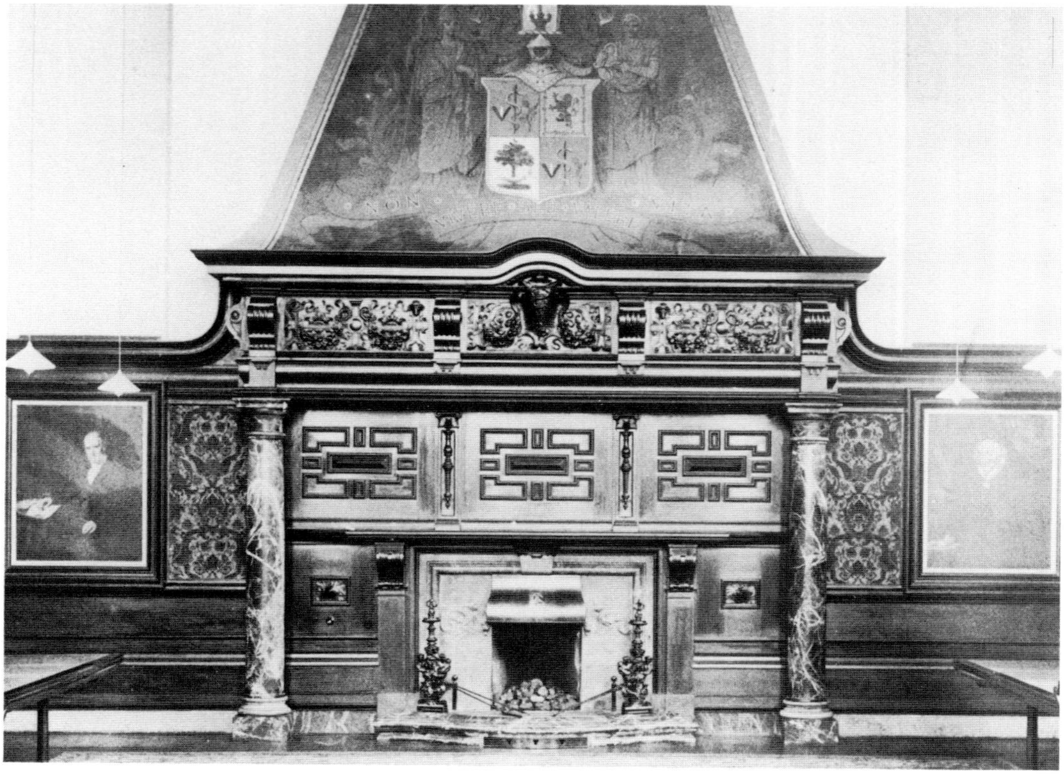

*The fireplace of the new Faculty Hall photographed probably at the turn of the 19th/20th centuries; electric lighting was introduced in the Hall in 1898. The portraits of Maister Peter Lowe and James Watson share equal prominence at the sides of the coal-burning fire which would then be the focal point of the room.*

greatest triumph was the Medical Act of 1858. On the 2nd of August of that year he reported to the Faculty that the 'new Medical Bill had passed both Houses of Parliament, and he congratulated the meeting that a medical reform measure had at last passed the legislature in which the Faculty had obtained all the privileges, and were confirmed in all the rights claimed by them, the same as enjoyed by any Royal College in the Kingdom'.

He was then appointed the first Faculty representative to the General Medical Council set up by the 1858 Act and held this office until ill-health forced his resignation. He lived for some ten years after he retired from active practice, returning to reading the classical authors of his student days. When he died on 30th May 1871 the funeral took place from the Faculty Hall 'to give the Fellows of the Faculty an opportunity of attending it'.

In the annals of the Faculty he must be reckoned as second only to Maister Peter Lowe.

# 8

## THE FIRST SPECIALISATIONS

*Ophthalmology*
William Mackenzie (1791 to 1868)
Andrew Freeland Fergus (1858 to 1932)

*Obstetrics*
James Wilson (1783 to 1857)
William Loudon Reid (1845 to 1931)

For at least two centuries there has been active resistance to any new specialisation. Even earlier it is probable that surgeons looked upon medicine as a branch of surgery, while physicians scorned the surgeons as technicians carrying out their instructions.

The main argument against specialisation has always been that it is a form of advertisement, however ethical, designed to attract patients from the general doctor. This was undoubtedly true in many early cases. The first specialist clinic in Britain is said to have been that opened in Holborn in 1771, called grandiloquently 'St. John's Hospital for Diseases of the Eyes, Legs and Breasts'. The wily general practitioner would often have a notice saying that he consulted on chest complaints on Monday, female ailments on Tuesday, arthritis on Wednesday, and so on. Such practices, and many others less ethical, were so widespread that in 1854 the Faculty adopted a 'Code of Ethics' which began:

> 'It is derogatory to the dignity of the profession, to resort to public advertisements, or private cards or handbills, inviting the attention of individuals affected with particular diseases, *publicly* [original italics] offering advice to the poor gratis, or promising radical cures; or to publish cases and operations in non-medical prints, or suffer such publications to be made; to invite laymen to be present at operations; to boast of cures and remedies; to adduce certificates of skill and success, or to perform any other similar acts'.

But there is always a way round the rules and one was the establishment of a special clinic offering free treatment. In 1870 we find John Reid (*q.v.*) in the *Glasgow Medical Examiner*, a journal which he himself edited, reporting a paper which he himself had given to the Glasgow Medico-Chirurgical Society on 'Gratis Special Dispensaries', 'whether they hold out for the *eye*, the *ear*, the *skin*, the *chest* or the *stomach*; the immediate and ultimate object is gain to the *quasi*-benevolent benefactor of the so-called Institution'. Since John Reid was his own reporter, his diatribe is liberally interspersed with '(Applause)', '(Hear, hear)' and '(Laughter)'. He recommended that the Faculty should remember its own Code of Ethics and deal with its Fellows accordingly. In the discussion which followed his paper, however, there were others who spoke more temperately and there was agreement that such institutions as the 'lying-in' hospital and the Eye Infirmary were acceptable although they treated the poor gratis.

The first accommodation to be reserved for special cases was undoubtedly the 'cells' in the Town's Hospital to house the insane. Two of the portrait subjects, Robert Cleghorn and John Balmanno, were respectively first and second physicians to the Glasgow Lunatic Asylum which opened in 1814. The patient care was then custodial rather than psychiatric, however, and since Cleghorn and Balmanno were two of Glasgow's last 'pure' physicians, they were described earlier under that heading.

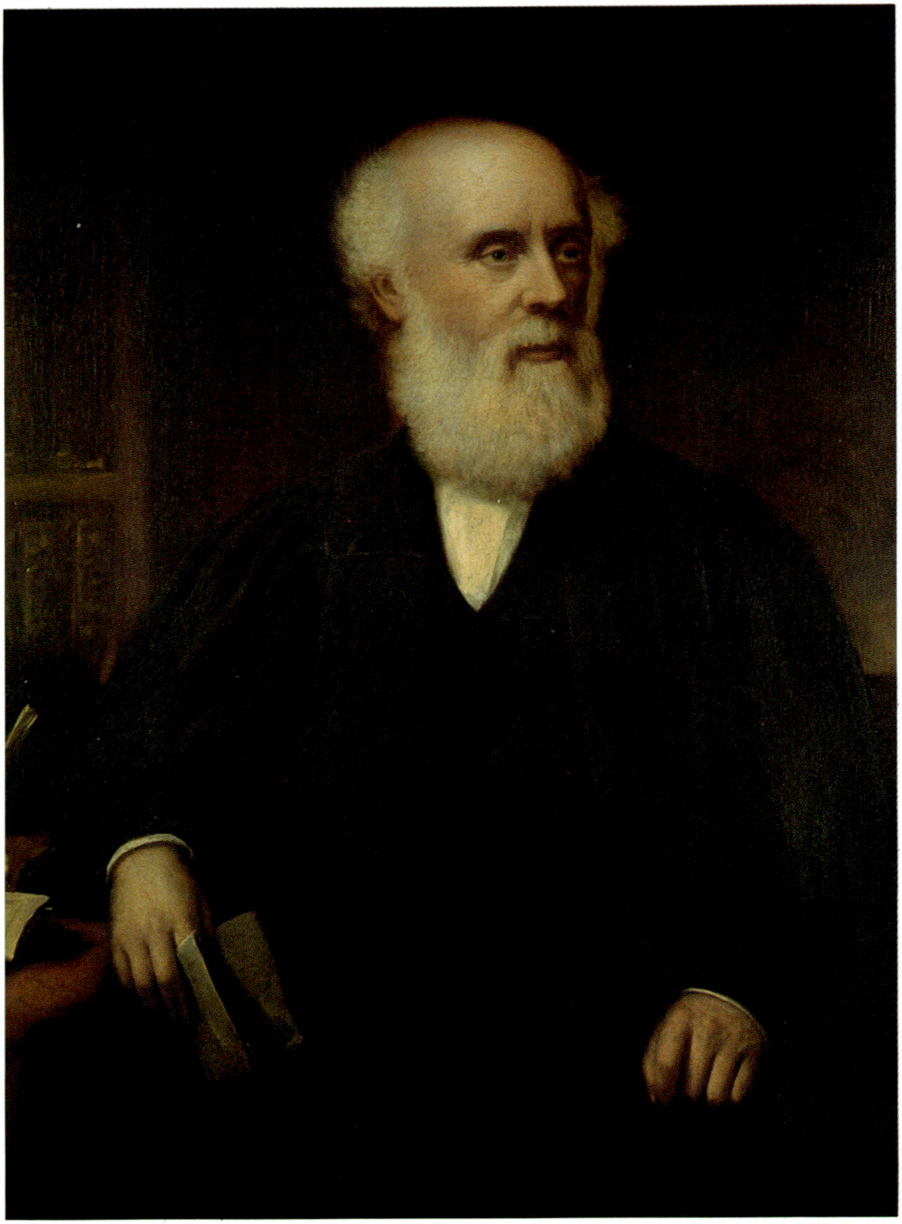

*William Mackenzie (1791 to 1868) was an internationally recognised ophthalmologist, the writer of a renowned textbook of ophthalmology and one of the founders of the Glasgow Eye Infirmary. He was also the first editor of the* Glasgow Medical Journal. *The portrait is a copy of one by A. Keith.*

## *Ophthalmology 1*

# WILLIAM MACKENZIE

1791 to 1868

*The portrait is a replica of one by A. Keith in the possession of the Mackenzie family and was presented to the Faculty by Mackenzie's widow in 1884.*

William Mackenzie was the only son of a prosperous muslin manufacturer and was born in one of the new villas with garden attached which had recently been built in Queen Street in Glasgow. He went to Glasgow Grammar School and thence to the University. At first he studied Arts in preparation for the Ministry but later changed over to Medicine and obtained his diploma from the Faculty in 1815. He was well provided for, and spent the next three years travelling first to London and then through the Continent of Europe in France, Germany, Austria and Italy. He learned much about many aspects of medicine and surgery but his interest in ophthalmology, which had arisen while he was still a student, was greatly strengthened during his stay in Vienna. Specialisation came earlier to the Continent than to Britain, and in 1817 Georg Josef Beer was already Professor of Ophthalmology there and probably the leading ophthalmologist of his day. Mackenzie was already fluent in French and German and made full use of his stay.

In 1818 Mackenzie came back to London and took his Membership of the Royal College of Surgeons in England. He set up in general practice there and tried to specialise as an oculist but had little success. An application for the post of Lecturer in

Anatomy in London University was unsuccessful, so a discouraged Mackenzie came back to Glasgow, sailing up the east coast to Leith and coaching across.

Glasgow seemed almost to be waiting for him. In 1819 he was appointed Professor of Anatomy and Surgery at Anderson's College. He took over a lecture room near the University in College Street and there he lectured on materia medica, medical jurisprudence and diseases of the eye. If this were not enough he soon had a busy general practice which he never quite gave up even when he had international fame as an ophthalmologist.

The eye, its abnormalities and diseases absorbed more and more of his time and energy and led to two outstanding events for which he will always be remembered: the founding of the Eye Infirmary in Glasgow in 1824, and the publication of his text book *Practical Treatise on Diseases of the Eye* in 1830.

One reason for the upsurge of interest in ophthalmology at this time was the high incidence of trachoma in the British Army during and after the Napoleonic Wars. Special hospitals for eye diseases began to appear in several cities after the first, Moorfields Eye Hospital in London, was founded in 1804. Mackenzie must have begun to plan an Eye Infirmary for Glasgow almost as soon as he returned, and he was ably assisted by Dr George Monteath, the foremost Glasgow oculist of the day. Between them, they seem to have had no difficulty in selling the idea to the Lord Provost and the local Member of Parliament. A committee was set up, subscriptions collected, and the Glasgow Eye Infirmary was opened in 1824 when Mackenzie was still only 32 years old. The original site not far from Glasgow Cross has long since been demolished. It was very small and at best had only four beds. In 1835 the Infirmary was transferred to 14 College Street, but the house was damp and the district deteriorating, and in 1852 it moved again to a house in Charlotte Street. This was an improvement, but soon the neighbouring University went west to Gilmorehill and a site near the academic centre seemed desirable. This time the Infirmary was built as such on the site at the corner of Berkeley Street and Claremont Street which it occupies today. It opened in 1874, six years after Mackenzie died, a lasting monument to his pioneering work for ophthalmology in Glasgow.

His *Practical Treatise on Diseases of the Eye* was published in 1830. It was enthusiastically received by the medical press who praised it for its comprehensiveness, its wealth of original observations, and its thorough review of the literature in Britain and the Continent. Four editions in English appeared, it was translated into German and French, and in 1866 a supplement, corrected by Mackenzie, was published in Brussels. It was and remained for some time the standard reference work on ophthalmology.

Mackenzie wrote many articles mostly on eye conditions and became the first editor of the *Glasgow Medical Journal* which began as a quarterly in 1828 and to which he was a copious contributor. At this time he gave up his Chair in Anatomy and Surgery at Anderson's College and became a lecturer in Glasgow University on 'The Structure, Function and Diseases of the Eye'. To accomplish all this, Mackenzie became an avid reader and collector of works on ophthalmology, and the Faculty Library was greatly enriched in 1885 when his collection was presented to it by his widow and son.

He graduated MD in Glasgow University in 1833 and was elected FRCS in 1843. His greatest honour, however, was his appointment in 1838 as 'Surgeon Oculist to the Queen in Scotland'.

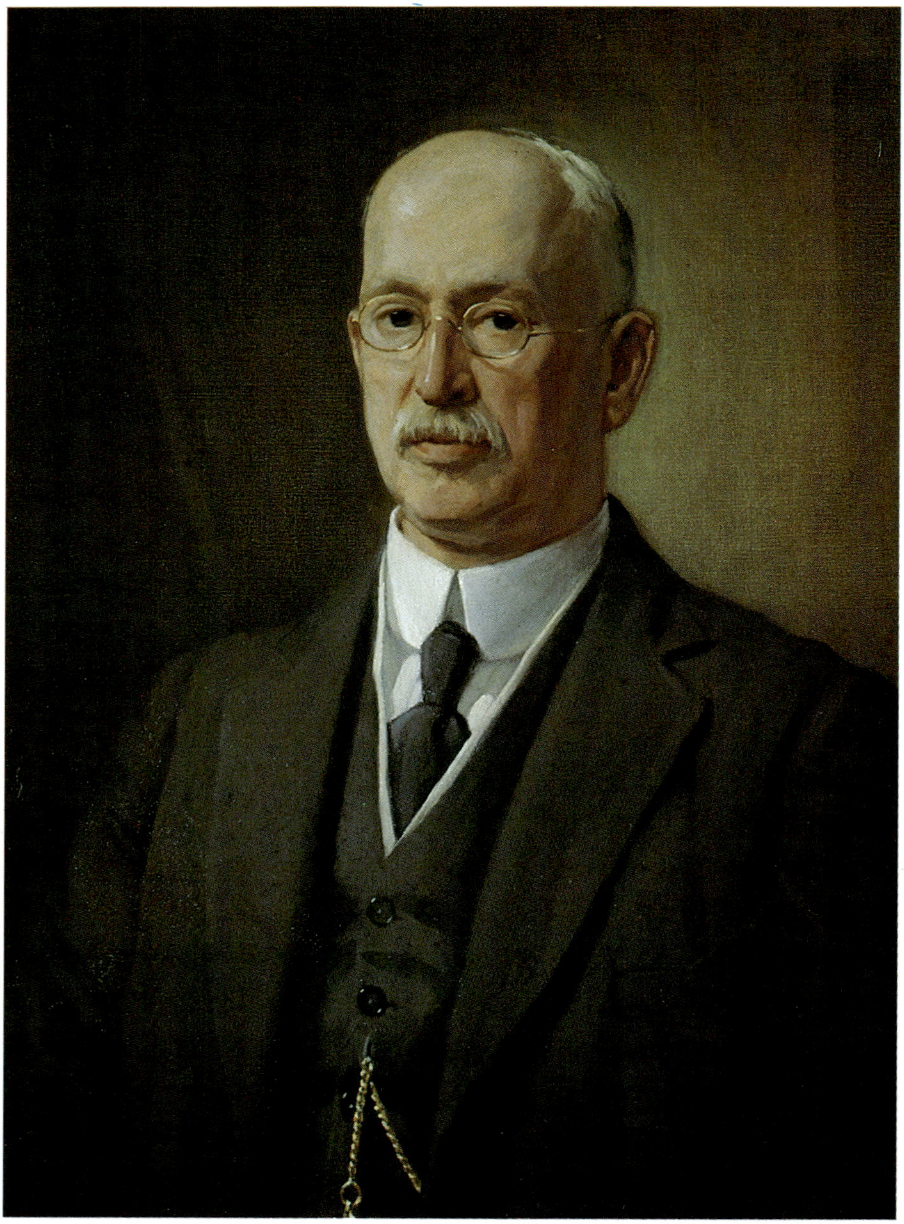

*Andrew Freeland Fergus (1858 to 1932) was a son of another President of the Faculty, Andrew Fergus (1822 to 1887), and devoted his life to ophthalmology and the Glasgow Eye Infirmary. The portrait is by Charles R. Dowell.*
*President, 1918 to 1921.*

# *Ophthalmology 2*

## ANDREW FREELAND FERGUS

1858 to 1932

*In the minutes of the Council of the Royal Faculty of 4th April 1921, there is a report that the then President, Dr Freeland Fergus, had presented to the Faculty a large number of medical works for the Library and also his portrait in oils by Mr Charles R. Dowell. This portrait was located in the basement in 1979 and was subsequently cleaned and reframed. There is also a framed photograph.*

Andrew Freeland Fergus was always known as, and signed himself, 'Freeland Fergus'. His father, Andrew Fergus, had been President of the Faculty from 1874 to 1877, and the son dropped the 'Andrew' presumably to distinguish him from his father. Freeland Fergus' brother John F. Fergus (*q.v.*) also became President of the Royal Faculty in 1929.

Unlike William Mackenzie who continued in general practice, Freeland Fergus practised for most of his life as a full time ophthalmologist. He was admittedly for some time the Professor of Physics in the Anderson College, but this was probably just an extension of the wide knowledge of optical physics which he stressed in all his teaching. Later he was given the Chair of Ophthalmic Medicine and Surgery in the same College, a post which he held from 1909 to 1915.

He graduated MB, CM in Glasgow University in 1881 and MD in 1891. After postgraduate studies in Utrecht and Paris he became an Assistant Surgeon in the Eye Infirmary in 1882 and a full Surgeon in 1890, a post which he held until 1919. He made many contributions to ophthalmology including: the bacteriology of ocular secretions and the introduction of sterilisation of instruments and dressings; excision of the lacrimal sac; tendon advancement rather than tenotomy to correct squint; a modified trephine operation for glaucoma.

During the 1914-1918 War he served as a Major, RAMC on the staff of the 4th Scottish General Hospital and was mentioned in dispatches. The welfare of the blind was a particular interest of Freeland Fergus and he played a leading part in promoting the Blind Persons (Scotland) Act of 1920.

As a member of a famous medical family he had a wide acquaintance with medical and other professional men throughout Scotland. His many interests outside medicine culminated in his Presidency of the Royal Philosophical Society of Glasgow and his election to Fellowship of the Royal Society of Edinburgh.

He had a love of small boats and adopted Rothesay first as his holiday home and later for retirement. He had a keen sense of humour which seems to have progressed to practical jokes on occasion. Thus, in 1904, already middle-aged, he wrote to the Directors of the Eye Infirmary that one afternoon he had heard loud screams coming from the Superintendent's office and on enquiry learned that the Matron had been caning the page boy! There seems to have been no substance to the complaint, however; perhaps Fergus had fallen out with the Matron!

In 1921 Glasgow University awarded him the honorary degree of LLD. He was President of the Royal Faculty of Physicians and Surgeons of Glasgow from 1918 to 1921.

H

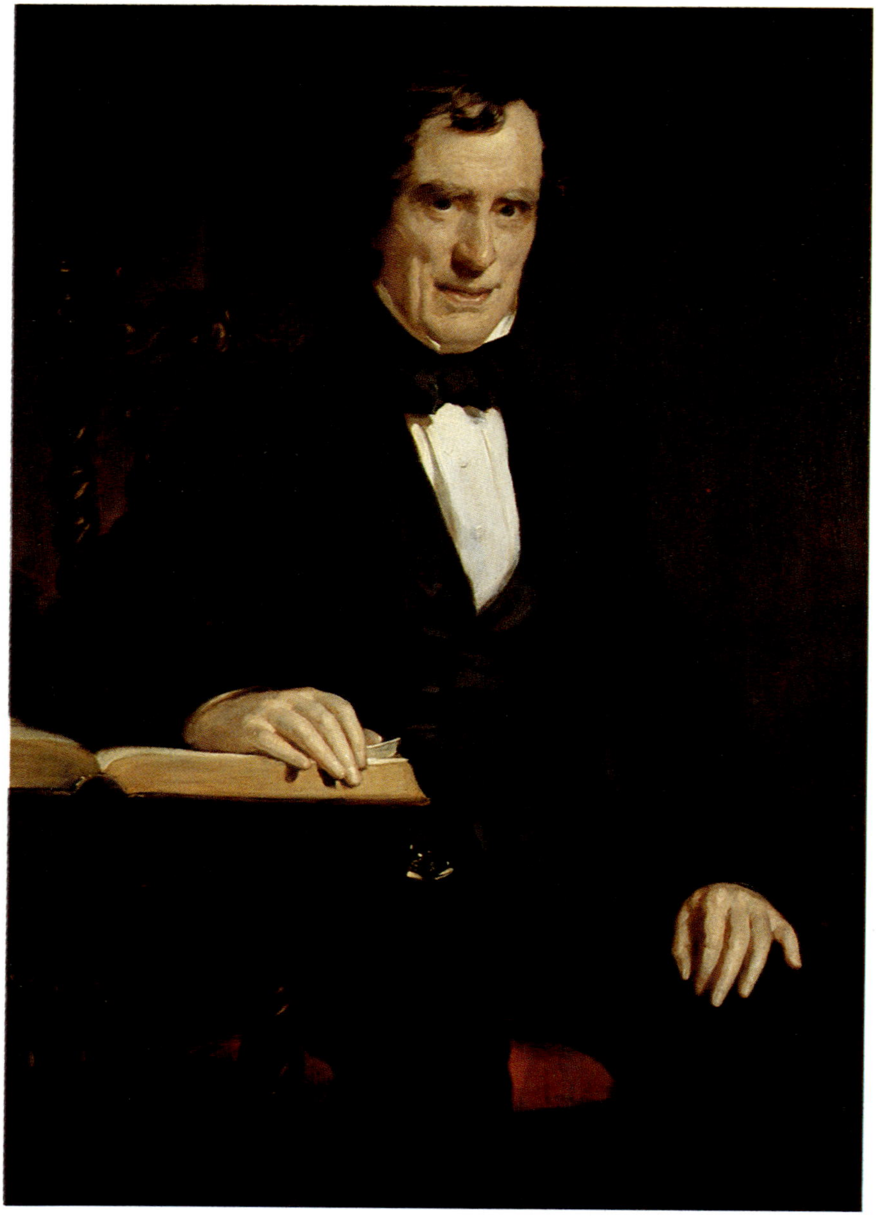

*James Wilson (1783 to 1857) was largely responsible for the founding of the Glasgow Maternity Hospital and was its first physician. The portrait is unsigned but is after the style of Sir Daniel Macnee.*

*Obstetrics 1*

# JAMES WILSON

1783 to 1857

*There is a possibility that the portrait attributed to James Wilson may not be his. It was one of those found in a basement cellar in 1979 which bore neither the name of the subject nor that of the artist. All the others have been positively identified from photographs either of the portrait or of the subject.*

*The reasons for believing this to be a portrait of James Wilson are:*

*In the Faculty Minutes of 1918 it is noted that 'Dr. J. Munro Kerr presented to the Faculty the portrait by Sir Daniel Macnee of Dr. James Wilson (1784-1857) who was mainly instrumental in founding the Glasgow Maternity Hospital and the President in name of the Faculty accepted the donation and expressed the cordial thanks of the Faculty to Dr. Munro Kerr for the gift as an excellent work of art and the portrait of a distinguished Glasgow Physician and Fellow of this Faculty.';*

*The portrait therefore came into possession of the Faculty 61 years after Wilson's death when none remembered him and few perhaps remembered even who he was. Unnamed, the portrait may soon have found its way into oblivion in the cellar;*

*The portrait is certainly in the style of Sir Daniel Macnee (1806-1882) and the College has several examples of his work for comparison. While most are signed, that of Robert Perry is not and it may be that he omitted his signature on occasion;*

*The style of dress is that of the 1840s and 1850s;*

*There are other portraits which the College is known to have possessed which no longer exist, but all of these can be excluded with a fair degree of certainty.*

*Meanwhile, therefore, let us accept him as James Wilson.*

The obituary notice in the *Lancet* gives the date of birth of James Wilson as 1783; the Faculty minute quoted above gives 1784; Finlayson says 1782. This variation was not uncommon at this period which was prior to the introduction of the registration of births and birth certificates. The place of birth, however, is known to have been Douglas in Lanarkshire and most of his medical education seems to have been obtained at Glasgow University. There is, however, a shortage of exact data about his early career and the following comes partly from his obituary in the *Lancet* and partly from Duncan's *Memorials*.

After qualifying, probably with the Licence of the Faculty, he went into practice in Carluke, but he enjoyed the friendship and patronage of the Glasgow University Professor of Anatomy, James Jeffray, became a full member of the Faculty in 1816 and then settled in practice in Glasgow. Gradually he acquired an extensive reputation as what was then called a 'physician-accoucheur' and held the post of Lecturer in Midwifery in the Portland Street School from 1830 to 1838.

The Faculty took unto itself in 1740 the right to examine and license all midwives within its bounds and to fine those who practised without such a licence £40 Scots. Some arrangements were made to give them a training and courses of lectures were later available as 'man-midwifery' became more acceptable, and more and more medical practitioners became experienced and proficient in it. The first 'lying-in' hospital in Glasgow began in 1791. It was a small private institution belonging to James Towers who became the first Professor of Midwifery in Glasgow University in 1815. It was originally supported entirely by himself with the aid of patients' and students' fees, but in 1795 an annual grant of £10 was given by the City Council to cover some of the expense incurred in treating poor patients. There is no further record of it, and where it was situated or for how long it flourished has not been discovered.

An attempt was made to found a public lying-in hospital in 1805 but was abandoned because of the Faculty objection that 'it appeared to be promoted for private ends'; as noted previously, there may well have been some truth in this attitude.

The population of Glasgow was now increasing rapidly, however, and the need for a Maternity Hospital was becoming ever more essential and so, at last, at a meeting in the Town Hall on 19th September 1834, James Wilson obtained the support he required to establish a public lying-in hospital not just for patient care but for teaching students. Committees were set up to obtain subscriptions and draw up a constitution.

The Hospital opened in December of the same year on a shoestring in a second floor flat and some attics of the old Grammar School in Greyfriars Wynd off George Street. There was no bath, no w.c.; the rent was £30 per annum. It moved to an equally unsuitable house in St Andrew's Square in 1841 and from there, in 1860, to an old house in Rottenrow on the site of which a new Maternity Hospital was built and opened in 1881. It too proved inadequate for the ever increasing needs of the now established specialty, and the present Glasgow Royal Maternity Hospital was opened next to it in 1909 and the old building used for nurses' accommodation.

It is with the older buildings, however, that James Wilson was first and senior physician until his death in 1857. His place was taken by his son, James George Wilson, who had been reared in an atmosphere of obstetrics and appears to have restricted his practice entirely to it. He became Professor of Midwifery in Anderson's College in 1863.

James Wilson's obituarist sums him up thus: 'Dr. Wilson's reputation had been long and firmly established and though, from his unobtrusive manners, he was little heard of beyond the circle of his profession, no name stood higher within it'.

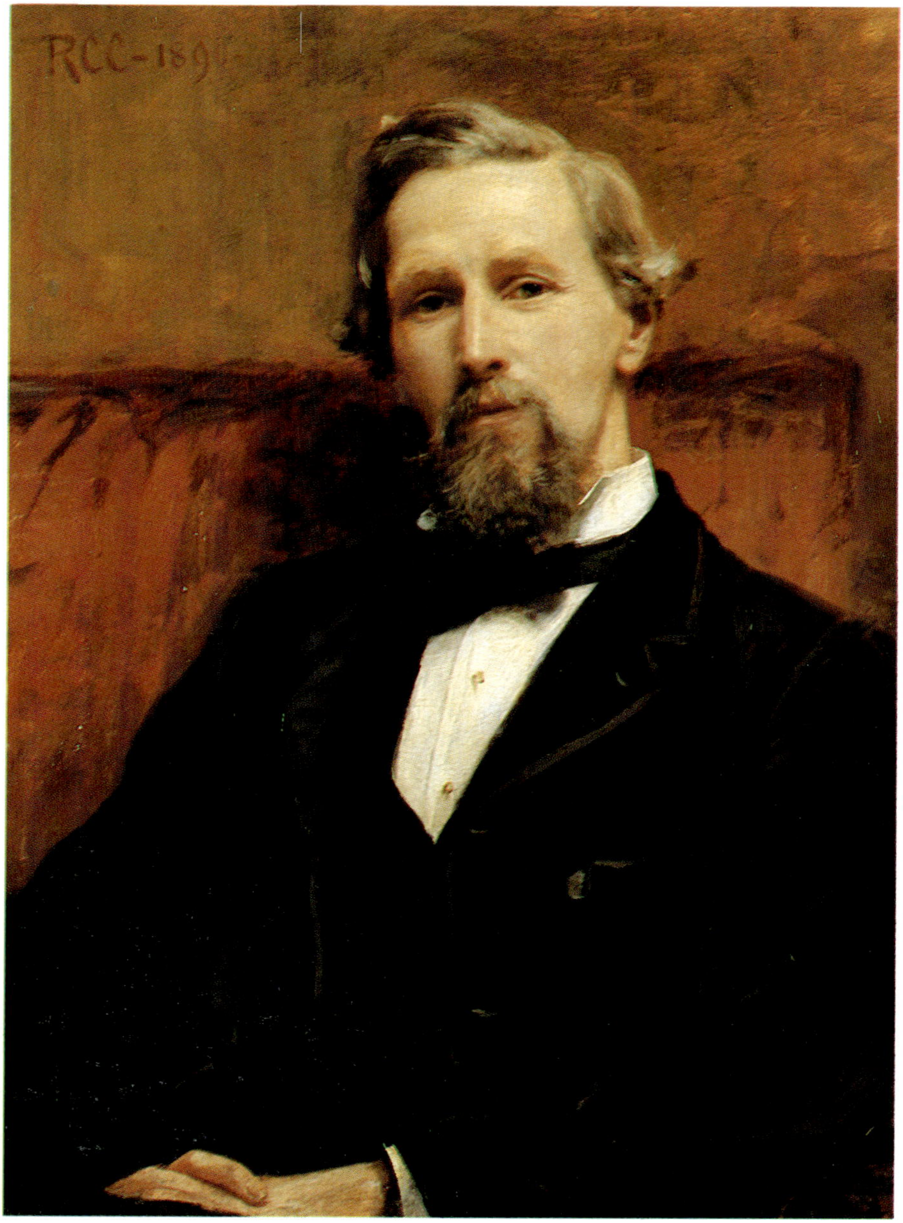

*William Loudon Reid (1845 to 1931) was a well known Glasgow obstetrician who combined a lust for salmon fishing with good works in the fields of religion and alcohol abstention. The portrait is by R. G. Crawford.*

*President, 1905 to 1907.*

# WILLIAM LOUDON REID

1845 to 1931

*The portrait is by Mr R. G. Crawford and was presented to the Royal Faculty in 1932 by Dr W. L. Reid's widow 'in order that it may be hung in the Hall among the portraits of other Presidents', and the minute of the Faculty meeting of 4th April 1932 concludes with the statement from the President that it has indeed 'been hung in one of the panels in the Faculty Hall'. It was removed for safe-keeping during the War years and on its return seems to have progressed no further than the basement cellar where it was found in 1979 and cleaned, restored and reframed.*

William Loudon Reid was born in Motherwell, went to school in Hamilton, studied at Glasgow University and graduated there MB, CM in 1866. As a senior student he had acted as 'dresser' to Joseph Lister. He began as a general practitioner in Glasgow and then spent some time abroad studying particularly obstetrics and gynaecology, which were to become his full-time, life-long specialty.

He took his MD in 1869 and became a Fellow of the Faculty of Physicians and Surgeons of Glasgow in 1877, the same year in which he obtained his first specialty appointment as 'Outdoor Physician-accoucheur' to the Royal Maternity Hospital and Women's Hospital.

Since its inception the Maternity Hospital has always stressed the value of attending births in the patients' own homes, only the more difficult cases being admitted. The 'outdoor' appointments were therefore usually held by juniors who might advance later to 'indoor' posts. So it was with Dr W. L. Reid. The posts which he subsequently held included: Obstetric Physician to the Royal Maternity Hospital; Professor of Midwifery and Diseases of Children in the Anderson College; Gynaecologist to the Western Infirmary; and Consulting Surgeon to the Royal Samaritan Hospital for Women.

Dr Reid wrote a number of papers, particularly about new or modified instruments: a long forceps; a vaginal speculum; a uterine dilator. He travelled extensively in Europe and America mainly in pursuit of game fish, although he did give a paper to the International Medical Congress in Washington in 1887 on 'The remote results of the operation of shortening the round ligaments for displacement of the uterus'.

Apart from being a compulsive fisherman and a tier of artificial flies, he was a life-long total abstainer and was active in the temperance movement and also in religious circles; for many years he was President of the Glasgow Medical Missionary Society. He was in fact a member of many boards and committees but latterly had to give them up because of increasing deafness. The last 20 years of his life were spent in retirement in Carmunnock where he had the leisure to devote more time than before to his temperance and religious work.

In 1931 the Royal Faculty of Physicians and Surgeons of Glasgow bestowed on William Loudon Reid their highest honour, that of Honorary Fellowship. He was their President from 1905 to 1907.

# 9

# PLAGUES AND PESTILENCES

Robert Perry (1783 to 1848)

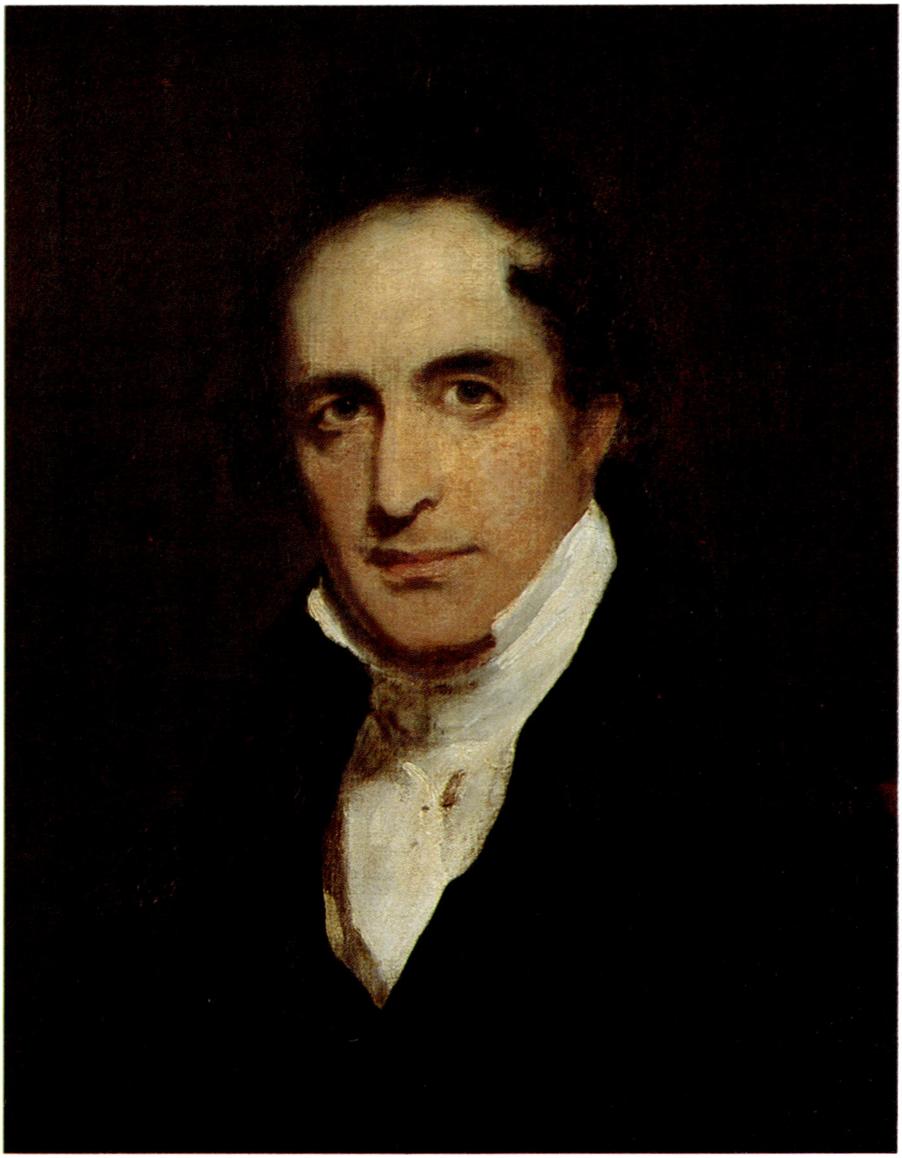

*Robert Perry (1783 to 1848) took a great interest in the epidemic fevers which ravaged Glasgow every few years, and played a significant part in the differentiation of typhoid from typhus fever. The portrait, although unsigned, is by Sir Daniel Macnee.*

*President, 1843 to 1845.*

The history of mankind and civilisation is intimately linked with bacteria and other minute creatures; some are harmless, some beneficial and indeed essential, others have destroyed more humanity than wars, floods or famines. The latter were always around, but every now and then they had bouts of epidemic ferocity particularly when people were crammed together in the ever enlarging cities. Every few years Glasgow would have another, and the bigger the city became the more awesome the mortality. The recognition of the part John Balmanno played in the 1818 epidemic has already been noted; the story of Joseph Lister's wards being built over a cholera pit will be told later. Here the life of Robert Perry illustrates many of the problems which existed before bacteria were identified and some measure of control effected.

## ROBERT PERRY

1783 to 1848

*The portrait was painted by Sir Daniel Macnee and was left to the Faculty by a holograph codicil to the will of Perry's son, also Robert, who was President from 1889 to 1891. On the 4th of February 1918 the Council recommended its acceptance and informed the widow of Robert* filius *of their pleasure at the gift.*

Robert Perry was born in Kilmarnock and received his medical education at Glasgow University where he graduated MD in 1808 and entered the Faculty in 1812. For over 30 years he was attached to Glasgow Royal Infirmary first as a surgeon and later, when the rules were changed, as a physician; he also worked in the old Fever Hospital in Clyde Street. He seems to have been a 'clubbable' man since he was one of the first members of the Glasgow Medical Society, founded in 1814, and a founder member and first Vice-President of the Western Medical Club which was founded in 1845 and continues to flourish today. He is most memorable, however, for two related topics: the differentiation of typhus from typhoid fever, and the close association of bad sanitation with disease and crime.

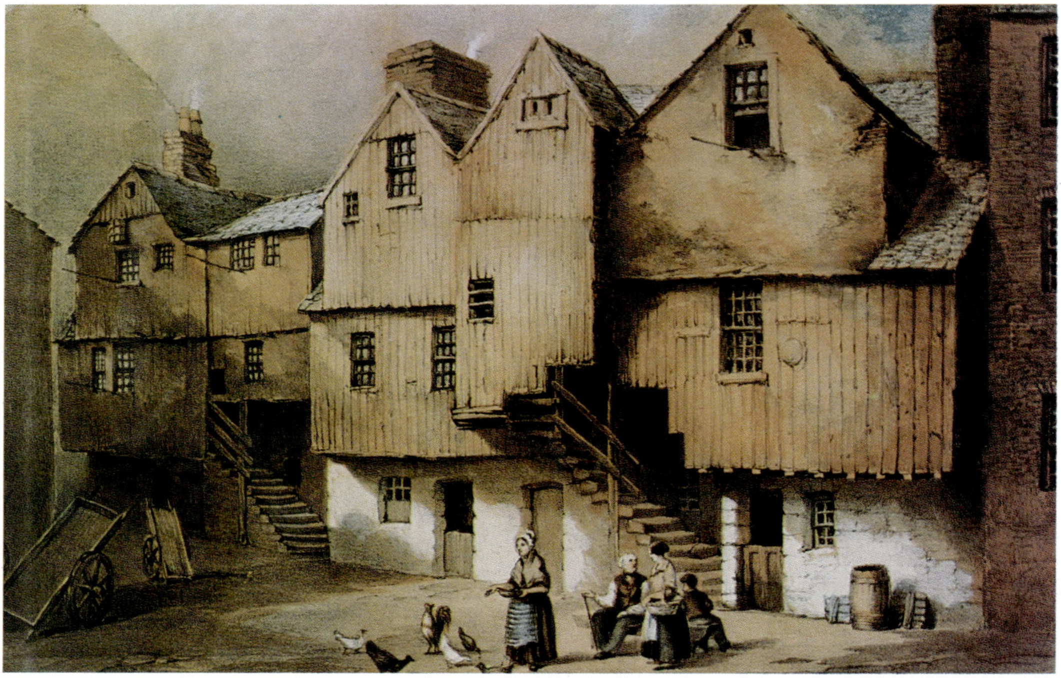

'WOODEN HOUSES IN CLOSS 77 SALTMARKET' (*Fairbairn*, 1850)

*To provide accommodation for the expanding population in the 17th and 18th centuries these wooden houses were built on top of single storey stone buildings by laying projecting wooden beams over the stone walls to support another one or two storeys of wooden houses. They obstructed light and ventilation and were cold and comfortless. They were in addition a great fire risk and by 1850 any further such constructions were prohibited.*

*In accommodation such as this epidemics of cholera, typhus, typhoid and other contagions were continually recurring.*

Before the turn of the 18th/19th century, those who perished in the epidemics which swept through the land every few years, died in their homes. Cases of bubonic plague and cholera were easily sorted out but many of the remainder were simply called typhus. However, as more hospitals were opened and more patients came under medical scrutiny, it became apparent that there were several different syndromes being admitted under this heading. In the social conditions then existing, and bearing in mind that epidemics had their major impact on the poor and underfed, all sorts of infections such as pneumonia, meningitis, erysipelas, measles and smallpox, and a variety of worsening deficiency diseases, could be admitted as victims of the typhus; many patients too had multiple infections. The gradual awareness that there were two separate major contagions became stronger in Britain, Europe and America during the 1820s and 1830s and it would be wrong to ascribe their differentiation to a sudden discovery by any one individual; but Perry's writings were a strong pointer in the right direction. It was Dr Louis in France who in 1829 coined the name 'typhoid'. Other French doctors called it 'dothienenteritis' and this was the term which Perry used. Perry first published his 'propositions' in manuscript form in the essays of the Glasgow Medical Society of 1835 but these were well received and were printed in the *Edinburgh Medical Journal* in 1836. They were based on over 4,000 admissions with about 400 deaths, on the great majority of which he carried out post-mortem examinations.

Reading his work today there is no doubt that he had gone far to establish that typhoid and typhus were quite separate diseases, but his colleagues were in such doubt about his claims that the Glasgow Medical Society went so far as to send a deputation of five of their members to Dr Perry's wards to see and discuss his work and supply a report to the Society; but, although there was some agreement, there was also dissension and the report was never written.

Another strange aspect of the affair was the paper by A. P. Stewart in the *Edinburgh Medical Journal* of 1840 entitled 'Some considerations on the nature and pathology of typhus and typhoid fever applied to the solution of the question of the identity or non-identity of the two diseases'. It had been read to the Parisian Medical Society and was mostly an analysis of the writings of previous workers in Europe and America rather than a study of his own cases. Stewart was an unusual man; he was born in 1813, studied in the Faculty of Arts in Glasgow University and from 1828 to 1830 travelled with his family extensively in France. Returning to Glasgow he graduated MD in 1838 and although he spent most of his subsequent career in London, he became house-physician to Robert Perry for some months after graduation, and it was during this period that he became convinced of the specific distinction of typhoid and typhus fever. The strange point of his paper is that in all its 30 odd pages he refers to Perry only once and that shortly, telling how a Dr Peebles who was familiar with typhus as it occurred in Italy had told Perry of its characteristic rash and 'from this time Dr. Perry taught the difference between contagious typhus and dothienenteritis and appears to have been the first in the country to do so'.

Garrison and Morton, the great source for medical innovators, names both Perry and Stewart as distinguishers of typhoid and typhus. The Sydenham Society of London did Stewart the posthumous honour of reprinting his paper in 1884. One of Perry's old students, on the other hand, wrote to the editor of the *Medical Times and Gazette* in 1857 of the precedence of Perry over Stewart: 'As long ago as the session 1835-6, Dr. Perry, then physician to Glasgow Royal Infirmary, was constantly pointing out at the bed-side the distinction between typhus and typhoid fevers . . .'.

Again and again in the evolution of medical knowledge there comes a time when a new discovery is inevitable and if one does not make it another must; arguments over precedence are tedious and often irrelevant.

Dr Perry was President of the Faculty at the time of the great epidemic of 1843. The first cases were seen late the previous year but from May to December 1843, when the fever was it its worst, there were 14,758 known cases in the 17 districts of central

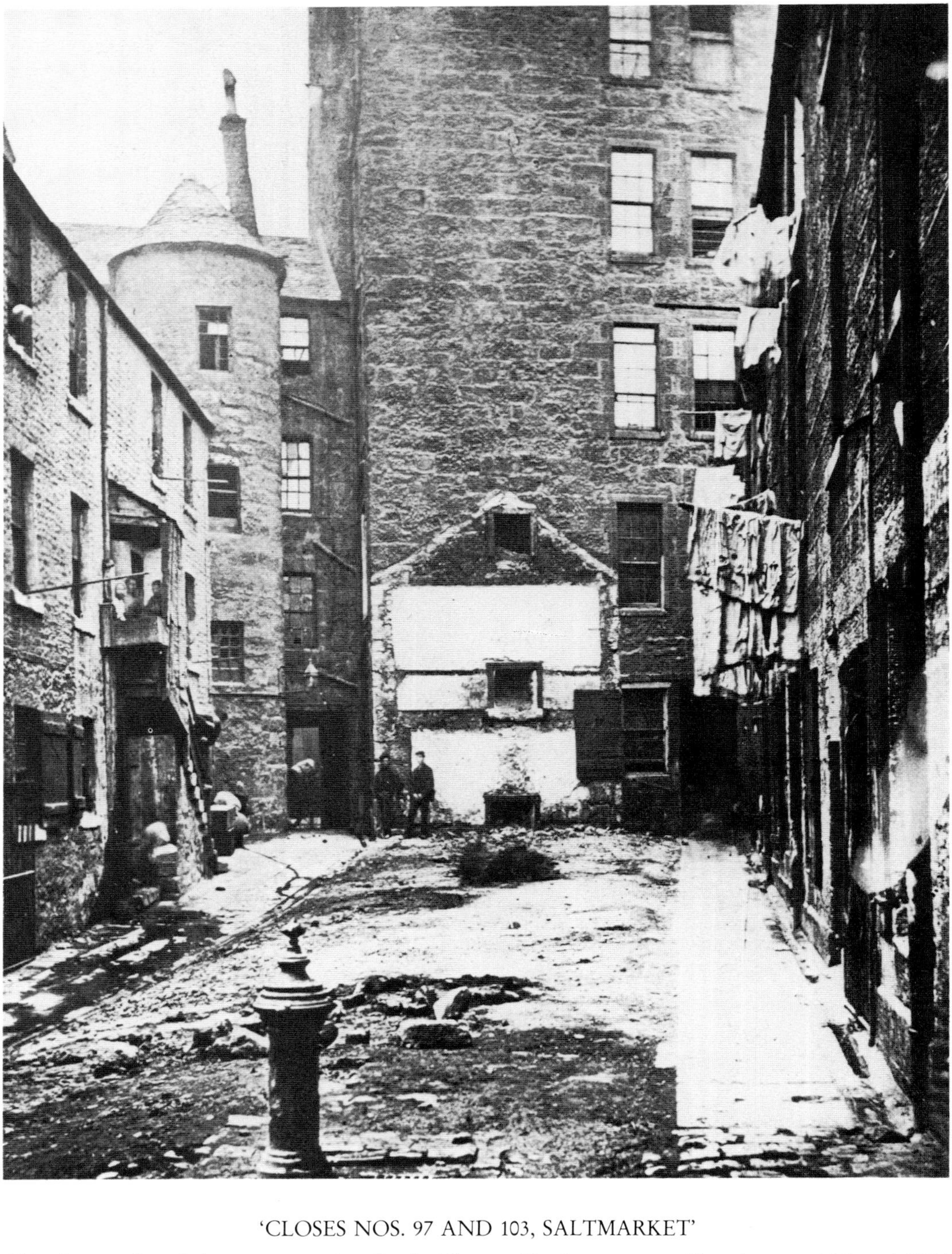

'CLOSES NOS. 97 AND 103, SALTMARKET'

*This photograph and the next were taken for the Glasgow City Improvement Trust between 1868 and 1877. Twenty-five years after Perry the squalor is still appalling.*

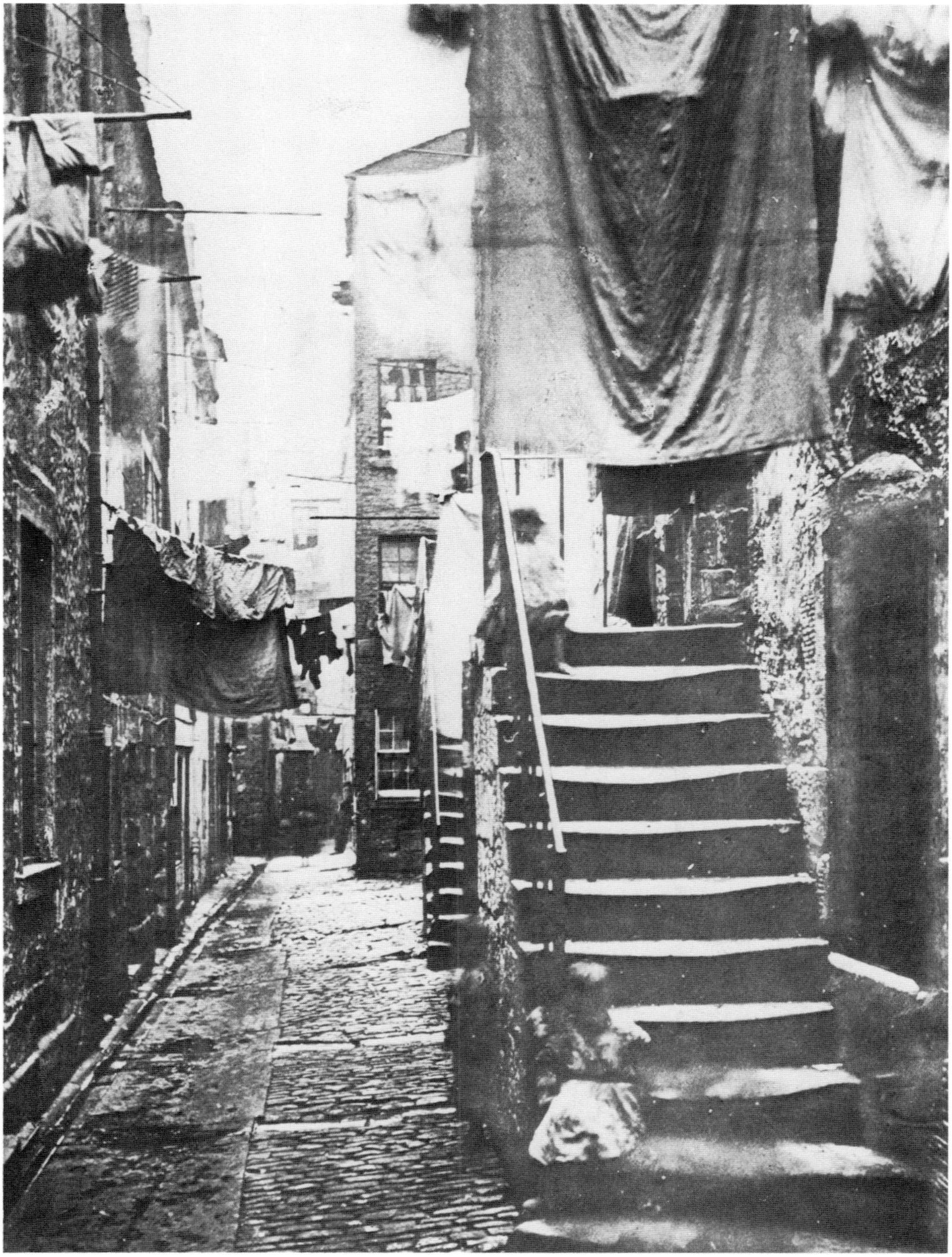

'CLOSE AT 193 HIGH STREET'

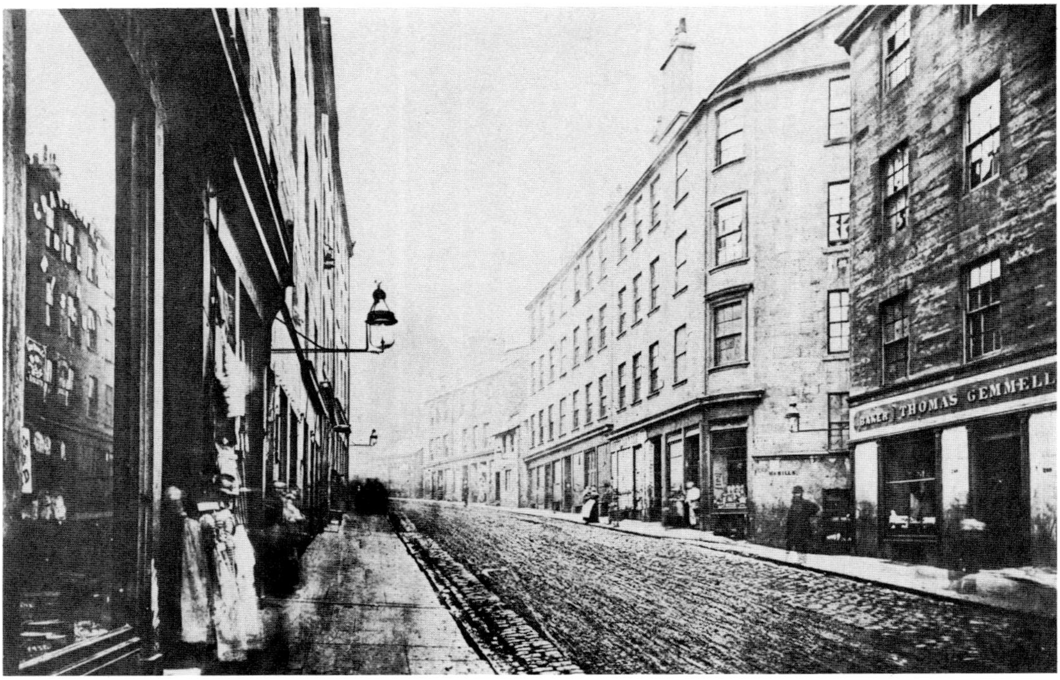


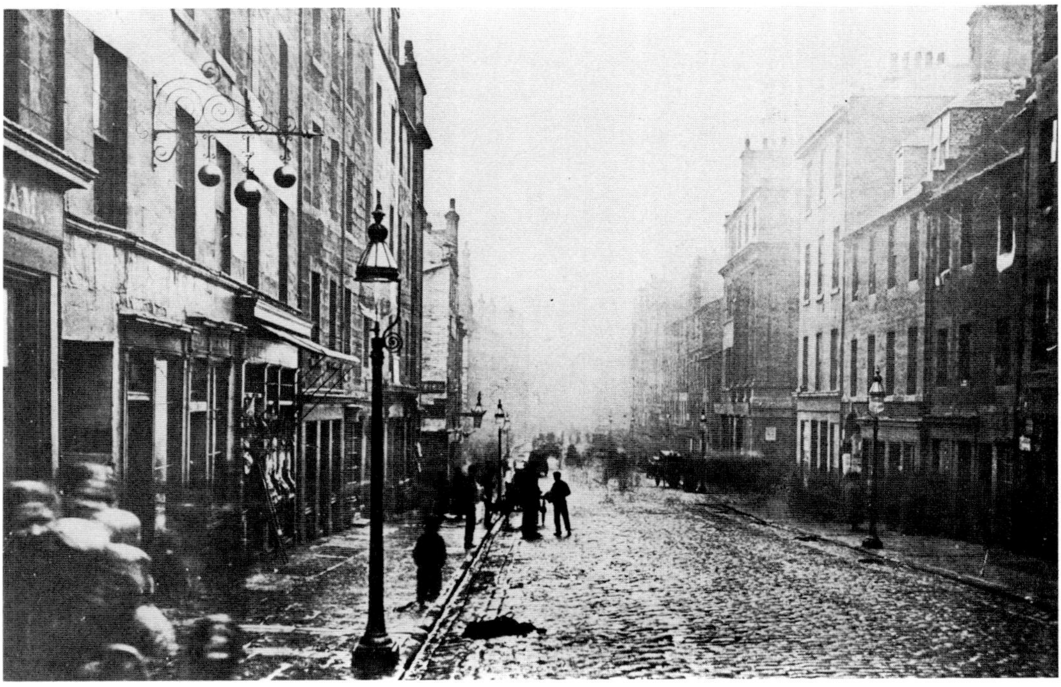

*These photographs, taken at the same time as those of the Closes, show much improvement in the High Street looking north (above) and south (below). But behind the facade the squalid closes remained.*

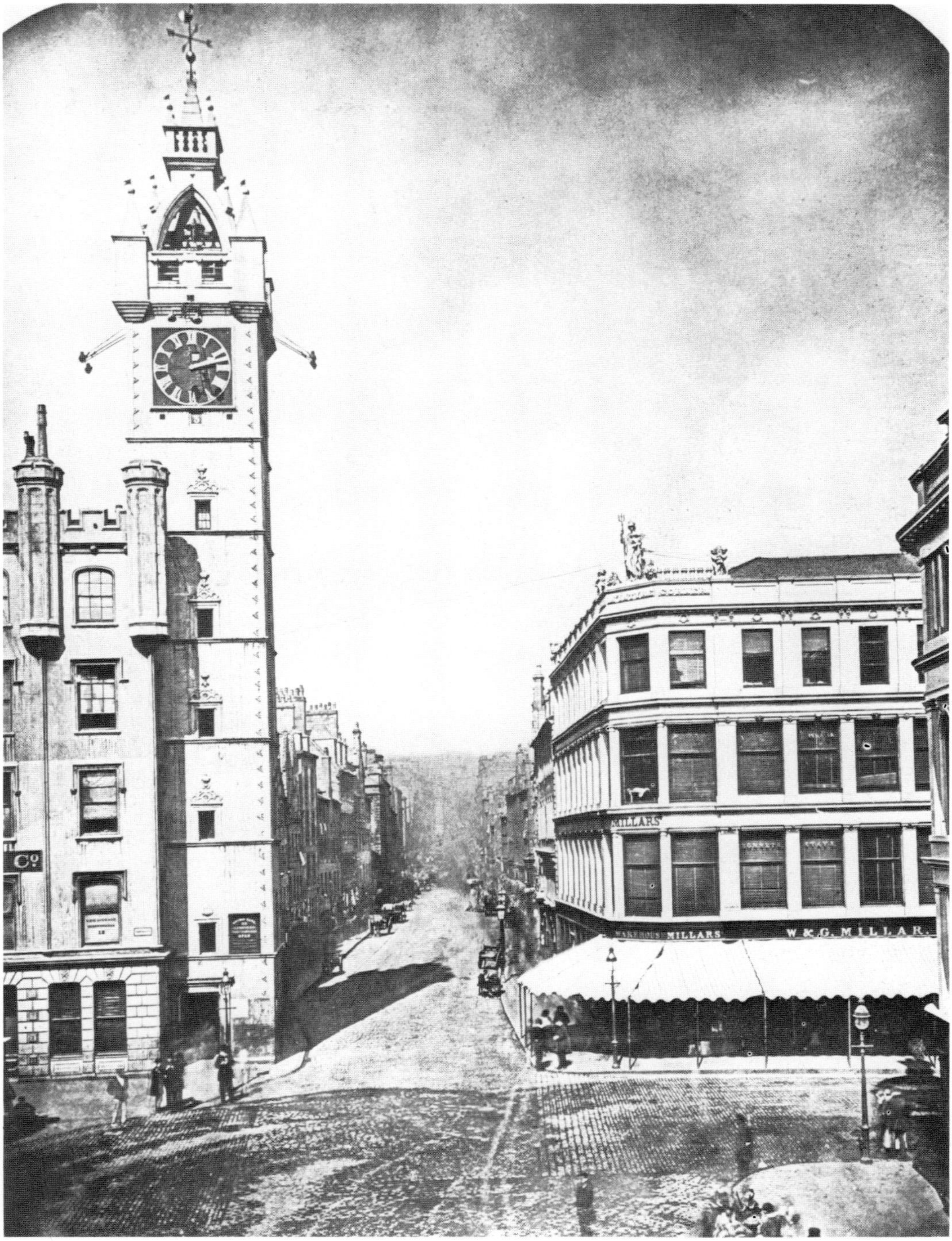


*A view from Glasgow Cross looking up High Street also taken between 1868 and 1877. Note the 'floodlighting' by gas lamps on the Tolbooth clock.*

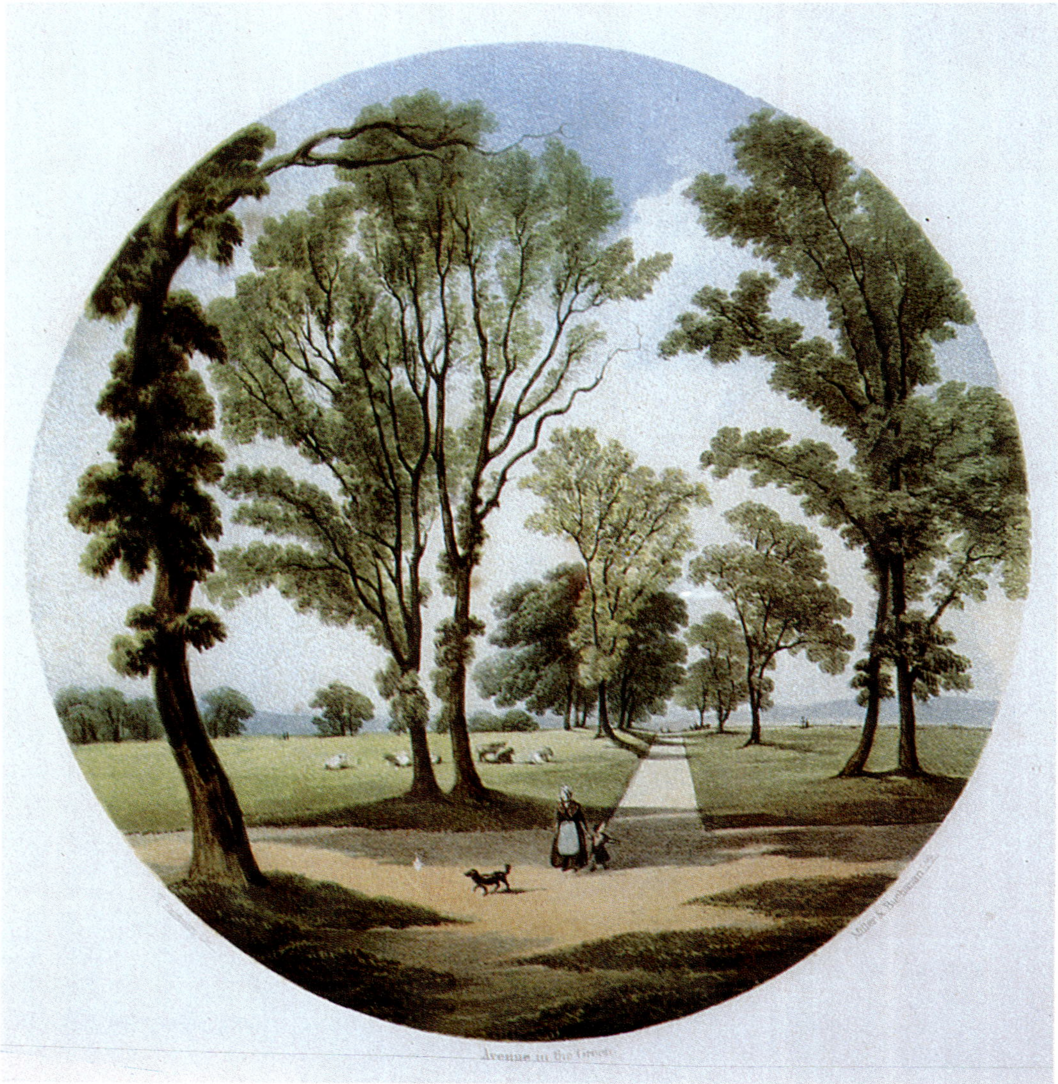

*Glasgow is rightly famous for its parks and even in Perry's time pleasant rural walks could be enjoyed near the city centre. This vignette by Fairbairn (1850) is entitled 'Avenue in the Green'. It looks south towards the river: 'the trees are redolent of leafiness; the green expanse is dotted with kine; the river rolls on its way'. But looking in any other direction 'the eye takes in the spires, steeples, domes, towers, and chimneys of a mighty city'. Take away the 'kine' and a similar rustic view* might *still be observed today.*

Glasgow with a population of 118,000. The number of coffins given out to the poor in these districts was 1,378 but not all the paupers asked for coffins and the death rate was probably between 15 and 20 per cent. The infection was unnamed, even by Perry with his extensive experience, although he says that it 'more closely resembles cholera in its mode and progress throughout the country than any other epidemic I have witnessed', but the symptoms were different. The Irish immigrants, preferring the hovels of Glasgow to death by famine in the bogs, were blamed and there is no doubt that the conditions under which many of them lived would have spread any infection; but not all the poor were Irish.

Whatever the disease was, Perry used the epidemic to highlight the appalling state of sanitation in parts of Glasgow in the work which he addressed in 1844 to the Lord Provost of Glasgow: 'Facts and Observations on the Sanitary State of Glasgow during the Last Year with statistical tables of the late epidemic showing the connection existing between Poverty, Disease and Crime'.

After describing the epidemic Perry tells how he asked the 17 District Surgeons for reports on the numbers of cases and the sanitary conditions. Most of them replied, describing the unbelievably appalling filth in which people lived, 'worse than pigsties and often shared with pigs and donkeys'. Two examples will suffice:

> 'In a lodging house in Parker Close [I] saw ten individuals lying with the fever at the same time in one apartment and that den without a window';
>
> '. . . five of which houses [*sic*] do not exceed five and a-half feet square, yet in one of those houses on the ground floor there was a man, his wife and four children all of whom had fever at one time. As they occupied the whole space as a bed I frequently could not gain admission and had to supply them with what was necessary through the window'.

From District after District the descriptions of disgusting squalor and deprivation recur. Perry linked such poverty closely with crime for many reasons, not the least of which was that the real poor were better off in prison than outside and many continued to commit offences just to return to the comfort of their cell.

Perry's report must have had a sickening impact on the municipal authorities and undoubtedly improvements to alleviate the poor have been continuing ever since; but perhaps it is inevitable that 'the poor always ye have with you'.

Read what Perry wrote in 1844: 'As to the causes which have led to this state of destitution and wretchedness among the poor, men will differ according to their prejudices and interests, one class ascribing it to restrictions on trade, another to the improvements in machinery, a third to the want of moral training and habits of intemperance, and a fourth to the amount of taxation, often mistaking effects for causes'.

*Plus ca change . . . .*

Robert Perry was President of the Faculty of Physicians and Surgeons of Glasgow from 1843 to 1845.

# 10

## TRAVELS AND EXPLORATION

Hugh Miller (1812 to 1879)
David Livingstone (1813 to 1873)

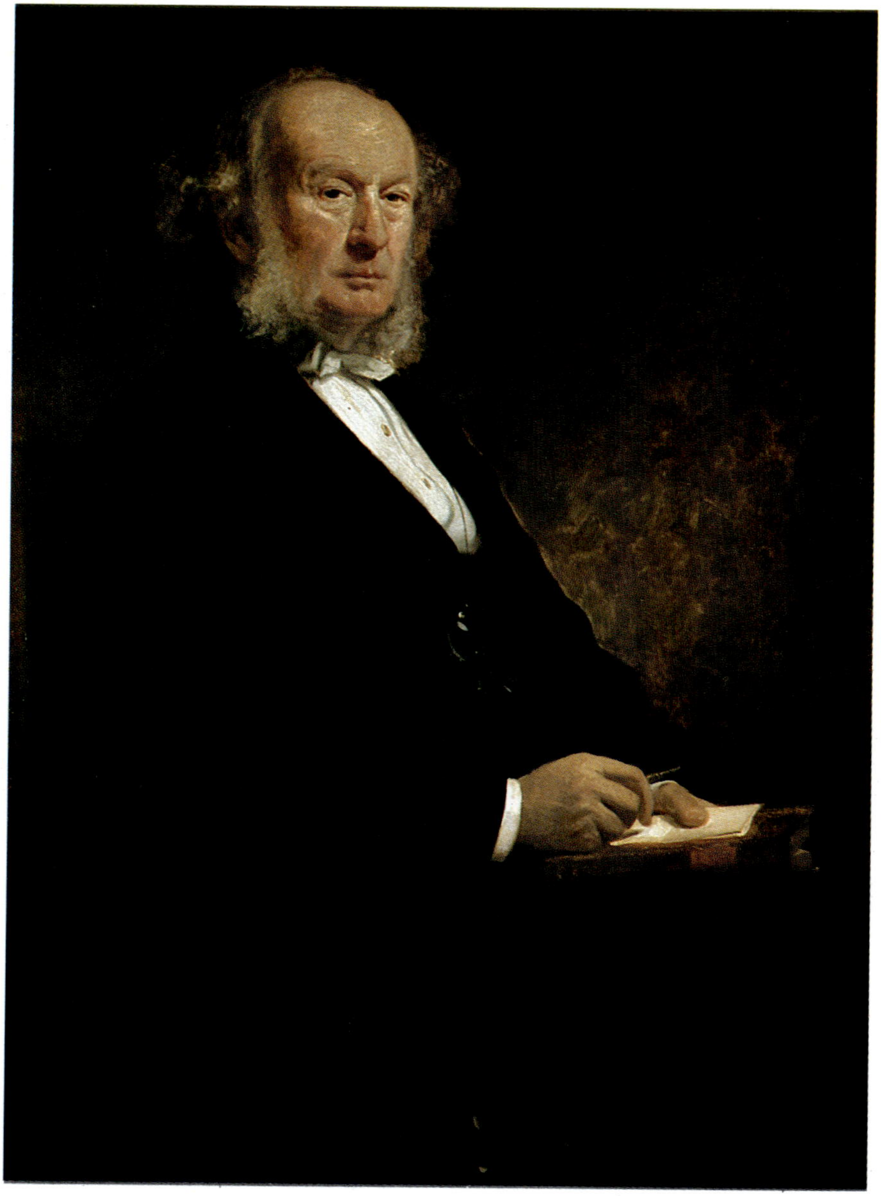

*Hugh Miller (1812 to 1879) was a successful upper class practitioner in Bombay and invested his savings partly in the expanding mission fields of India and partly in a coffee plantation in Ceylon. The portrait is by Norman MacBeth and did not reach the Royal Faculty until 1939.*

The Scottish doctor has often shown a desire for travel and it will be noted how often the subjects of the portraits made a postgraduate tour of medical centres in Europe. But there were other reasons for going abroad in the 19th century. The British Empire was burgeoning and fortunes were to be made in overseas stations, sometimes by doctoring alone, at others by helping to exploit the natural wealth of the countries being 'developed'. At the other extreme were the Christian Missionary doctors who began early in the century and continued in increasing numbers to take their religion and their medical skills to the most primitive parts of the world.

The first of the subjects, Hugh Miller, combined the desire to make his fortune with a devoutness which made him give much of his money to missionary endeavours. David Livingstone's missionary fervour led him to become one of the greatest explorers of continental Africa.

# HUGH MILLER

1812 to 1879

*This portrait at first presented a puzzle. A relatively modern label stuck on the back of it said '? Andrew Buchanan (much mildewed)'. Andrew Buchanan was a distinguished physician who was Professor of the Institute of Medicine in Glasgow University and President of the Royal Faculty of Physicians and Surgeons of Glasgow from 1879 to 1880. The portrait might well have been accepted as his had there not been found in the Council minutes of 1939 a letter from Mitchells, Cowan and Johnston, Solicitors, saying that subsequent to the death of a Mrs Steel, the portrait of Dr Hugh Miller which was to come to the Royal Faculty on her death could now be collected. This was wartime and, as there was no record of the portrait having been collected, the solicitors were contacted. It so happens that the firm of Mitchells, Cowan and Johnston are now Mitchells, Johnston, Hill and Hoggan and by a coincidence also the lawyers of the Royal College. An enquiry there produced from one of the partners not only a short summary of the life of Hugh Miller but a privately printed biography of him by the Rev. W. W. Peyton, in the frontispiece of which there is a reproduction of his portrait. There can be now no doubt that the College portrait which might have been Andrew Buchanan's is undoubtedly that of Hugh Miller.*

*The portrait, which we now know to have been painted by Norman MacBeth, reached the Royal Faculty 60 years after Miller died. Although it was left to the Faculty, his wife had it for her lifetime and then their adopted daughter Agnes, who married the Reverend John Steel, had it for hers. By the time it reached the Royal Faculty there can have been no Fellow who remembered Hugh Miller and it is doubtful if the portrait has ever hung on the College walls.*

*It is a noble portrait, however, and one of the few examples we have of many who emigrated to seek their fortune in the first half of the 19th century, to foreign countries about which they knew very little. Many died of disease, drink or despair. Hugh Miller prospered and came home and enjoyed almost 15 years of comfortable retirement on the Firth of Clyde.*

Hugh Miller was the youngest of eight children born on a farm called Gallowayford near Dunlop in Ayrshire. His father died when he was 14 months old and his mother brought up the family until the eldest son could work the farm. Hugh went first to the local school and, when the family moved to a larger farm at Maybole, to the school there. He started off to be a lawyer and was articled to a Kilmarnock firm for three years after which he moved to a firm in Glasgow. But he was bent on medicine and by means of classes at Glasgow University, Anderson's College and privately, he was able to take the Licence of the Faculty of Physicians and Surgeons of Glasgow in 1835.

He went first to Belfast to practise and then came back to Glasgow to help out his elder brother Alexander, who was also a doctor but 'enjoyed ill health', and with whom Hugh's future career was intimately bound. Alexander made trips to Madeira for his health, and many years later died and was buried there. Hugh looked after the practice while he was away. Then Alexander went to Bombay and soon Hugh followed him. The immediate reason seems to have been that his application for the post of surgeon to the Town's Hospital was turned down.

That Alexander cared more for his environment than for his brother is illustrated by the fact that as soon as Hugh arrived in Bombay, Alexander left for Poona to avoid the coastal monsoon rains. Indeed, although Alexander was responsible for setting up Hugh in a good practice in Bombay, the relationship between the brothers deteriorated and ended in a law suit at the end of which Hugh was awarded damages against his brother. The Reverend W. W. Peyton, Hugh's biographer, was a man full of Christian charity and gives no details of the misunderstandings between the brothers, but tells how in the end they were 'forgotten and forgiven and the family circle made whole again' when Hugh erected a family gravestone and inscribed Alexander's name upon it!

Hugh Miller's practice in Bombay was among the British community, the Parsees, already wealthy industrialists, and the higher caste Hindus. He made money, his fees in one six-month period being over £1,000, and spent it either in supporting the Christian Missions which were now gaining impetus in India or investing it in a coffee plantation in Ceylon. At first the latter venture swallowed capital but by 1869 the boom in coffee was such that his profit from it was running at about £10,000 per annum.

The Indian Mutiny of 1857, while it did not involve Bombay to any great extent, must have been unsettling and in 1860 Hugh Miller came home on furlough. He took further classes at Glasgow University and graduated MD, became a Fellow of the Faculty of Physicians and Surgeons of Glasgow, and made a long trip through Europe. He went back to his practice in 1862 but two years later decided finally to leave India. He was given a lavish presentation of silver plate valued at 5,000 rupees (about £2,500), and an address signed by many eminent people including the Aga Khan.

Once home in Scotland he bought the estate of Broomfield on the shores of the Gareloch not far from Rhu. The old house was demolished and a new mansion built and there the Millers lived for the rest of their days.

The Millers were intensely religious and Hugh served on many committees on Church of Scotland affairs both for home and missions overseas. In 1873 he accompanied the Rev. Narayan Sheshadri of Bombay, one of the first Brahmin ordained ministers of the Free Church of Scotland, to an Evangelical Conference in New York and spent some weeks with him touring America and Canada.

Miller's brother-in-law, William Taylor, was a director of the City of Glasgow Bank which crashed in 1878 and he, with the other directors, was arrested and tried for fraud the following year. Miller sat through the 11 days of the trial, heard his brother-in-law sentenced to eight months' imprisonment and returned home a sick, unhappy man; he died ten days later.

The coffee plantation had been sold for £33,000 in 1877 and Hugh Miller left about £100,000, a quarter of which was bequeathed to missionary enterprises. The Rev. Mr Peyton, who wrote the biography really to please Mrs Miller, described him as 'an ordinary man, who attained more than average success. . . . Here is no master mind or extraordinary gifts of nature to picture and present . . . he rose into wealth by the force of average ability and mediocre faculties'.

One detects a faint trace of envy.

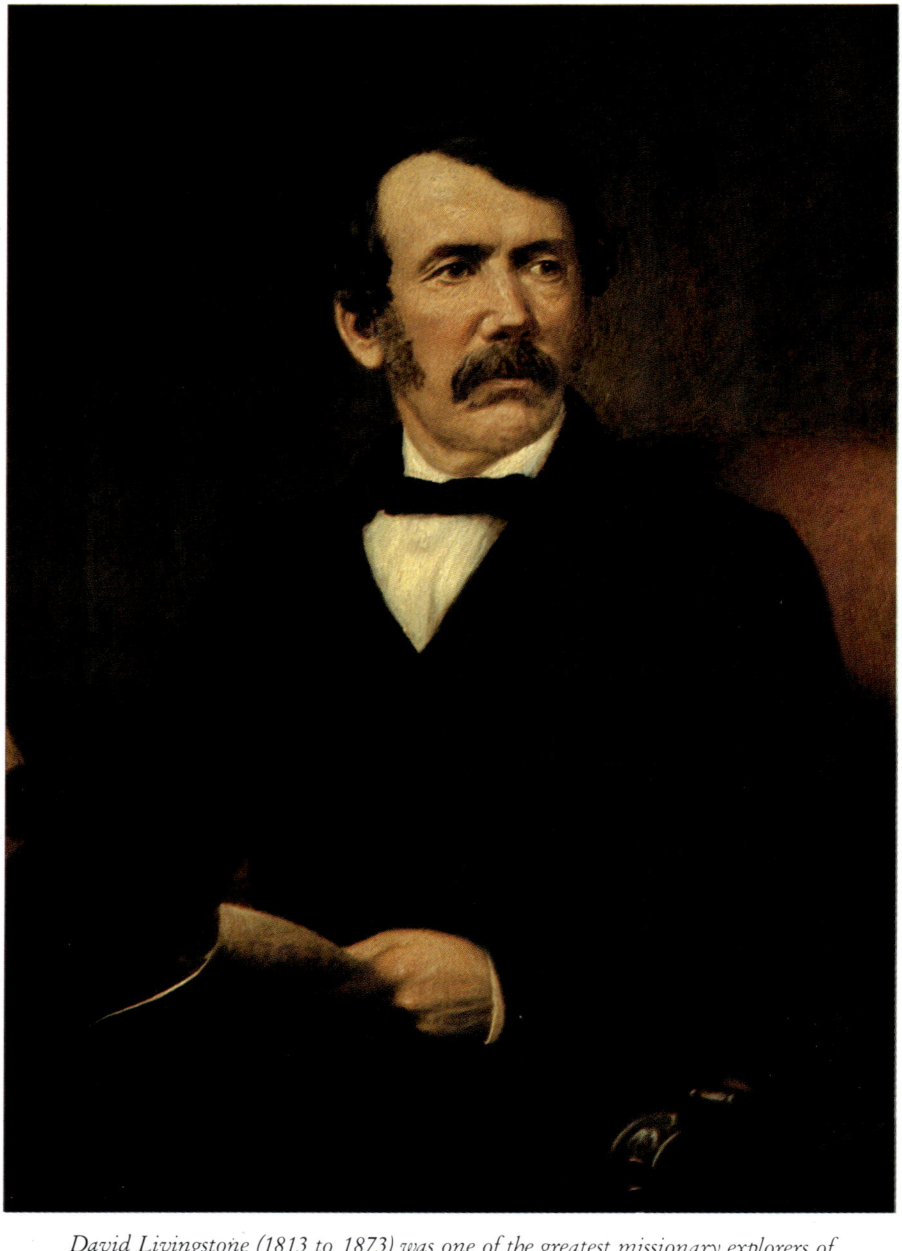

*David Livingstone (1813 to 1873) was one of the greatest missionary explorers of Africa. He obtained the Licence of the Faculty before going overseas and on his return was made an Honorary Fellow. The portrait was created from a photograph taken by Annan in 1864.*

# DAVID LIVINGSTONE

1813 to 1873

*The portrait was purchased by the Faculty in 1875. It is 'an enlarged photograph by Mr. Thomas Annan coloured in oil' and cost 30 guineas. The photograph was taken in 1864 and a black and white version was until recently displayed in the shop window of T. & R. Annan & Sons Ltd., the Glasgow photographers.*

David was the second son in the family of seven of Neil and Agnes Livingstone. Neil was a tea merchant in a small way of business in Blantyre and Hamilton, and David at the age of 10, after some basic 3-R's schooling, was sent to work at the local cotton factory six days a week at 6 o'clock each morning. He furthered his education at evening school and by reading books propped on the spinning-jenny at work. When about 19 years old he developed strong Christian religious convictions and, on hearing a missionary from China appeal for help, determined to be a medical missionary in that country. He was now a tradesman cotton spinner and his summertime wages were enough to pay for his first medical studies in the winter months at Anderson's University.

The London Missionary Society, after a preliminary examination and a period of probation, accepted him and helped him to pursue his medical studies in the London hospitals. He became a licentiate of the Faculty of Physicians and Surgeons of Glasgow in 1840. Such a licence gave him the right of practice within the bounds of the Faculty, but no corporate rights. It was acceptable to the London Missionary Society and he was ordained a missionary later the same year.

The Opium War in China prevented his going there and he went instead to South Africa, having come under the influence of Dr Robert Moffat who was already active in the mission field there and whose daughter later became Livingstone's wife and the

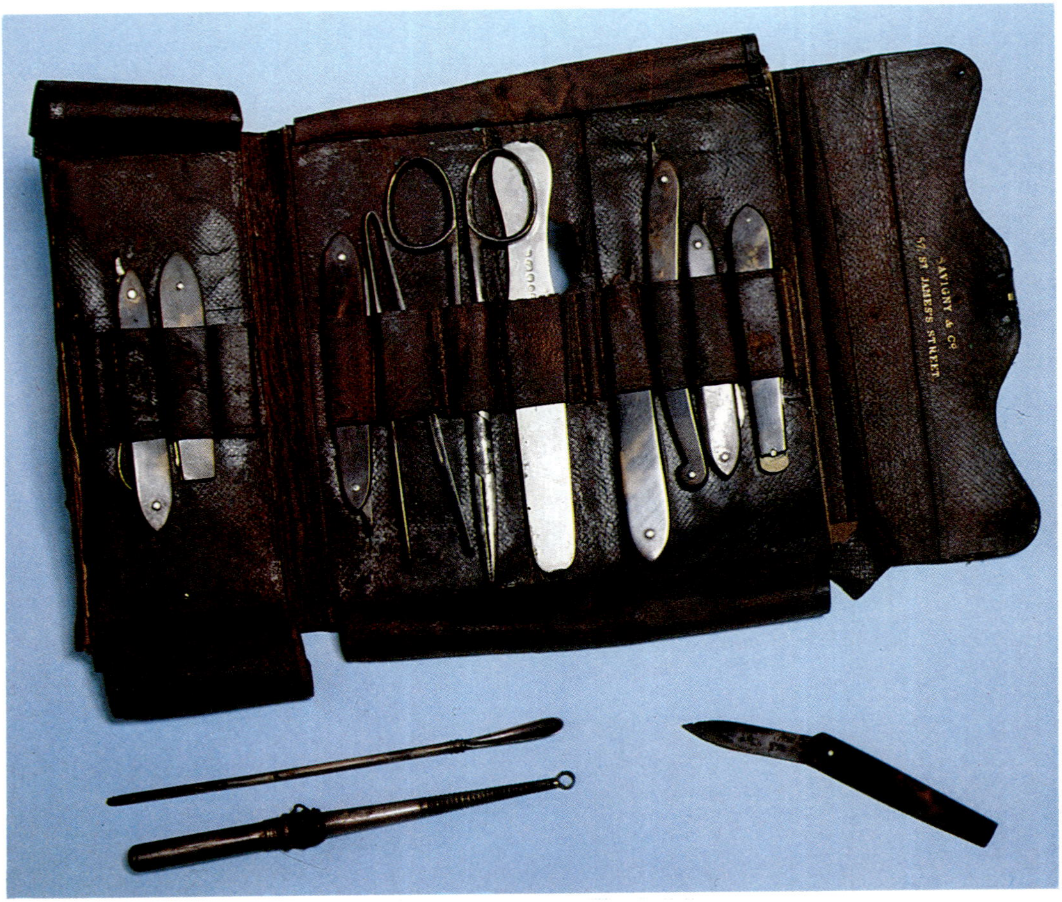


*The small leather pocket case of surgical instruments which David Livingstone carried on his explorations.*

mother of his six children. Although he started teaching and preaching in missionary stations, he soon came to believe that the greatest Christian impact in heathen Southern Africa would come from converted natives in their own tribes. This in turn led to his enthusiasm to learn the native languages and to explore and open up more and more of the dark continent.

His explorations in the face of disease, deprivations, attacks by wild animals, and the enmity of the Arab slave traders and the Boers, who also sought slaves, are a matter of history. He came home twice.

On the first occasion, late in 1856, he was reunited with his wife and children whom he had sent home in 1852. In the following year, he was feted by many learned

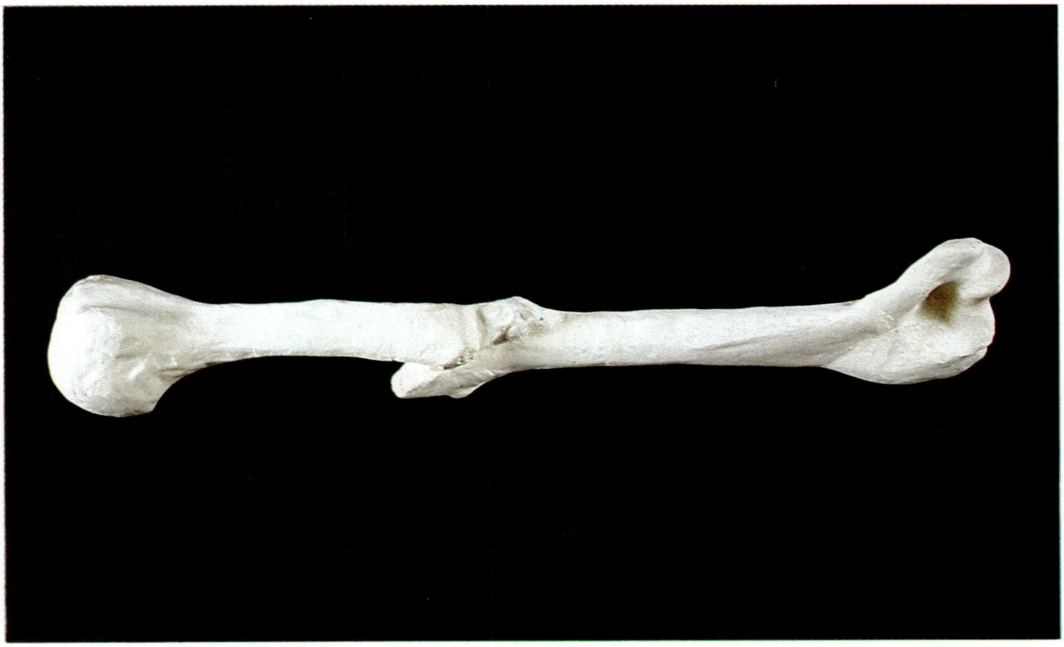

*A replica cast of David Livingstone's left humerus which was presented to the College by the Livingstone Memorial Trust in 1973 on the anniversary of his death. The compound fracture occurred when he was mauled by a lion on his first travels. Although the shaft is badly rotated the deformity caused him little disability. The cast was made when the body was examined prior to interment in Westminster Abbey, and the old healed fracture proved that the remains were indeed those of David Livingstone.*

societies, made a Freeman of the City of London and of the town of Hamilton. Oxford gave him the honorary degree of DCL, and the Royal Society created him a Fellow. In Glasgow, the University made him LLD, a public subscription raised £2,000 to help with his work, and the Faculty conferred on him their Honorary Fellowship. During this furlough, he completed and published his first account of his explorations, *Missionary Travels and Researches in South Africa*.

He returned to Africa the following year and spent six years in further exploration before coming home for the second time in 1864. He was again made much of but managed to retreat for some months to Newstead Abbey where he wrote his second great work, *Narrative of an Expedition to the Zambesi and its Tributaries and of the Discovery of the Lakes Shirwa and Nyassa, 1858 to 1864.*

He disappeared for long periods after he went back to Africa in 1865. The Royal Geographical Society sent out a search party in 1867 and were assured of his safety. The search by H. M. Stanley in 1871, financed by the *New York Herald*, is one of the great epics of history, not only because of its difficulties and dangers, but because of its success. The Royal Geographical Society sent out a second party in 1872 to which the Faculty contributed £10; they met Stanley's party coming back and were reassured about Livingstone's survival.

But he was already a sick man and although he would not go back with Stanley, and tried to continue his explorations, he died in 1873. His native companions Susi and Chuma brought his body and belongings to the coast whence they were shipped to London. His remains were finally buried in Westminster Abbey on 18th April, 1874. The expenses incurred by the Faculty in attending the funeral were £21.

# 11

## GLASGOW MEDICAL SCHOOLS OTHER THAN THE UNIVERSITY

John Gibson Fleming (1809 to 1879)

In the early days of the Faculty, apart from those *rarae aves*, the pure physicians with their MD's, all medical practitioners had to pursue a period of apprenticeship training and examination before the Faculty would grant them a diploma. As the University Medical School developed, attendance and attested performance at lecture courses were accepted more and more in lieu of apprenticeship time *so long as the lecturers were members of the Faculty*. By the turn of the 18th/19th centuries, however, because of the increasing population, the Napoleonic Wars and the developing colonies, the demand for doctors had increased beyond the capacity of the University to teach them.

Chronologically Anderson's University, founded in 1796, was the first to plan alternative courses but it was many years before its medical school had achieved the status which its founder had planned. John Anderson had held the Chairs of Oriental Languages and Natural Philosophy in Glasgow University and had been frustrated in trying to reform the academic abuses he found there. He therefore left in his will all his property to found an alternative university in which the professors 'shall not be drones or triflers, drunkards or negligent of their duty'. The will was a highly detailed document providing for faculties of Law, Divinity, Arts and Medicine, each with nine professors who were named. Unfortunately, all the property he left to launch this ambitious venture came to only £1,000 and the medical faculty had little to offer the medical student for two or three decades.

Dr John Burns, who was named in Anderson's will as the Professor of Anatomy and the Theory of Surgery, actually came to occupy a chair, the only one of the 36 so named who did so; but the position was largely titular. So John Burns went ahead on his own and in rooms in College Street taught anatomy, surgery and midwifery, was joined first by his brother Allan, then by Robert Watt (*q.v.*) who lectured in medicine and by others, and a group was formed known as the College Street School which flourished into the mid-1830s, by which time the Andersonian school was attracting more and more students and lecturers.

A similar group formed the Portland Street School. Portland Street ran parallel to, and to the east of, the present Montrose Street and is now incorporated in the Strathclyde University complex. The building itself was unprepossessing; 'everything that met the eye about the school was dingy and uninviting tending to repel more than attract'. Yet it numbered many brilliant men among its lecturers: for example, William Weir (*q.v.*) and James Wilson (*q.v.*). Perhaps the most outstanding was Thomas Graham who lectured there in chemistry in 1828, who became internationally known subsequently for his original work on the diffusion of gases and liquids, who was appointed Master of the Mint in 1854, and who is one of the few Glasgow men commemorated by his statue in George Square.

The Portland Street School, like the College Street School, gradually dwindled and died. One of its last lecturers in 1844 was Dr Robert Knox, the anatomist who, disgraced in Edinburgh by the Burke and Hare exposures of 1828, came to Glasgow with a forlorn hope to re-establish himself.

By now the Anderson University Medical School was thriving and in the 1840s and 1850s it was enrolling 100 to 150 students each year into its Anatomy course alone and was offering courses in Botany, Materia Medica, Physiology, Medical Jurisprudence, Natural History, Chemistry, Surgery, Medicine and Midwifery. It was the most successful faculty of the University and yet its teachers got nothing from it directly but their title and the use of rooms, and even for those, they latterly paid rent. But the good successful lecturer attracted students and their fees and the reputation he gained attracted patients and theirs.

In the 1860s Glasgow University and Anderson's University both had successful medical schools attracting students from abroad as well as home, and both were dependent on Glasgow Royal Infirmary for clinical training. Glasgow University, however, was planning to move West to Gilmorehill and did so in 1870; the Western Infirmary was about to be built to house the

University's medical school and opened its doors in 1874. It seems strange now that the Andersonian Medical School did not remain in George Street and use the clinical facilities which it had possessed for years round the corner in the Royal Infirmary, but it too decided to follow the University. Anderson's University was soon afterwards divided into the Technical College, which remained in George Street and became first the Royal College of Science and Technology and finally the University of Strathclyde, and the independently incorporated Anderson's College Medical School which found itself a site on Dumbarton Road next to the Western Infirmary and constructed there a 'handsome and well-arranged building' some of which still exists. It opened in 1889.

There is no doubt of the close symbiosis between Anderson's College and Glasgow University. The former never quite achieved the status of the latter and indeed occupied a lower rung on the academic ladder. Thus we find Sexton, who wrote about 'The First Technical College' in 1894, saying quite seriously that the very high reputation of Anderson's College was proved 'by the fact that since its commencement no less than seventeen Professors have passed from its chairs to those of the University'!

Had it not been for the active dedication of the subject of our next portrait, all medical training facilities would have been concentrated in the west, and Glasgow Royal Infirmary, already internationally famous as a centre of medical education, would have become a non-teaching municipal hospital.

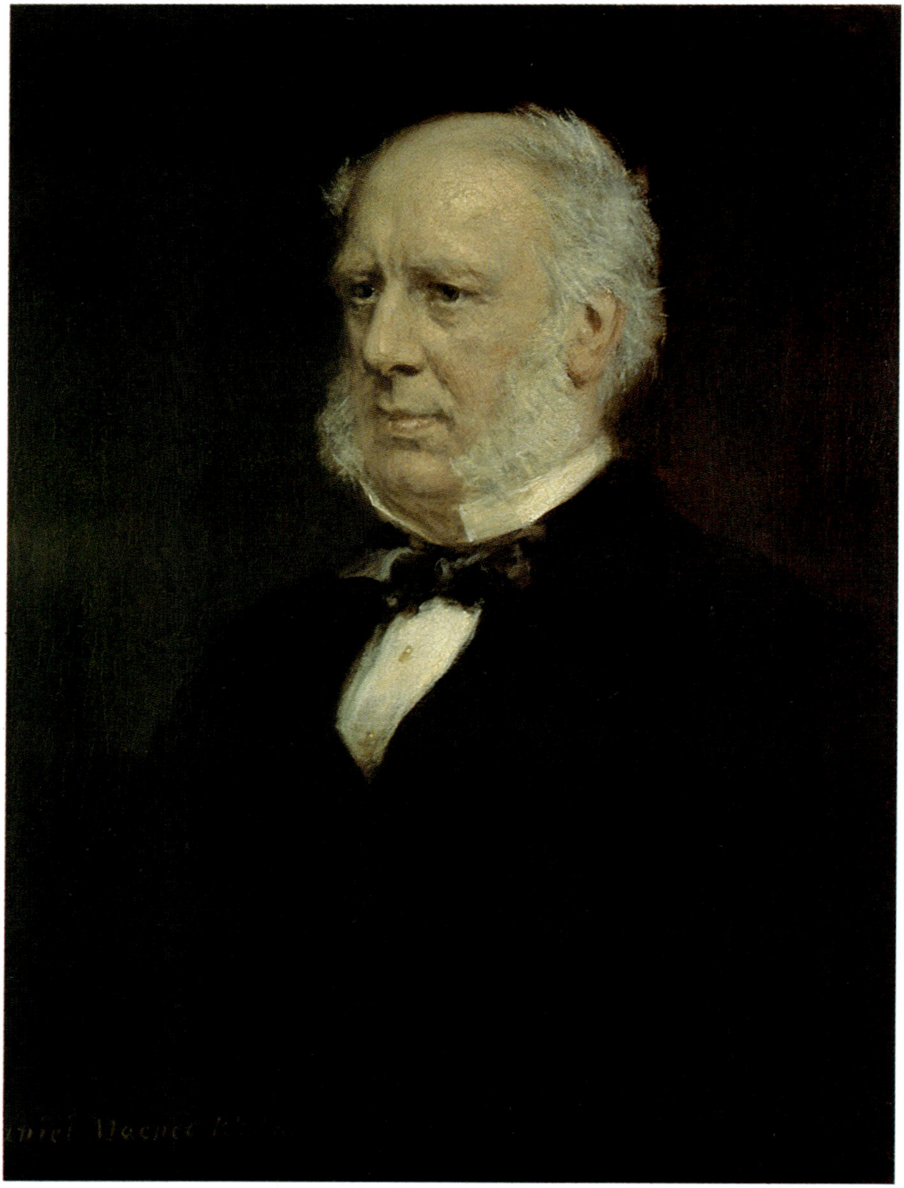

*John Gibson Fleming (1809 to 1879) was a member of a distinguished medical family and was responsible for the continuation of Glasgow Royal Infirmary as a teaching hospital with its own medical school when the University moved to Gilmorehill and the Western Infirmary. The portrait is by Sir Daniel Macnee.*
*President, 1865 to 1868; 1870 to 1872.*

# JOHN GIBSON FLEMING

1809 to 1879

*The portrait was commissioned posthumously by the Faculty from Sir Daniel Macnee in 1880 and was presumably painted from a photograph.*

John Gibson Fleming was one of a distinguished line of Glasgow citizens and Glasgow doctors said to be descended from 'Flemings of Flanders' of the 17th century. His medical connections have already been referred to in the sketch of John Balmanno. John Gibson's father, William Fleming, was a cousin of John Balmanno. John Gibson's son was William James Fleming, a surgeon in the Glasgow Royal Infirmary, and his son was Professor Geoffrey Balmanno Fleming who was President of the Royal Faculty from 1946 to 1948.

From Glasgow Grammar School, John Gibson Fleming went to Glasgow University and graduated MD in 1830. He came of a prosperous family and after graduation went on a continental tour and studied for some time in Paris. He passed the Faculty examination in 1833 and settled in central Glasgow as a general practitioner. In 1846 he was appointed a surgeon in the Royal Infirmary. The period of such an appointment at that time was four years followed by one year of ineligibility. In fact, Fleming had to wait for a further three years for a suitable vacancy before he was appointed in 1853 for his final four years as a surgeon. His surgical ability seems to have fallen short of brilliant, but he had a sense of humour to disarm his critics. After much fumbling around trying unsuccessfully to remove a coin stuck in a man's throat, he cried, 'Send for Dr Lyon. If there is anyone can get a half-crown out of a poor man, it is he'.

He took much to do with the Faculty and was one of those responsible for the passing of the 1850 Act which gave the Faculty parity with the Scottish Colleges and discontinued the Widows' Fund contributions. When the 1858 Medical Act was passed and the General Medical Council came into existence, James Watson was the first Faculty representative on the Council. Fleming took over from Watson in 1862 and remained the Faculty's representative until 1878, the year before he died. He is also recorded as saying that the best thing he ever did for the Faculty was his 'discovery of Duncan' (*q.v.*).

For 35 years Fleming was the chief medical adviser of the Scottish Amicable Life Assurance Society whose head office was in Glasgow, and in 1870 he published his main literary work, *The Medical Statistics of Life Assurance.*

When his first term of office as a surgeon in the Royal Infirmary expired in 1850 he was appointed a Manager of the Infirmary and it was as such that he made his greatest contributions to Glasgow medical history. From the first he campaigned against the limited terms of appointments of a physician or a surgeon and more particularly the period of ineligibility which followed. This interrupted continuity of patient care, the pursuit of clinical research, and often led talented men to seek employment elsewhere. It took a long time but the necessary changes were finally made.

It has already been noted that the University move to Gilmorehill, taking with it the professors in the Faculty of Medicine to the Western Infirmary, would have destroyed the Royal Infirmary as a clinical teaching hospital. It was John Gibson Fleming who persuaded the Managers to set up a committee of which he was made chairman to see that this did not happen. They 'memorialized' Her Majesty Queen Victoria to amend their original charter of 1791 so that the managers might 'afford facilities and accommodation to individual teachers for instructing students in medicine, surgery and the collateral sciences usually comprehended in a medical education, in addition to encouraging the clinical instruction of students as hitherto'. The Queen gave her gracious consent, the Managers cooperated to the full and sufficient accommodation and equipment was available by November 1876 to open THE GLASGOW ROYAL INFIRMARY SCHOOL OF MEDICINE.

John Gibson Fleming gave the inaugural address and until his death superintended the development of the school. Although the accommodation first provided was barely adequate, the school increased in numbers, the managers appealed to the public for funds and donations were soon received sufficient to justify 'the erection of buildings worthy of the hospital and the city', according to the *Glasgow Herald* of 1st November 1882. The Editorial goes on to describe the new lecture rooms and laboratories for anatomy, physiology, forensic medicine, chemistry and surgery. The anatomy lecture room could seat 150 students and one of the features of the School was a students' room where they might 'smoke, read or chat'. It was a pity that J. G. Fleming did not live to see the birth of the offspring with whose conception and gestation he had so much to do.

John Gibson Fleming was President of the Faculty of Physicians and Surgeons of Glasgow from 1865 to 1868 and again from 1870 to 1872.

The Royal Infirmary School of Medicine in 1889 was converted by licence of the Board of Trade into an incorporated college known as St Mungo's College and now comprised a complete medical faculty with professors and all necessary accommodation and equipment for a medical course. At this time there were in the Western Infirmary two Chairs in both Surgery and Medicine: the Regius Chairs and the Chairs of Clinical Surgery and Clinical Medicine. In 1911, the clinical professorships were renamed the St Mungo Chair in Surgery and the Muirhead Chair in Medicine and transferred to the Royal Infirmary where their patronage was vested in 11 curators, chosen jointly by the University Court, the Managers of the Royal Infirmary and the Governors of St Mungo's College.

After the 1914-1918 War the numbers at St Mungo's and Anderson's Colleges diminished and they were used mainly by those who for one reason or another could not get places in University schools; in the 1930s, for example, many were American Jews denied admission to many American medical schools. Both Colleges were wound up in 1947 when all undergraduate medical teaching became the direct charge of the University.

Throughout their existence the Faculty was directly and indirectly involved with the extra-mural schools. In the early days at least all teachers had to be Faculty members; as a licensing body they had to supervise closely the courses of lectures and other teaching provided and they had representatives on the Boards of Management of the Royal and Western Infirmaries.

The Faculty's litigation with the University in the early 19th century over its licensing powers has already been described. After the Medical Act of 1858 there were changes: the Faculty and the Royal College of Surgeons of Edinburgh had each the right to license in surgery. At the same time each body could combine with the Royal College of Physicians of Edinburgh to give the so-called Double Qualification which, when registered, permitted its holder to practise all branches of medicine in every part of Her Majesty's dominions. This arrangement was tidied in 1884 when the three bodies joined to produce the Triple Qualification which was for many years an honourable alternative to the Universities' MB,ChB. Although the extra-mural schools have long been abolished, the Triple Qualification still exists and may be taken by examinations today. It is almost entirely used to allow overseas medical graduates to obtain a registrable qualification to practise in the UK or its directly controlled territories.

# 12

# JOSEPH LISTER (1827 to 1912) AND THE RAPID GROWTH OF SURGERY IN THE SECOND HALF OF THE 19TH CENTURY

*Lister's Sceptics:*
James Morton (1820 to 1889)
John Reid (1809 to 1881)

*Lister's Disciples:*
William Macewen (1848 to 1924)
Hector Clare Cameron (1843 to 1929)

Enough has already been written to show that, for over two centuries, surgeons in the Faculty belonged to a caste inferior to that of physicians, but the divide between the two was already narrowing in 1820 when the Faculty agreed that a surgeon, or at least a non-pure physician, could become its President. But the amount of surgery, excluding such minor procedures as venesectomy, which was carried out in Glasgow at that time was not great. Moses Buchanan, who published the first history of Glasgow Royal Infirmary in 1832, listed a total of 2,189 operations performed since surgery began there in 1795; in other words about 60 per annum.

The reason was obvious; Buchanan himself warned his students about the difference between the class of operative surgery on the dead, 'where all is smooth, all natural, and most easily dissected', and 'the amphitheatre of this Hospital . . . where all is agitation, and the parts about to be the subject of operation, are, it may be, confounded, displaced, and imperfectly seen through the surrounding disease—all the frame of the unfortunate and sensitive sufferer is unsteady,—and cries, which would melt the most obdurate, too often pierce the heart, and unnerve the hand, of the most skilful and determined'.

The range of surgical operations available, however, was much more extensive than commonly thought. In 1844, just before the introduction of general anaesthesia put an end to much of the pain and terror of an operation, Joseph Pancoast published his book on *Operative Surgery* which runs to 650 pages of finely detailed and beautifully illustrated surgical procedures.

Most ablative types of operation and some reconstructive procedures had been carried out, but the body cavities were usually regarded as inviolable although there had been the rare success. When Ephraim McDowell in Kentucky in 1809 incised Mrs Crawford's belly to remove her ovarian tumour, her intestines immediately spilled out on the table and lay there for 25 minutes while he removed 15 pounds of gelatinous material from her cyst. She survived and outlived McDowell for several years. The ignorant have claimed this as the first successful ovariotomy, but Dr Robert Houston, a member of the Glasgow Faculty, had also been successful more than a century earlier in 1701 when he removed an even larger mass from Mrs Millar 'in the shire of Renfrew ten miles from Glasgow, North Britain'. He was luckier than McDowell, for his incision passed straight into the tumour and he had no trouble with extruded gut. After twisting a stick in the glutinous contents he removed '2 yards' of them followed by '9 quarts'. Mrs Millar survived for 13 years.

But these were rarities to be recorded and remembered. Until the painful horrors of surgical operations could be abolished little further progress was feasible. Chemistry had advanced far during the century after Joseph Black and it was inevitable that some would sniff the new substances and note their effects; thus, in the 1840s, nitrous oxide, ether and chloroform came into use to produce insensitivity during operations. Immediately the number of operations increased, but so did the mortality. J. Y. Simpson, writing after he had introduced chloroform to a grateful profession, was well aware of the paradox: 'a man laid on the operating table in one of our surgical hospitals is exposed to more chances of death than the English soldier on the field of Waterloo'. A plethora of pathogens potentiated by plentiful *passages* through patient after patient, packed into overcrowded wards, produced every possible wound infection. The appearance of pus was 'laudable' because it indicated resistance and a chance of the patient's survival. Surgery had taken a major step forward, but infection had to be controlled before real advances could be made. Lister and Macewen, who showed how wound infection could be reduced to an acceptable level, both carried out their initial clinical research in Glasgow Royal Infirmary.

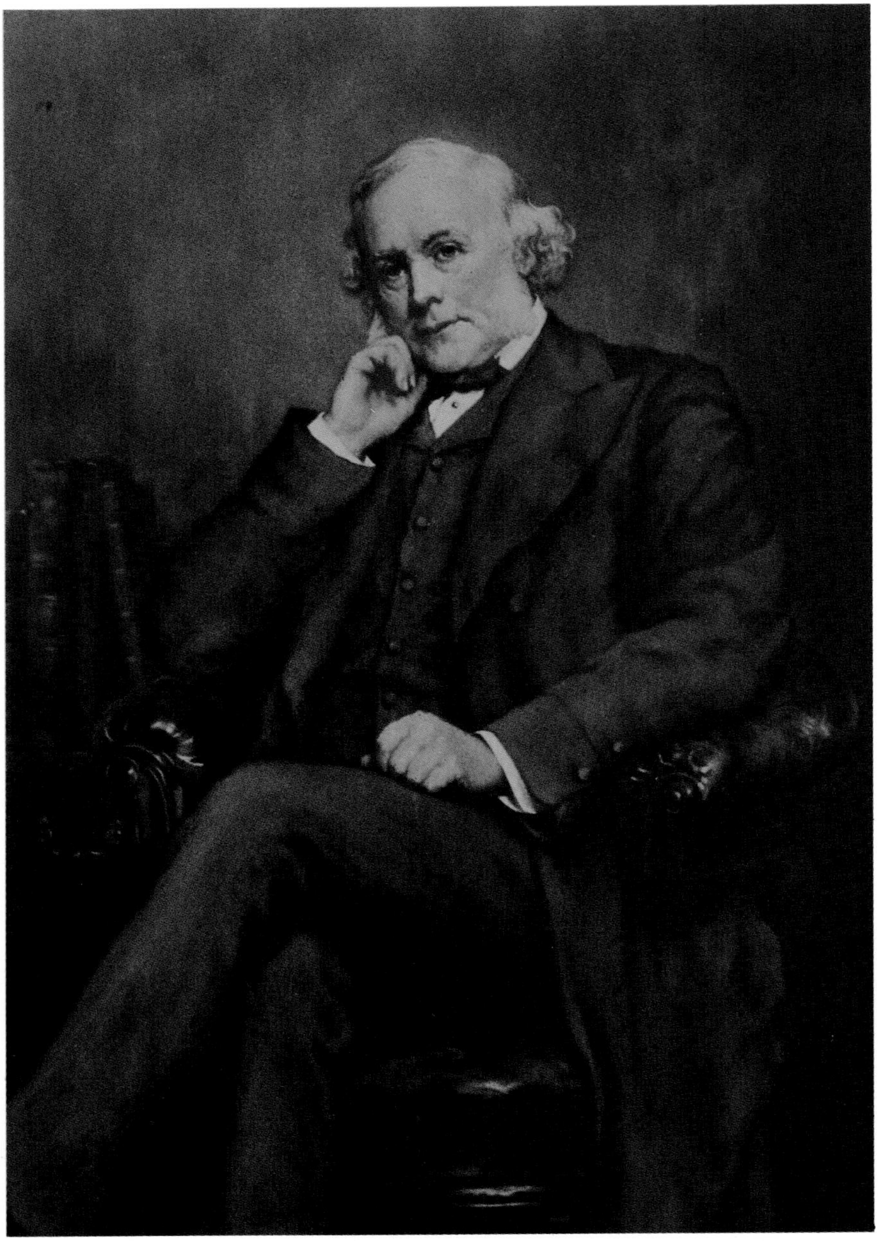

*Joseph Lister (1827 to 1912).*
*Mezzotint by T. Hamilton Crawford after W. W. Ouless, R.A.*

# JOSEPH, BARON LISTER

1827 to 1912

*The College has two copies of an 'Original etching of Lord Lister by Wilfred C. Appleby'; one was presented to the Royal Faculty about 1951 by the late Dr T. J. Honeyman, the other appears to have been purchased by the Royal Faculty. There is also a 'Mezzotint in colour by T. Hamilton Crawford after W. W. Ouless, R.A.'.*

Joseph Lister was born in 1827 at Plaistow, then a village some five miles from central London. He was the second son of four children in a prosperous middle class Quaker family and attended the Quaker School at Tottenham. Oxford and Cambridge were closed to him because of his religion and in 1844 he went instead to University College in London which was known as the 'godless' college since it accepted denominations other than the Church of England. He studied Arts for three years and graduated BA in 1847, but seems to have had a nervous breakdown and been unhappy until he took up medicine, again at London University, where he graduated MB in 1853. He went to Edinburgh shortly afterwards to spend a month of postgraduate study with James Syme, the Professor of Clinical Surgery; he stayed there for seven years. At first he was only a 'supernumerary clerk', but so impressed Syme that he soon became Syme's resident house surgeon and was supported by Syme when he applied successfully for the post of Lecturer in Surgery in the Royal College of Surgeons of Edinburgh in 1855. Next year he became an Assistant Surgeon in Edinburgh Royal Infirmary and also married Agnes, Professor Syme's daughter, who although childless was a constant help and companion throughout his career.

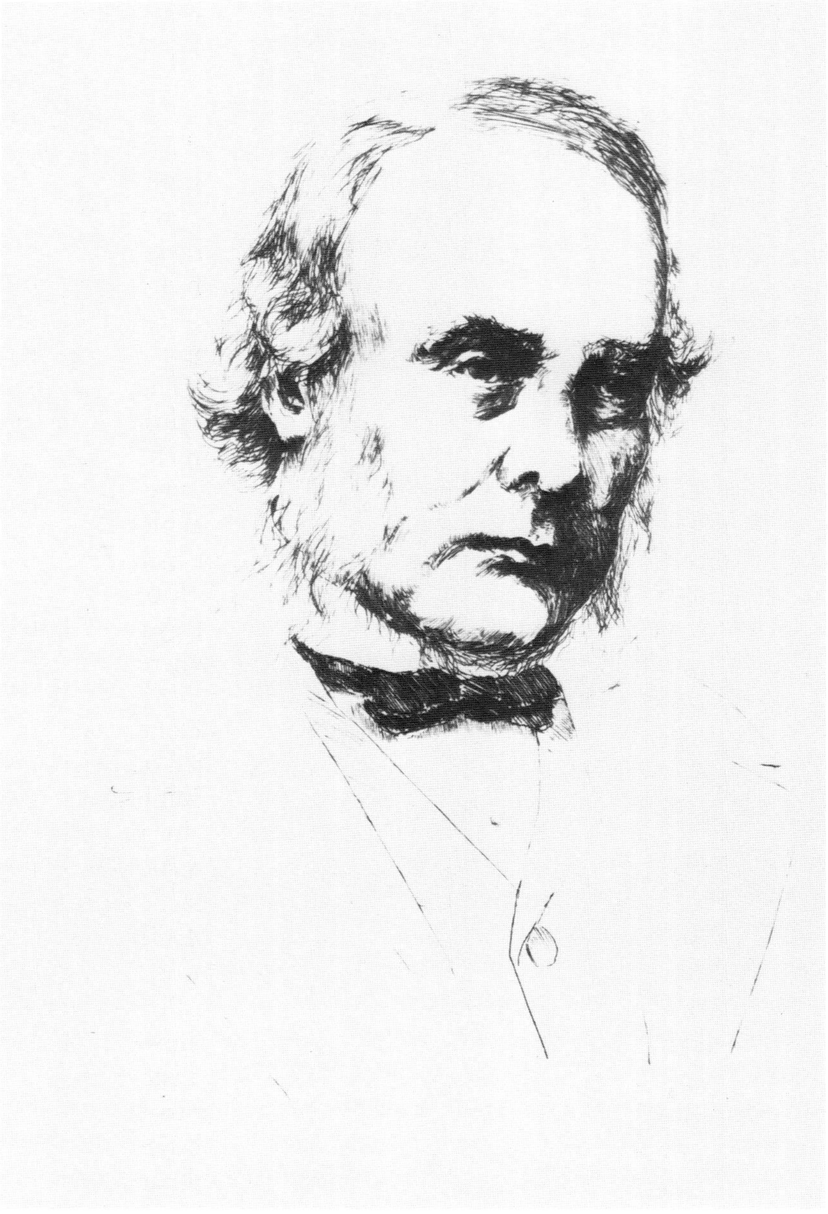

*Joseph Lister (1827 to 1912).*
*Etching by Wilfred C. Appleby.*

Lister's father was an enthusiastic amateur microscopist and young Lister acquired an early liking for the instrument. He studied the phenomenon of inflammation as it occurred in the foot web of a frog caught in Duddingston Loch and began his surgery course with a lecture on inflammation, a practice still common today in surgery and pathology.

A Regius Chair of Surgery had been established in Glasgow University in 1815; the first incumbent was John Burns and he was succeeded on his death in 1850 by James Adair Lawrie who in turn died in 1859. There were seven applicants for the vacancy and Lister was chosen; he took up the post early in 1860. Glasgow was still expanding with a population now close to half a million and the scope for surgery was greater than in Edinburgh; Lister in fact seems to have been the first surgeon in Glasgow to limit his practice solely to surgery.

It is doubtful if Lister's stay in Glasgow was altogether happy. To begin with he had no beds, since none then went automatically with the Chair. These had to be applied for when a vacancy arose in the Royal Infirmary. Lister was unsuccessful on his first application and over a year elapsed before he was appointed in charge of Wards 24 and 25; even then the tenure was for a maximum of 10 years, when he must leave the hospital for at least a year. The wards were in the new surgical block and Ward 24, his male accident ward, was on the ground floor built over a pit containing thousands of bodies from the cholera epidemic of 1848 with no great depth of soil to cover them. There were tales of rat infestations and the death rate from pyaemia, erysipelas and hospital gangrene was appalling, perhaps no worse than elsewhere, but still distressing to the young surgeon.

Although the Regius Chair of Surgery in Glasgow was one of the best Chairs in the country, Lister's discontent is shown by the fact that he applied on three occasions for posts elsewhere. He failed to obtain the Chair of Surgery in Edinburgh in 1864, or the Chair at University College in 1866, but his final application for the Chair of Clinical Surgery in Edinburgh, vacated by the ailing James Syme, was successful in 1869.

But there were compensations in Glasgow, such as his friendships with men like William Tennant Gairdner (later knighted) the Professor of Medicine, Allen Thomson the Professor of Anatomy, and William Thomson (later Lord Kelvin) Professor of Physics. It was another of his friends, Thomas Anderson the Professor of Chemistry, who drew Lister's attention to Pasteur and his work which showed that fermentation was due to tiny living organisms. The association in Lister's fertile mind of fermentation with putrefaction and the sepsis of wounds led to his use in wounds of carbolic acid which was known to prevent putrefaction in substances of animal origin. His first attempt was a failure but his success with the second patient, the 11 year old boy James Greenlees, who had a compound fracture of his tibia, is a medical historical milestone. On the day of the accident, the 12th of August 1865, pure carbolic acid on a piece of calico was applied to all parts of the wound, the wound itself was covered with two overlapping layers of lint soaked in undiluted acid and the lint in turn was covered with a sheet of thin tin fixed by strips of plaster. The wound cicatrised and healed; there

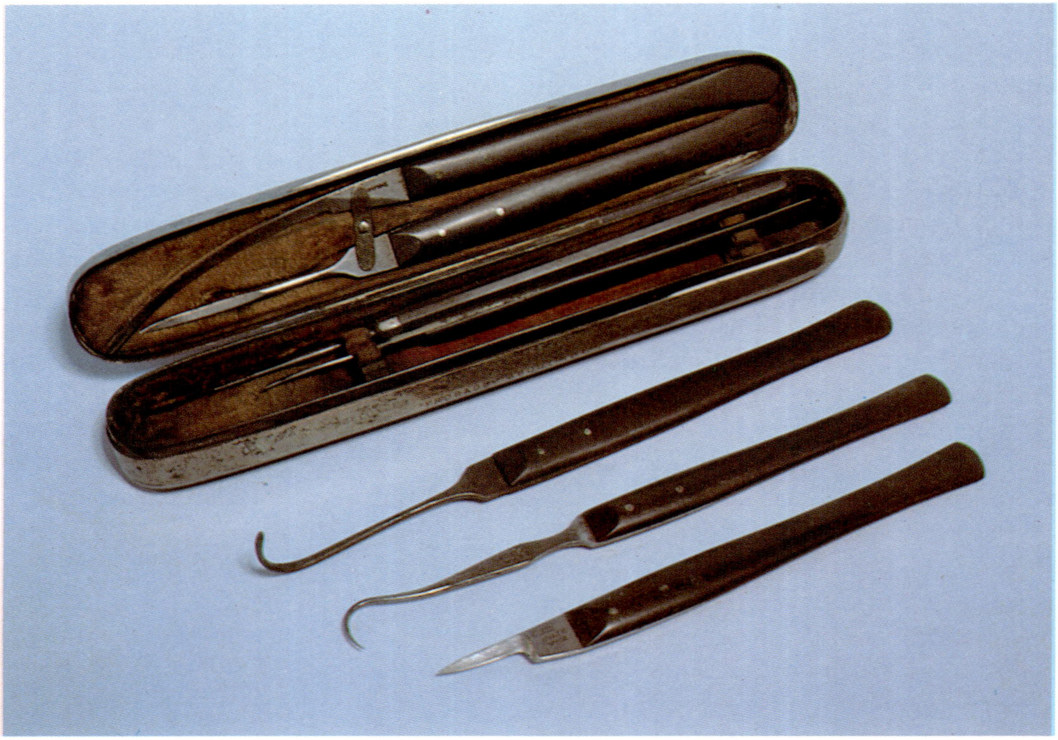

*A pocket case of lancets, bistouries, probes and hooks which belonged to Joseph Lister.*

was no infection, no gangrene and the often inevitable amputation was avoided. Ten more compound fractures were treated with only two mishaps; one developed hospital gangrene when Lister was away from home, the other died from haemorrhage caused by perforation of the femoral artery by a sharp fragment of bone some weeks after the injury. His results were first printed in the *Lancet* in 1867, and a series of papers followed. Their reception was mixed and varied from condemnation through tolerance to enthusiastic support. Their impact on Glasgow and the Faculty Fellows is dealt with in some detail below. But it was the same story in Edinburgh when he went there in 1869. The great Sir James Y. Simpson and James Syme were often in contention and it is not surprising that Simpson was anti-Lister. But Lister's second spell in Edinburgh became the busiest and happiest years of his professional life. Developing his antiseptic techniques, lecturing in the classroom and in the wards, gave him an international reputation and following. By 1877 when he accepted the invitation to take up the Chair of Clinical Surgery which had been created for him at King's College Hospital, his class

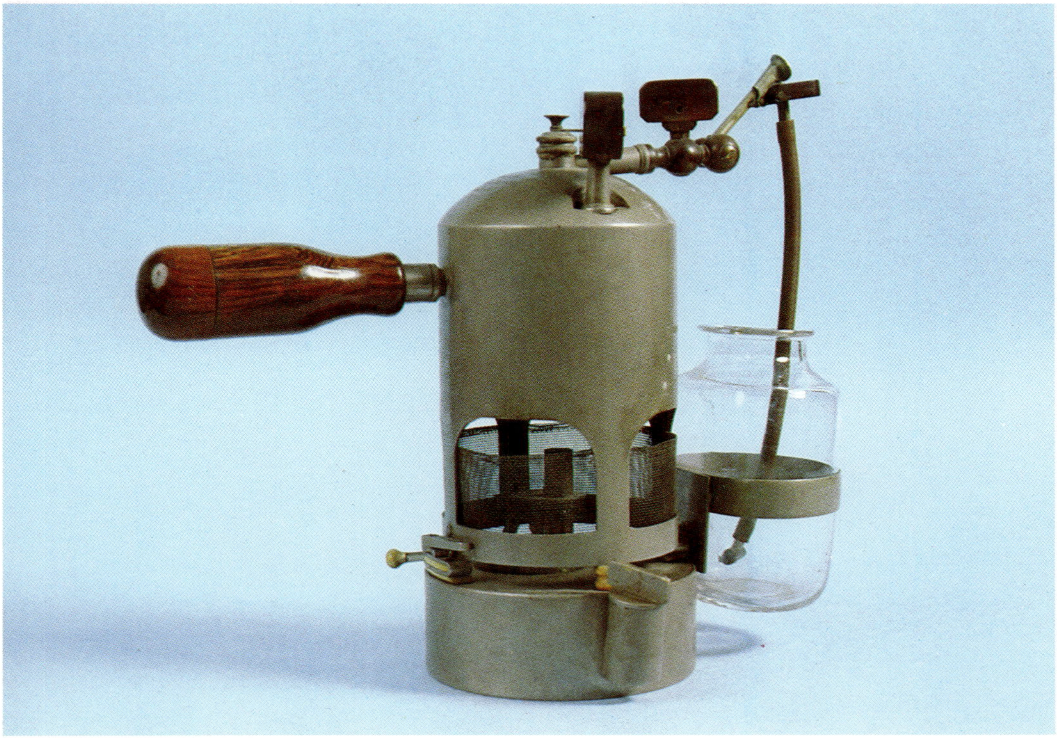

*Lister's carbolic acid spray. Water in the upper container was boiled by a spirit lamp in the lower and the steam produced was emitted across the tube leading to the bottle of carbolic acid. This was drawn up and mixed with the steam according to the Venturi principle.*

often numbered 400 students. London, however, gave him a chilly reception and he was fortunate at first if 20 turned up to hear him. But he lived not only to see his work universally acclaimed but to have honours showered upon him at home and abroad, including the Freedom of the City of Glasgow in 1908.

Several full biographies of Lord Lister are readily available and the data given above are only those most germane to his revolutionary work in Glasgow with carbolic acid and antisepsis. Most professions meet radical change with a varying degree of conservative inertia and Glasgow surgeons were no exception. To begin with Lister had many sceptics, but their voices were finally silenced as national and international acclaim increased. But there were also those who worked with Lister and saw the fundamental truth in his works and went on to develop much of surgery as we know it today.

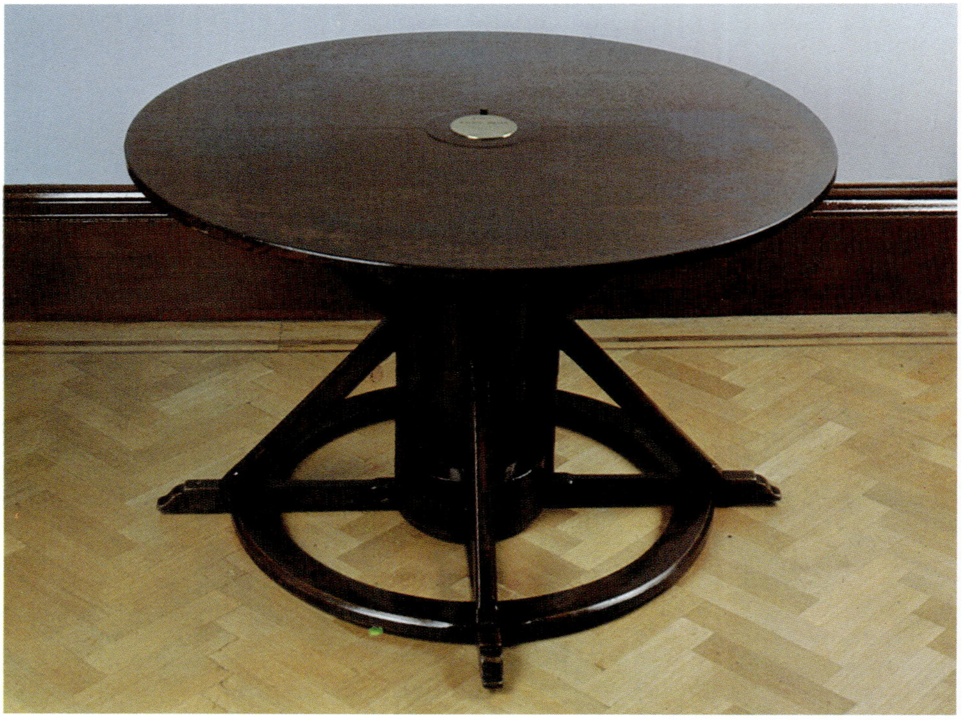

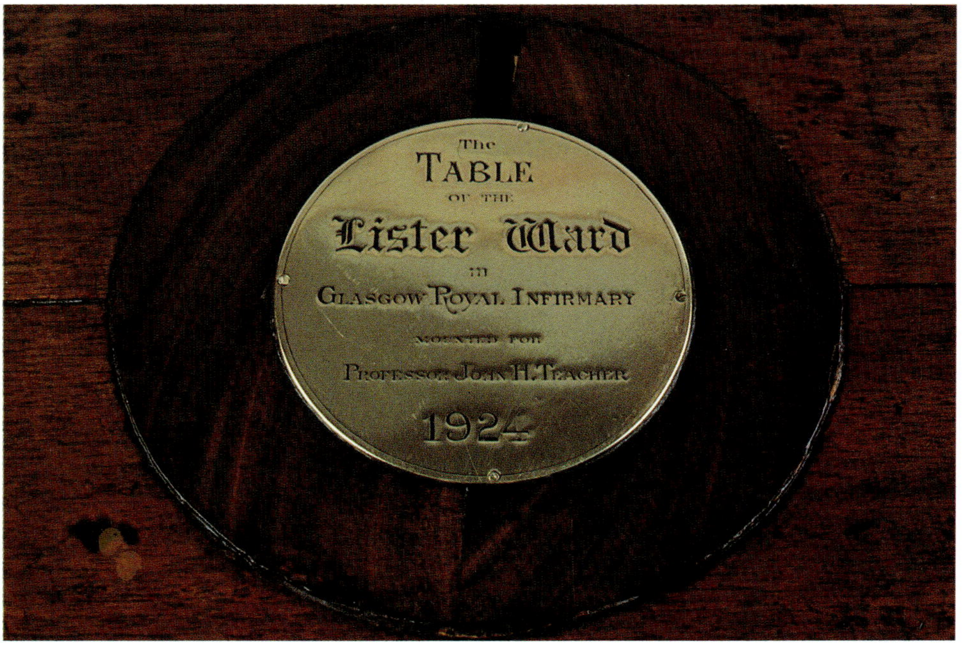
The
TABLE
OF THE
Lister Ward
IN
GLASGOW ROYAL INFIRMARY
MOUNTED FOR
PROFESSOR JOHN H. TEACHER
1924

*A table rescued from the Lister wards demolished in 1924. It was originally built around a pillar which ran through the central aperture.*

## *The Sceptics*

On 17th April 1868, Lister spoke to the Glasgow Medico-Chirurgical Society on 'the atmospheric germ theory of putrefaction'. Unfortunately his talk lasted nearly two hours and there was no time left for discussion. However, one month later Dr Ebenezer Watson (the son of Dr James Watson, the 'Father of the Faculty') gave a paper on 'The Theory of Suppuration and the use of Carbolic Acid Dressings'. He greatly doubted the germ theory of putrefaction and attributed the good effects of carbolic acid to coagulation of albumen and the production of a firm cover impervious to air. At least he admitted to some 'good effects'.

## *The Managers of the Royal Infirmary and Lister*

In the issues of the *Lancet* of 1st and 8th January 1870 there appeared a two-part article by Lister entitled 'On the Effects of the Antiseptic Treatment upon the Salubrity of a Surgical Hospital'. In order to show just how good was his antiseptic method, he described the insalubrious state of his wards in very strong terms and how his techniques had converted his wards 'from some of the most unhealthy in the kingdom into models of healthiness'. He tells of the cholera burials under the floor, and of the pits for pauper funerals in the neighbouring Cathedral grounds. His wards had not been cleaned for three years and were much overcrowded. 'I was engaged in a perpetual contest with the managing body who . . . were disposed to introduce additional beds beyond those contemplated in the original construction'.

Even more damnatory was: 'my patients suffered from the evils alluded to in a way that was sickening and often heartrending so as to make me sometimes feel it a questionable privilege to be connected with the institution'. The figures he gave in support were suggestive but not conclusive; comparing the death rates following amputations in a two year period before the antiseptic regime and a similar period during it, he found:

Pre-antiseptic period, 35 cases, 16 deaths;

During antiseptic period, 40 cases, 6 deaths.

However, taking other factors into account, they are certainly highly suggestive.

Obviously the Managers of the Glasgow Royal Infirmary could not ignore this attack, and a long letter to the *Lancet* from their Secretary, Henry Lamond, dated 18th January 1870, was published in the *Glasgow Herald*. The Managers refuted Lister's statements point by point. They quoted statistics of deaths following surgery to show that the Royal Infirmary was as good if not better than other similar hospitals. They strongly denied he was engaged in a perpetual contest with them about overcrowding, and indeed he had treated in his ward fewer cases than a colleague in a neighbouring ward. The letter ends by saying that, while they have no intention of discussing antiseptic treatment, 'in their opinion, which is shared by those of their number belonging to the medical profession, the improved health and satisfactory condition of the hospital which has been as marked in the medical as in the surgical department, is mainly attributable to the better ventilation, the improved dietary and the excellent nursing, to which the directors have given so much attention of late years'.

An editorial accompanied this letter and underlined most of the points, stating again that while they did not pretend to judge the merits of antiseptic treatment 'Professor Lister . . . has laid himself open to a crushing reply from his opponents'.

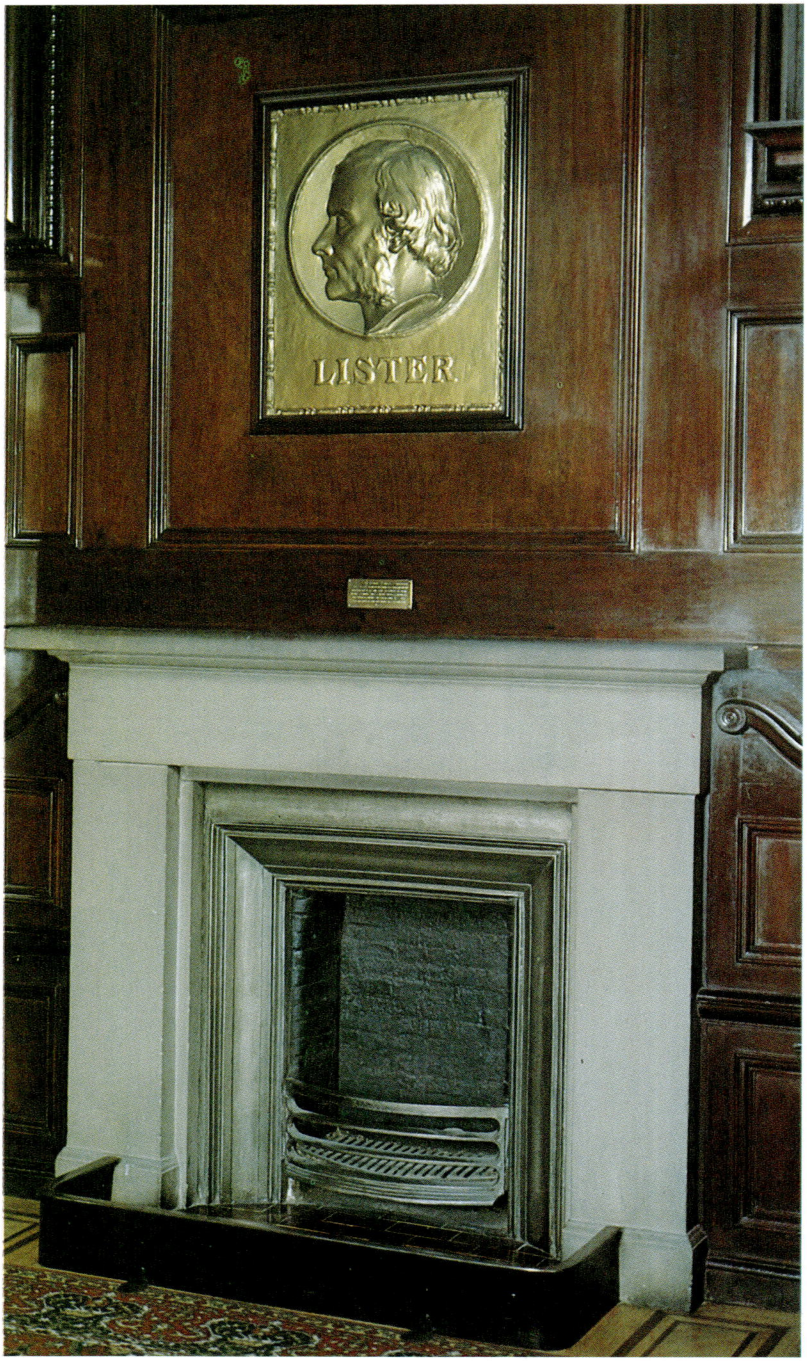


*A fireplace from Lister's wards and a copy of the plaque which hangs in Glasgow Royal Infirmary which are now built into the Council or Lister Room.*

Lister was now safe in Edinburgh but memory of his unnecessary attack lingered long in the Royal Infirmary in Glasgow. In 1924, in spite of world-wide protests, the Managers demolished Lister's wards in the Glasgow Royal Infirmary. *Post hoc, ergo propter hoc?* Who can say.

The subjects of two of our portraits were sceptical of Lister's ideas. James Morton treated them seriously and carried out a 'comparative' trial; John Reid held them up to ridicule.

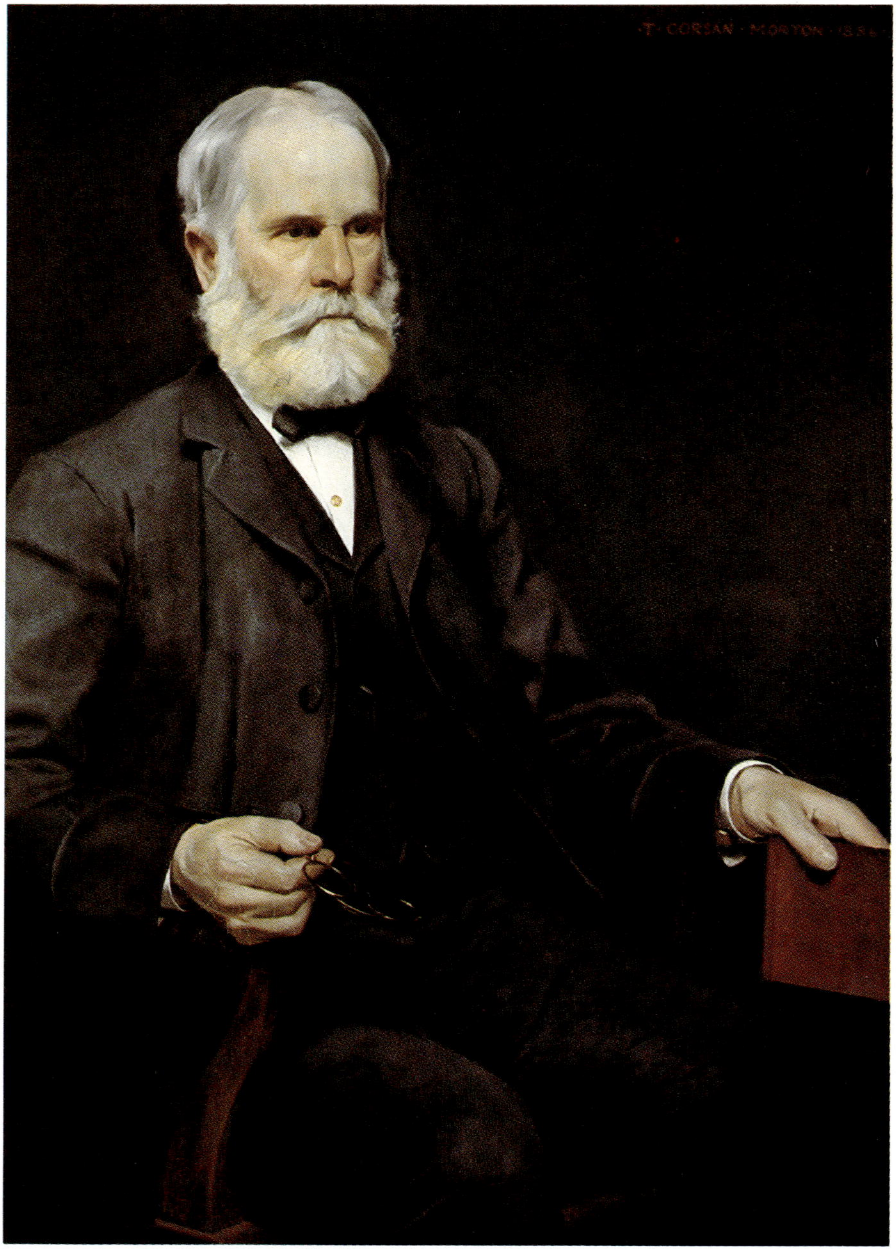


*James Morton (1820 to 1889) was a surgical contemporary of Joseph Lister in Glasgow Royal Infirmary who tried to evaluate the use of carbolic acid in wounds but found no significant advantage.*
*President, 1886 to 1889.*

# JAMES MORTON

1820 to 1889

*The portrait was painted by James Morton's son, T. Corsan Morton.*

James Morton was born at Ochiltree in Ayrshire apparently into a poor family. Little is recorded of his early days but he was largely self-educated and the monies for his medical education he earned with his own hands. He entered the medical school of Anderson's University when he was about 21 and in 1844 was admitted a Licentiate of the Royal College of Surgeons of Edinburgh. He obtained his MD in 1845 from the University of St Andrews. Thereafter he settled in Glasgow, became a Fellow of the Faculty of Physicians and Surgeons of Glasgow in 1851, and Professor of Materia Medica in Anderson's University in 1855. His teaching was interesting and popular with his students and he continued in the Chair until 1888.

In 1859, at about the same time as Lister came to Glasgow, Morton was appointed Surgeon to the Royal Infirmary and, except for an obligatory break of two years, continued in this post until 1885. He was thus working in the New Surgical Block at the same time as Lister was pursuing his studies there with carbolic acid. Morton, however, believed that the premises on which these were based were wrong and carried out what he called a comparative study to try to arrive at a true value of carbolic acid in wounds.

His paper, which he had read to the Glasgow Medico-Chirurgical Society in October 1869, appeared the following year in three weekly parts in the *Lancet* one month after the paper of Lister which so upset the Royal Infirmary Managers. Morton starts by saying that Pasteur's theory of germs or spores in the air has not been satisfactorily established and ridicules the idea that 'the air is always full of these vicious agents or materials'. In any case putting antiseptics into wounds is no new idea; the Good Samaritan poured in oil and wine.

His 'comparative' study consisted in treating open wounds in one of five ways:

Carbolic acid in oil or carbolic acid putty;

Pure oil (presumably olive);

Putty without carbolic acid;

Lint alone;

Water as wet dressings or by irrigation.

He does not say how many patients were treated but describes seven 'illustrative' cases in detail and concludes 'that carbolic acid was certainly not superior and barely equal to some of the other antiseptics in common use'.

Perhaps Morton was later convinced, but he makes no mention of it in his major work *The Treatment of Spina Bifida by a New Method* which was published in London in 1877. He started treating cases of closed meningocoeles in 1871 by injecting them with a solution of iodine and potassium iodide in glycerine. His results were impressive, the method was taken up by others, and a second edition of his book apeared in 1887 in which 71 cases are described, more than half of which were contributed by other surgeons throughout Britain. A Special Committee of the Clinical Society of London endorsed his method as the best and only method they felt justified in recommending.

Glasgow University conferred upon him the LLD in 1888.

James Morton was President of the Faculty of Physicians and Surgeons of Glasgow from 1886 to 1889.

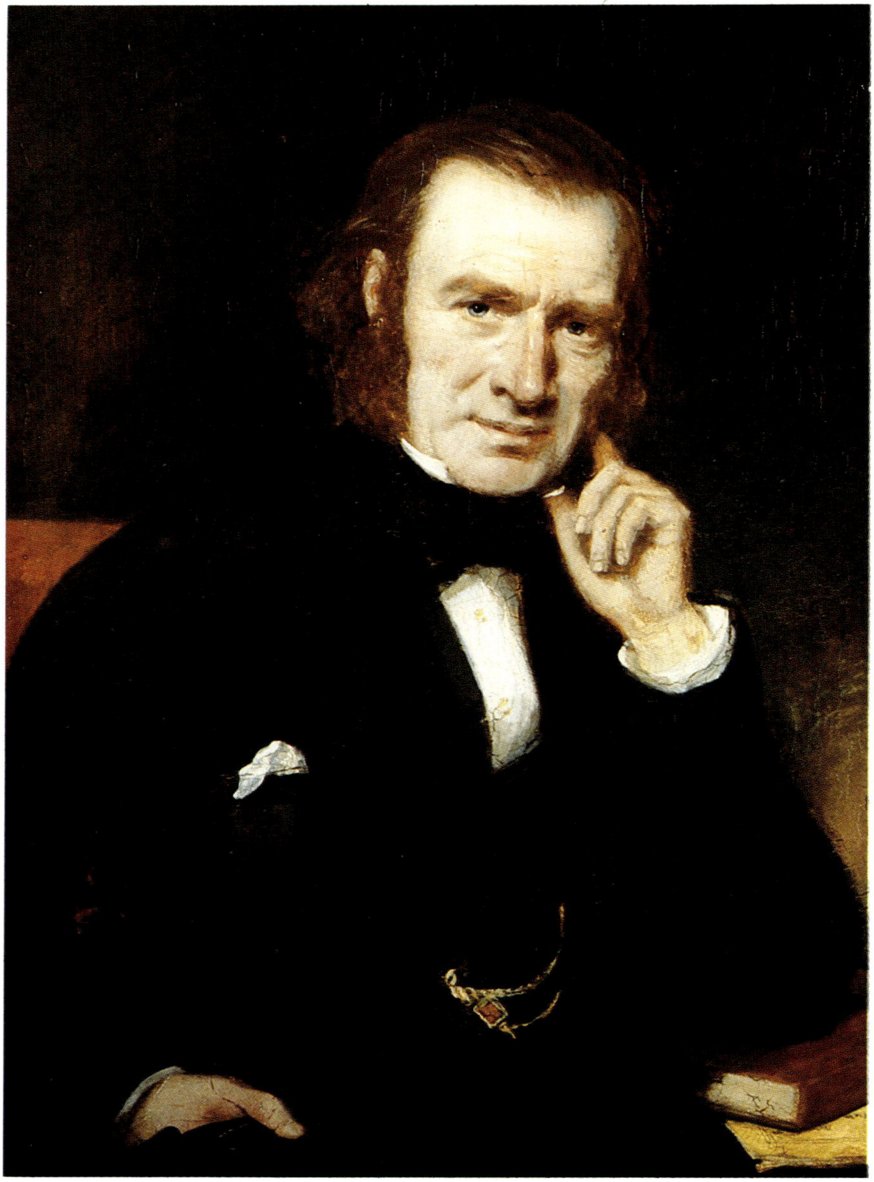

*John Reid (1809 to 1881) was never more than a Licentiate of the Faculty and is best known for two literary works:* The Philosophy of Death, *a treatise on the causes and incidence of mortality in the early 19th century, and his resurrection of the* Medical Examiner, *a journal which had perished 37 years before and which he used for his reactionary iconoclastic views. The portrait is unsigned but is in the style of Sir Daniel Macnee.*

# JOHN REID

1809 to 1881

*The portrait was found in the basement in 1979. It was in poor condition and although it bore neither the name of the subject nor that of the painter, it was decided to have it cleaned and restored by Mr Ian McClure. It then became possible to read the words 'The Philosophy of Death' on the spine of the book on which the left elbow was resting. Thereafter the subject was readily identified but no artist's signature emerged; it is of the style and period of Sir Daniel Macnee and one other College portrait, that of Perry and known to be by Macnee, is also unsigned.*

John Reid was born to a cabinet-maker and his wife in Hutchesonstown in Glasgow. Although he was first apprenticed to his father's trade, he began the study of medicine when he was 19 by enrolling in the class of Anatomy run by Dr William Thomson in the Anatomical Theatre in College Street. The Irish porter there also performed the duty of 'resurrectionist', and Reid described years later how he had outwitted the Sheriff's officers by concealing a corpse recently acquired by the porter in a secret recess behind a window shutter during one of their raids. Reid subsequently attended courses at Glasgow University and at Portland Street School, a voluntary association of medical teachers which was in existence from 1828 to 1844, and qualified by becoming a 'licenciate' of the Faculty in 1833.

The grade of 'licenciate' was first introduced in 1785 for country members. The Faculty permitted at that time only 'indwellers in Glasgow' to have any share in their government and the country members had jibbed at paying the full fees. By 1811 the

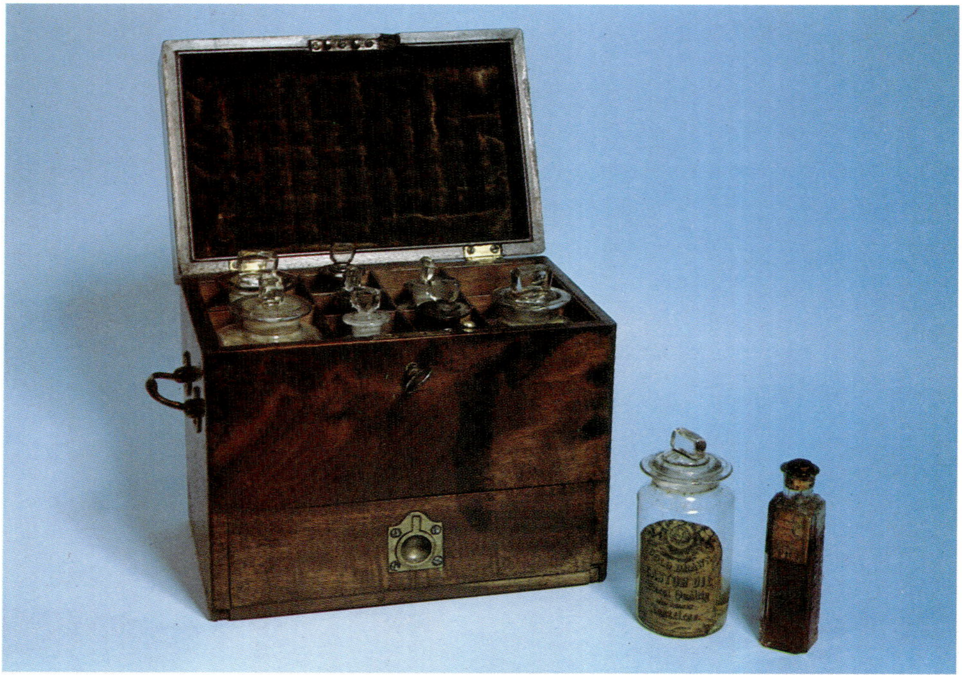

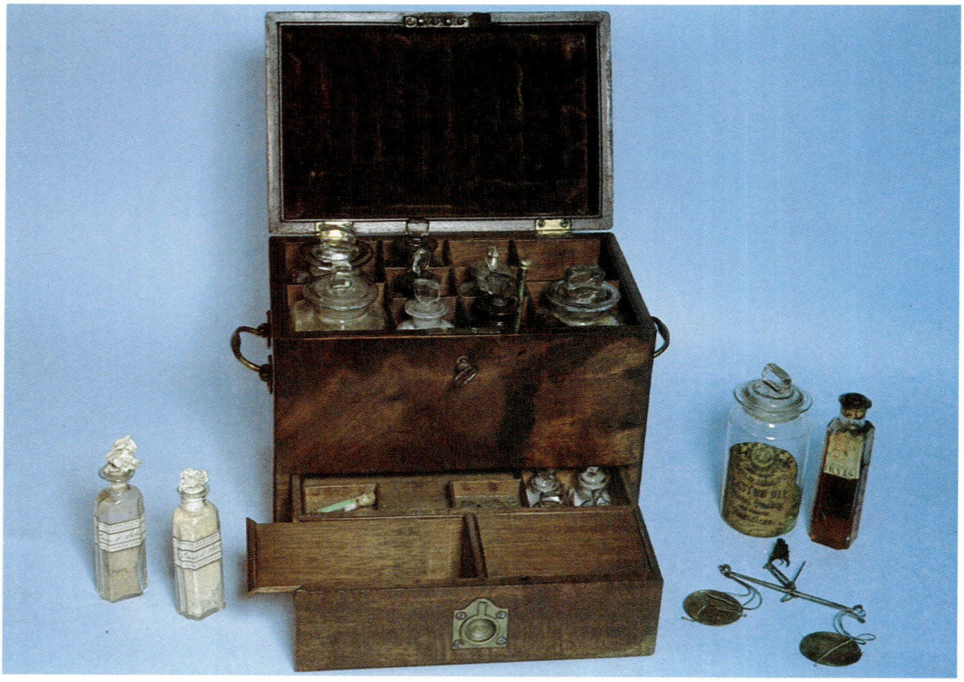

*A typical 19th century country practitioner's medicine case. It contained not only the essential available medicaments but also the necessary scales and weights.*

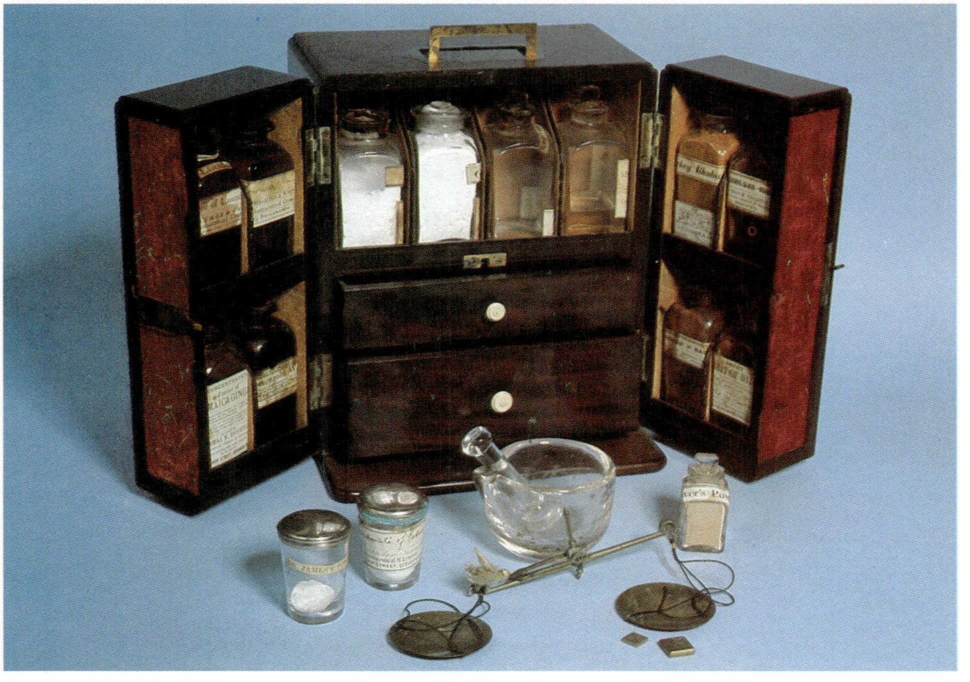

*A differently designed medicine case with its own pestle and mortar, scales and weights and drugs.*

qualification had been extended also to Glasgow practitioners who did not wish to pay the ever-rising fees for full membership. It allowed them freedom to practise but little else. The first volume of the *Glasgow Medical Examiner*, edited by J. P. Glen in 1831 and 1832, campaigned strongly against the degree. 'Licentiates are a species of members who have nothing to do with the Faculty laws but to obey them . . . a species of serfs who, upon payment of a certain tribute, are permitted to exist'. The licentiate grade disappeared with the later Medical Acts but it was enough for David Livingstone and many others including John Reid who never became a full member and always wrote 'Licentiate of the Faculty of Physicians and Surgeons of Glasgow' after his name.

John Reid spent the first 12 years of his professional life as a general practitioner in the Fifeshire village of Markinch, and it was here that he wrote *The Philosophy of Death* which was published in 1841. The word 'Philosophy' is used in its older connotation as in 'natural philosophy', and not its more modern sense as in 'moral philosophy'. Indeed the book is subtitled 'A General Medical and Statistical Treatise on the Nature and Causes of Human Mortality' and contains many interesting statistics of mortality particularly in Glasgow. In one way it resembles his later work in the *Glasgow Medical Examiner* by its use as a vehicle for criticising others. Here the main target is Malthus and his belief in 'the constant tendency in all animal life to increase beyond the nourishment prepared for it'. His criticisms are lengthy and often specious, but he concludes nevertheless that the 'fears of Mr. Malthus are mere chimeras of imagination founded on premises which have no general existence'. John Reid had difficulty in accepting new ideas.

He returned to Glasgow in 1845 where he spent the rest of his life as a general practitioner. The Glasgow Medico-Chirurgical Society was founded in 1844, Reid joined it in 1846 and was always one of its more devoted and loyal members.

For some strange reason, in 1869 Reid resuscitated the *Glasgow Medical Examiner*, a periodical which had perished as a one year old infant 37 years previously. This issue he called Volume II and it appeared irregularly until 1871 when it too expired. It was known as 'The Mustard Plaster', not only because of its yellow cover but for its often pungent contents. Reid's comments in it on specialisation are noted elsewhere; here we are concerned about his views on Lister.

In most of the issues there are derogatory remarks about Lister and his antiseptic method. It is tempting to quote him again and again, but one sentence which he wrote at the end of his review of Lister's 1870 *Lancet* paper will suffice to show his style, his enmity to the new ideas and his frequent non-sequiturs:

> 'The whole theory and the inferences of its learned apostle [i.e. Lister] are such a jumble of *ipse dixit* egotistical jargon that only a following F.R.S. of the famous Sir Joseph Banks could have come up to it; but poor Sir Joseph was modest compared with plain Mr. Joseph for when he found that his experimental fleas did not become red upon boiling, he at once abandoned his theory and like a man merely said "... Fleas are not lobsters".'

But it was not just against the 'sporules' of Lister that he inveighed. On Lister's work with ligatures he writes, 'How Mr. Lister can make such a mountain of success out of a midge of results we cannot understand', and he wrote a seven-page article on the coagulation of the blood mainly to refute Lister's early theories of 1864.

He was undoubtedly, for his time, a good reliable doctor. Appended to the 'Biographical Sketch' which Dr Lindsay Steven wrote for the *Glasgow Medical Journal* in 1895, there are 31 glowing references from colleagues and patients which he used when applying for the post of Medical Referee to the United Kingdom Life Assurance Company in 1846. Even when the false eulogies of references are partly discounted, he was still a well respected man.

He continued to attend the meetings of the Glasgow Medico-Chirurgical Society but as he aged he became more and more garrulous so that the Society invested in a clock which chimed every 10 minutes. After his death his sister (he never married) founded the John Reid Prize of £25 which was open to all medical students in the University.

John Reid never held office in the Faculty; his main connection with it seems to have been through the Glasgow Medico-Chirurgical Society.

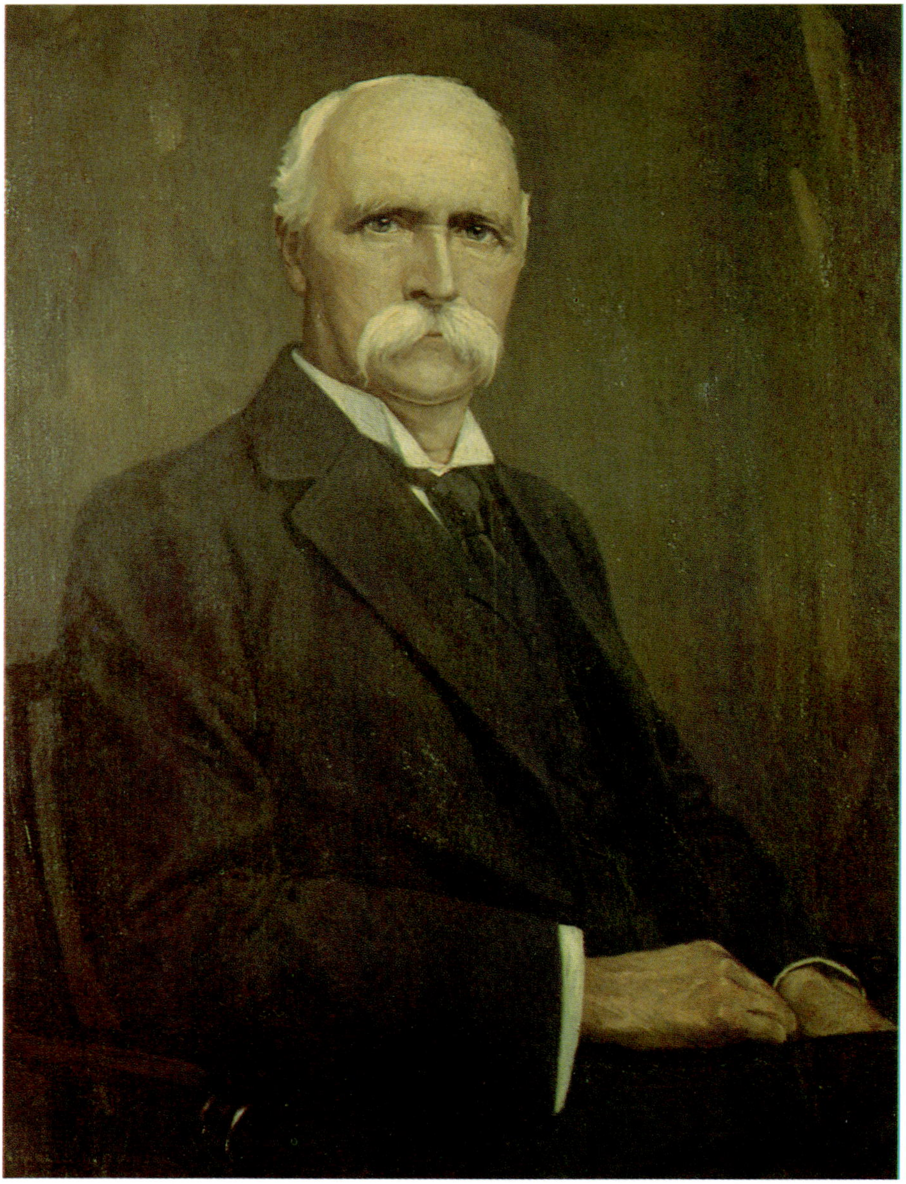

*Sir William Macewen (1848 to 1924) was one of the greatest innovative surgeons, when the discoveries of antisepsis and anaesthesia made so much possible for the first time. His international reputation was immense and he was feted wherever he travelled in Europe, North America or Australia. At home he remained strangely aloof from his colleagues.*

*He became an Honorary Fellow of the Faculty in 1913.*

*The Disciples*

Many who at first doubted Lister's work, or even scoffed at it, would boast in later years of having been his 'dresser' or even of having taken his lectures. Macewen and Cameron were devotees from the outset and surgery was immeasurably enhanced thereby.

## WILLIAM MACEWEN, KCB

1848 to 1924

*The portrait was painted posthumously; the following extract from the Royal Faculty minutes of 6th October 1924 explains:*

*'Dr. Freeland Fergus presented to the Faculty a portrait of the late Sir William Macewen. He explained that Sir William Macewen had never given sittings to an artist although often asked to do so, and that just before he left on his Colonial tour, he had given his consent and, had he survived, the work no doubt would have been put into the hands of some artist of note.*

*'In these circumstances Dr. Fergus had given to Mr. Charles R. Dowell, a gentleman of whose draughtsmanship he entertained the highest opinion, a cabinet-sized photograph by Messrs. Annan of Glasgow with the request that he would do his best to evolve a likeness of Sir William. He had considered whether he should offer the portrait to the Royal College of Surgeons in London or to this Faculty, but it seemed to him that no body had such strong claims as the Faculty which had supported Sir William at several important junctures in his career.*

*'The Fellows present declared the portrait an excellent likeness and the President expressed the gratification of the Faculty at being presented with so interesting and valuable a Memorial of Sir William Macewen for which, on their behalf, he thanked Dr. Fergus most cordially and stated that after consultation with him it would be hung in a suitable position in the Faculty Hall.'*

In 1892 William Macewen applied for, and was appointed to, the Regius Professorship of Surgery in the University of Glasgow and this is the curriculum vitae he gave:

'I am forty-four years of age.

'I graduated in medicine at the University of Glasgow in 1870, and since then have devoted myself to the study of surgery.

'In 1876 I was appointed Surgeon to and Lecturer in Clinical Surgery at the Royal Infirmary, Glasgow, which appointments I have the honour of still holding. Last year on the expiry of the usual term of office in the infirmary, the managers as a "mark of their appreciation of the distinguished services rendered" reappointed me for a second term.

'In 1881 I was appointed Lecturer on Systematic Surgery in the Royal Infirmary School of Medicine which lectureship I held for eight years, and at the amalgamation of this school with St. Mungo's College I was appointed Professor of Clinical Surgery.

'In 1883, I was appointed Surgeon to the Royal Hospital for Sick Children, Glasgow to which institution I am still attached. In 1884 I was invited to prepare a paper on Osteotomy to be read at the International Medical Congress at Copenhagen. In 1888 a special invitation was given me to address the British Medical Association on my "Recent Surgical Investigations".

'In 1889 I was invited to accept the Professorship of Surgery in the Johns Hopkins University of Baltimore, where every facility was provided for scientific research.* In that year I was appointed President of the Medico-Chirurgical Society of Glasgow.

'In 1890 the honorary degree of Doctor of Laws was conferred upon me by the University of Glasgow. In the same year I gave the inaugural address to the Midland Medical Society at Birmingham.

'In 1891 I was elected a Corresponding Member of the *Societé de Chirurgerie de Paris*. In the same year I delivered the inaugural address to the Royal Medical Society of Edinburgh, of which I had previously been elected a member. Also in 1891 the students of the University of Glasgow elected me President of the Medical Society of their University.

'Since the amalgamation of the Conjoint Boards of the Royal College of Surgeons, Edinburgh, and the Faculty of Physicians and Surgeons, Glasgow, I have been an examiner in surgery and clinical surgery.'

He appended 'a few testimonials'. There were 16 in all: from England, 6, including Sir J. Spencer Wells, Bt. and Sir Joseph Lister, Bt.; from Germany, 5, including such names as Mikulicz and Von Esmarch; from the United States, 2; from France, 1; from

* Macewen was offered *carte blanche*: money, laboratories, equipment, beds, even his own assistants and nurses. He refused!

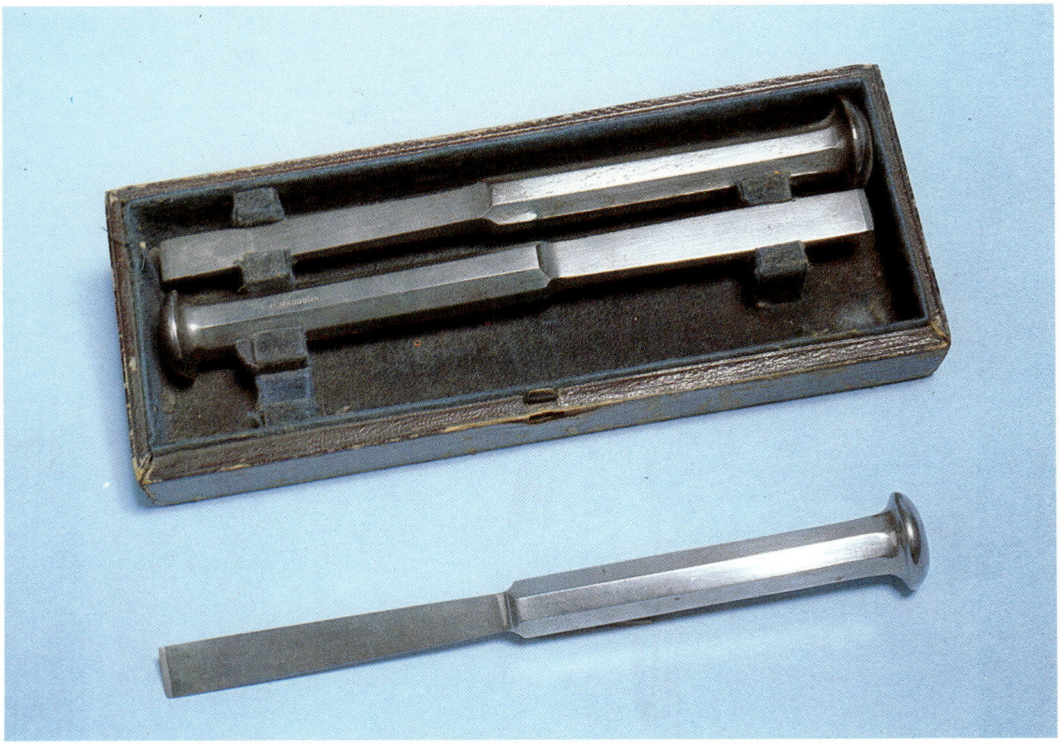

*Macewen's original osteotomes. The edge had to be sharp enough to pare one's nails!*

Scandinavia, 1; from Russia, 1. No colleague in Glasgow, indeed no one in Scotland, was mentioned.

This epitomises what Macewen had become and was to remain: a surgeon with an immense international reputation who treated his colleagues at home with disdain.

Macewen's international fame dated from his invited paper to the International Medical Congress in Copenhagen in 1884, 'Osteotomy for genu valgum'. He reported no less than 1,800 osteotomies without a single instance of pyaemia or other fatal wound infection. Since each operation produced a compound fracture, this work vindicated once and for all Lister's techniques. In a letter to Mrs Rebecca Strong, the Matron of Glasgow Royal Infirmary, Macewen wrote about the reception his paper received and how the German 'Hochs!' mingled strangely with the English cheers as he left the rostrum.

This was of course the era when anaesthesia and antisepsis opened up for any competent surgeon previously unexplorable paths of surgery. But Macewen towered over them all literally and figuratively. He was 6′ 2″ tall, slim and agile, with a good speaking voice and above all a 'presence'. His original works were manifold. His studies on the growth and transplantation of bone, the first excision of a lung, his pioneer explorations of the brain for abscesses and tumour and his many publications on diverse

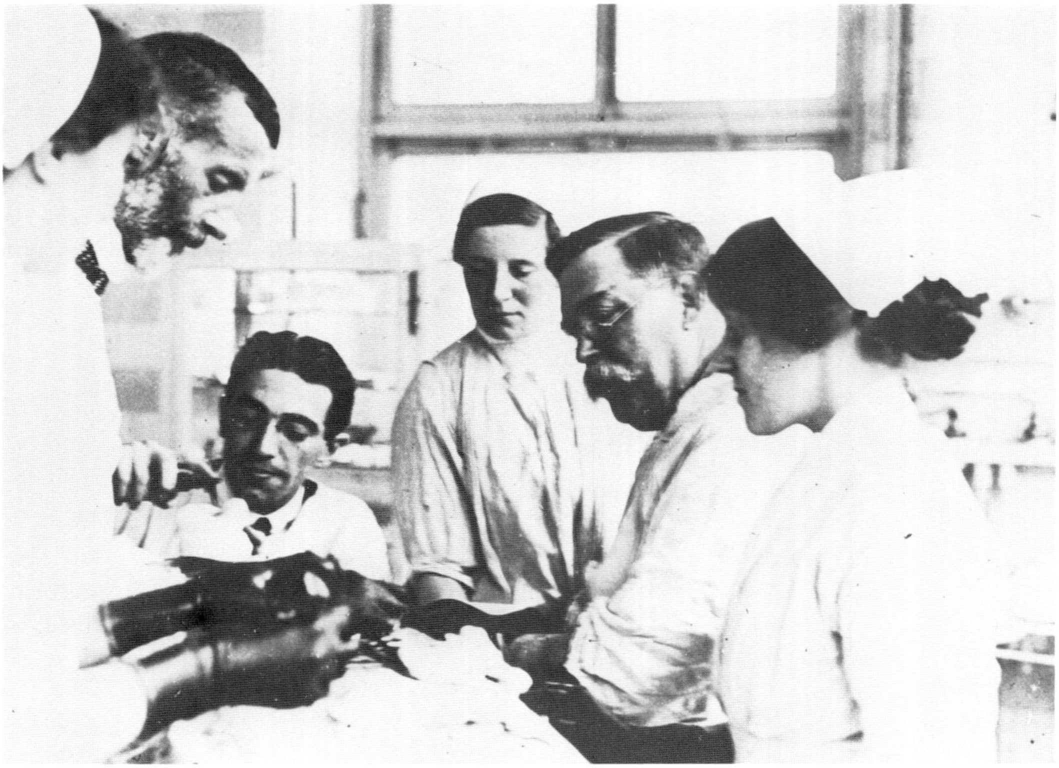

*Sir William Macewen operating in the Western Infirmary. Photograph taken probably in the first decade of the 20th century. His beard later became quite white and he finally shaved it off.*

aspects of surgery are well known. He helped Mrs Rebecca Strong, the Matron of the Glasgow Royal Infirmary, to found the first student nurses' training school in the world in 1892. As a Surgeon Rear-Admiral in the Great War he was called to look after 'Bertie', later King George VI, who had appendicitis, and his stay at Windsor led to his friendship with Princess Louise, Duchess of Argyll. This, in turn, led to the establishment of the Princess Louise Hospital for Limbless Soldiers and Sailors, beautifully situated on the shores of the River Clyde in Erskine House which had belonged to Princess Louise.

But he was anything but popular in the Western Infirmary. In his early period in the Royal Infirmary, he had been on good terms with the management who, recognising his worth, had acceded to many of his requests. The letters which he preserved from Mrs Strong showed a deep bond of sympathy between the matron and himself. But when he became Regius Professor all seemed to have changed. Since he was now based on Gilmorehill he should have beds for clinical teaching in the Western Infirmary. The managers, instead of making these immediately available, waited for

Macewen to apply for them—in order, it is thought, to make certain conditions to keep this ambitious, thrusting man under control. Macewen made no move and after some months when approached said that he would just retain his beds in the Royal Infirmary and the students could come there. The Management of the Western Infirmary were virtually forced to ask him to take their beds. Again, he wouldn't use their operating theatre and made use of an open space at the end of his wards; so they had to build new theatres. And so it went on; stories true or invented abound about his quarrels with the management and in particular with Colonel Mackintosh, the Medical Superintendent. Surgeons came from all over the world to see him operate, but as soon as he entered his wards the doors were closed to all 'management' until he left.

He was a good didactic teacher but was not averse to denigrating his colleagues. He referred repeatedly to Sir George Beatson, the discoverer of the hormonal dependency of some mammary cancers and at the same time the Chairman of St Andrew's Ambulance Association, as 'that ambulance man'.

He wrote letters of great tenderness to his family but could tell his students of the drunk who entered a railway carriage in Glasgow in which were two ladies and himself. The drunk, sitting opposite Macewen, was being objectionable and Macewen leant forward and shouted, 'Open your mouth!' The man, startled, did so. Macewen put both thumbs in his mouth, grasped his jaw and dislocated it. At the next station, Carlisle, he reduced the mandible and the drunk was bundled off. It sounds an absurd tale, but A. K. Bowman, Macewen's biographer, affirms that he heard Macewen tell it.

When speaking to students, patients or colleagues, he always referred to himself in the plural: 'we', 'us', 'our'. Admittedly when he travelled to Europe, across North America, to Australia, he was treated like royalty, but this mannerism did not endear him to many.

The smear has been repeatedly made that Macewen left behind no 'school of surgery'. If this is meant in the usual sense—'Sir Tom Richard-Harry always said . . .' or 'When I was his registrar, Sir Tom always did it this way and what was good enough for Sir Tom, my boy, . . .'—it is to his credit that he did not. What Macewen did was to build a solid basis for surgery and above all to give confidence to surgeons and surgery to forge ahead.

Sir William Macewen did not hold any office in the Faculty. He became a Fellow in 1874, and in 1913 the Royal Faculty conferred on him its Honorary Fellowship.

*Note:* It is impossible in a short sketch to give any but the most meagre details of this great man who had such a fully constructive and successful life. Dr A. K. Bowman's book *Sir William Macewen* runs to over 400 pages and tells most if not all. All is still to be, and may never be, told. Sir William and his family were compulsive collectors and storers of every document relating to him. The late Dr A. L. Goodall rescued some from Macewen's daughter, Daisy, when he found her tearing up document after document in a saleroom prior to the sale of some of Macewen's effects. The present writer, at the invitation of Mrs McDonald, Macewen's last surviving daughter, obtained for the Royal College most of the remaining papers of professional interest. The residue of the papers, on family matters, passed into the hands of Macewen's great-grandson, Mr Allan McDonald. In October 1981 he offered them to the College but when they were about to be inspected and collected, it was discovered that he had given them to Glasgow University!

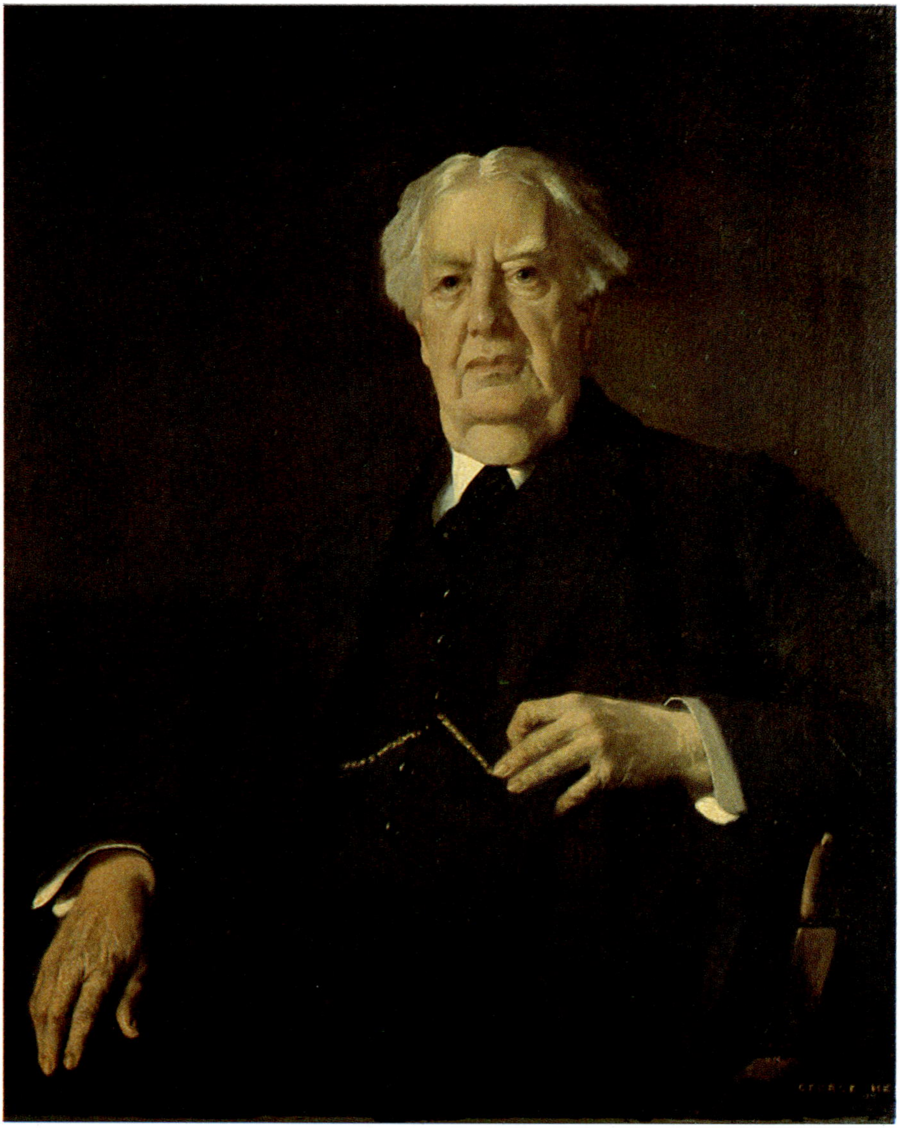

*Sir Hector C. Cameron (1843 to 1929) was an assistant of Joseph Lister and did much to confirm and promote Lister's ideas of antisepsis in surgery, becoming Professor of Clinical Surgery in the Western Infirmary from 1900 to 1911. The portrait is by George Henry and is a fine example of the artist's work.*

*Hector Cameron was President from 1897 to 1900, during which time the Tercentenary Celebrations were held and he was knighted.*

# HECTOR CLARE CAMERON, Kt.

1843 to 1929

*The portrait is by George Henry, R.A. and was bequeathed to the Royal Faculty by Sir Hector.*

Hector Clare Cameron was born in Demerara in British Guiana, the son of a sugar planter. As a young boy he was sent home to Scotland for his schooling at Madras College in St Andrews. He went on to spend several sessions in the Arts Faculty of the University there, but, deciding on medicine as a career, proceeded first to Edinburgh and then to Glasgow where he graduated MB,CM in 1866 and obtained his MD in 1868.

As a medical student he was taught by Lister and acted as one of his 'dressers'. After graduating he became Lister's house surgeon and in 1868 he became Lister's assistant. These were the formative years of his professional life and, as will be seen, he could still remember and describe them with clarity 60 years later. When Lister left for Edinburgh in 1869, Hector Cameron was the only one left in Glasgow Royal Infirmary who was not only thoroughly versed in Lister's methods and their underlying principles, but enthusiastically convinced of their rightness. His voice is not recorded as having been raised against the criticisms of the Reids and the Mortons but he was still only 26 years old. He seems rather to have proceeded quietly and patiently applying the new techniques and before long his results spoke for themselves; this was an impressive young surgeon and Glasgow Royal Infirmary Managers, however anti-Lister they may have been, recognised it and appointed him Visiting Surgeon in 1873.

He went across to the Western Infirmary in 1881, also as Visiting Surgeon, and in 1900 succeeded George Buchanan as Professor of Clinical Surgery there. He held this post until his retirement in 1911 when the chair was, in effect, transferred to the Royal Infirmary. At that time the University bestowed upon him the LLD.

Cameron was devoted to the Faculty: he became a Fellow in 1878 and was for 15 years the representative to the General Medical Council. At the tercentenary celebrations of 1899 he was then President and was knighted by Queen Victoria.

Although he did not write much, he was a good teacher with a memorable epigrammatic style. 'You must not make your light shine at a patient's cost', and 'To open an abdomen without a constructive diagnosis is the height of surgical curiosity' are two of his quotable remarks.

His most important publication was his last: *Reminiscences of Lister and of his Work in the Wards of the Glasgow Royal Infirmary, 1860-1869*. The University held a reception in the Bute Hall on 1st April 1927 in 'Celebration of the Centenary of the Birth of Lord Lister', and a copy of Cameron's 45-page recently published book was presented to every guest. It is one of the most important documents in the history of surgery; it gives a first hand description of Lister's most innovative period and, had it been written 60 years earlier, it would have silenced much criticism.

Cameron tells of the impression Lister made on his students and how his first class presented him with an appreciative address at the end of the course; of Lister's obvious physical distress at the appalling mortality in his wards from pyaemia and hospital gangrene; of his courage in helping to free a coachman when a brougham had plunged into a sunken area in front of the surgical wards and lay on its side pinning the driver, and with the horses kicking and plunging.

It is a common oversimplification to say that Lister invented antisepsis and Macewen modified it to asepsis. In the sense that there was a gradual change of emphasis from chemical disinfectants to other methods of killing germs, this is so; if, however, by 'asepsis' is implied complete sterility of everything at a surgical operation, this is an ideal yet to be achieved. Cameron writes, 'The word "Aseptic" was introduced into English by Lister to indicate the condition of a wound from which Sepsis is absent. . . . To speak of "the aseptic treatment of wounds" is as confused and as inelegant as to speak of "the antiseptic condition of wounds" since every method of avoiding sepsis is of course an antiseptic method'. It is largely a question of semantics, but Cameron affirms that Lister was the first to use dressings sterilised by heat, the first to experiment with tincture of iodine to sterilise the skin.

Lister's methods were undoubtedly more than the use of carbolic acid. If the following two cases which Cameron witnessed and described in his *Reminiscences* had been more widely publicised at the time . . . :

The first was a young man with four-months-old malunited fractures of his fibula two inches above the ankle joint and the tibial malleolus, and a backwards and outwards dislocation of the whole foot; the limb was useless. 'The whole region operated on, the hands of the operator and his assistants, as well as the instruments were thoroughly cleansed and immersed in a watery solution of carbolic acid'. Lister, through separate incisions, divided the callus around the fractures, opening of necessity the ankle joint, and a solution of carbolic acid in four parts of olive oil was dripped into the wounds. The dislocation was reduced by a system of pulleys and belts and the usual carbolic acid dressings applied. Some months later, after a secondary tenotomy of the tendo Achillis, the man was walking firmly and well with only some remaining ankle stiffness.

The second case is even more impressive: a 45-year-old man had an 18-month-old extracapsular fracture of the neck of the femur with 1⅛ inch of shortening and could only walk with crutches. Under chloroform anaesthesia Lister forcibly broke down the adhesions, 'the pulleys were applied', and the fracture exposed through a long incision. The bone ends were roughened with a powerful gouge and the bone chips left in the depth of the wound. Antiseptic dressings and external splints were then applied. The wound healed and in time the man walked again.

These operations took place between 1866 and 1869; they were surgically produced compound fractures, at a time when most of such injuries came to amputation or death. But it was only when Macewen, nearly 20 years later, reported 1,800 compound fractures produced at operation with virtually no morbidity or mortality, that the surgical world was finally convinced.

Sir Hector Clare Cameron was President of the Faculty of Physicians and Surgeons of Glasgow from 1897 to 1900.

# 13

## BIBLIOGRAPHERS, HISTORIANS AND LIBRARIANS

Robert Watt (1774 to 1819)
William Weir (1794 to 1876)
Alexander Duncan (1833 to 1921)
James Finlayson (1840 to 1906)
John Lindsay Steven (1858 to 1909)
Ebenezer Henry Lawrence Oliphant (1860 to 1934)

As soon as the Faculty had erected their first home in the Trongate in 1698, they set up their library which ever since has been one of their proudest and most valuable possessions. They began by seeking donations from the members, their friends and notable Glasgow citizens. Duncan, writing in 1896, said that there was a large folio manuscript volume in the Faculty Library giving the names of all the donors, but this can no longer be found; Duncan, however, lists the names in his *Memorials*. Some of their books are still there; others, particularly those of non-medical interest, have gone.

At first the office of Bibliothecarius was combined with that of Collector or Treasurer but by 1755 the Bibliothecarius or Librarian had become a Faculty dignitary in his own right. Most of them, although the position was honorary, seem to have taken it seriously. A Library Committee was formed in 1768 and the first printed catalogue appeared in 1778. The next catalogue was printed in 1817 and the number of books was then about 3,500. Dr John M. Pagan, the Honorary Librarian in 1842, directed the publication of a new catalogue, and a successor, Dr James Adam, added a supplement in 1861.

To begin with at least, the Honorary Librarian seems to have been the only librarian and had to attend at the monthly meetings to hand out books; by 1801 he was required to attend twice monthly! Later this task was taken over by the Faculty Officer and Mr Nathaniel Jones, who was the son of one Officer and also University Librarian, attempted to compile an Index of Subjects in 1842. But the first step of appointing a non-medical graduate as a full-time salaried Librarian, in addition to the Fellow who was Honorary Librarian, occurred in 1865 when Alexander Duncan was appointed Secretary and Librarian and served the Faculty faithfully for 55 years.

The subsequent history of the Library will emerge through the stories of the subjects of the following portraits. All of them were connected in one way or another with the Library, but outstanding is Robert Watt for whom the Faculty Library was only one small source of the material for his incredible single-handed achievement, *The Bibliotheca Britannica*.

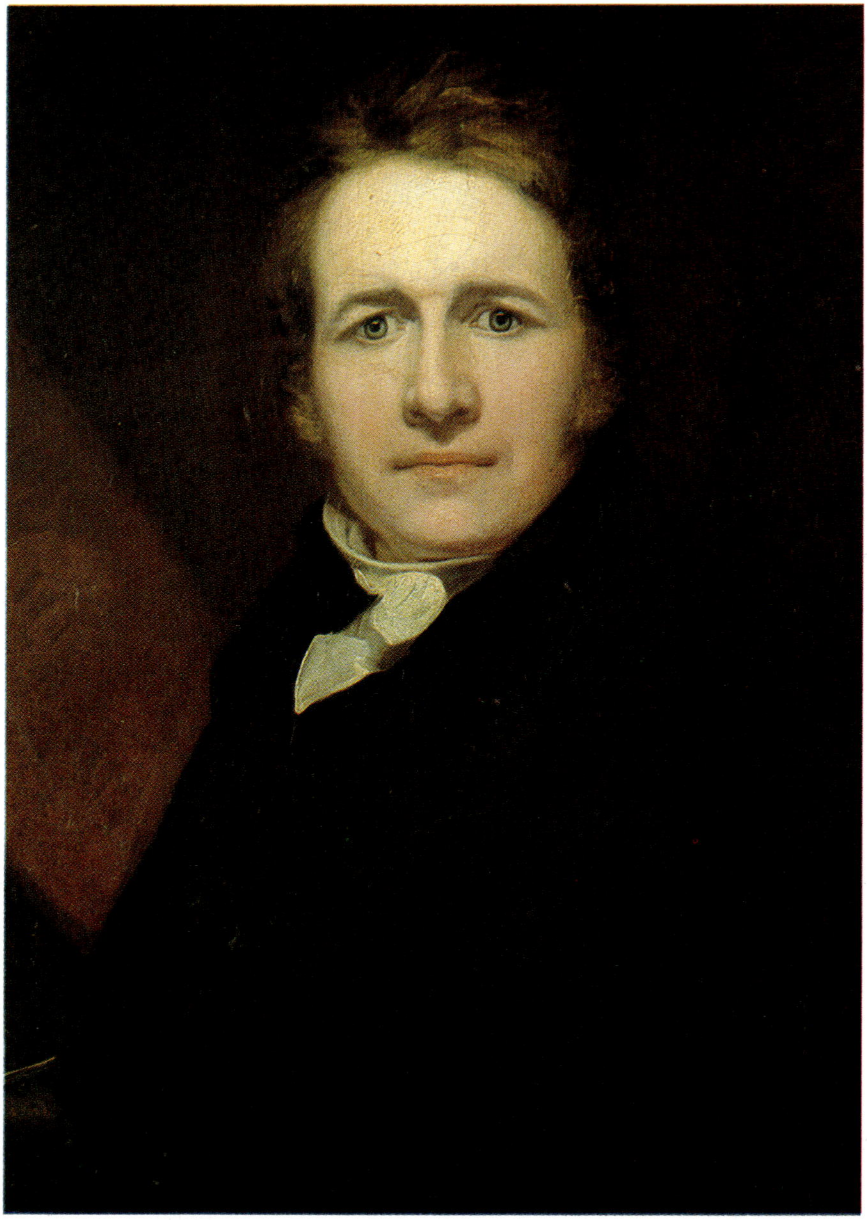

*Robert Watt (1774 to 1819) was one of the Faculty's most outstanding Presidents. Of humble origin he lived just long enough to complete the greatest bibliography ever written single-handedly, the* Bibliotheca Britannica. *The portrait is unsigned and the artist unknown.*

*He was President from 1814 to 1816.*

# ROBERT WATT

1774 to 1819

*There were two portraits. The first, which has hung for many years in the College Hall, was presented to the Faculty by Alexander Whitelaw in 1869 and was at one time attributed to Henry Raeburn, but there is no proof of this. The second was painted by Tannock of Kilmarnock and was apparently among the effects of Mary, Robert Watt's daughter, who died in Govan Asylum in 1864. Its delivery to the Faculty was authorised by a Mr Kirkwood, Inspector of Poor to the Parish of Govan in 1868. It appears to have degenerated beyond repair and been disposed of. A reproduction is in Goodall and Gibson (1963).*

Robert Watt was the son of a small farmer in Ayrshire. He had some local schooling until the age of 12 when he successively tried farm labouring, cabinetmaking and dyke and road building. In this last employment he went with a party into Dumfriesshire and was lodged for a short time in Ellisland, the farm which belonged to Robert Burns. He met the great poet and was allowed to borrow books from his library. When he was 18 a local schoolmaster gave him private lessons in Latin and Greek, and in 1793 and 1794 he was able to attend Glasgow University and take the classes in Greek, Latin and Logic. The following year, 1795, he went to Edinburgh to study moral and natural philosophy.

For the next year or so he seems to have hesitated between divinity and medicine as a career and took classes in both, but a local divine, for reasons unknown, persuaded him to abandon the ministry, so he completed his medical studies and became a Licentiate of the Faculty in 1799. This allowed him to practise outwith Glasgow and he set up a practice in Paisley.

Watt was a restless, ambitious man with a tremendous capacity for hard work.

Within a year he had published two papers describing a 'New Instrument for Operating for the Stone' and a 'New Machine for Curing Distorted Limbs'. His practice flourished and in 1802 he took as partner James Muir, to whom he dedicated his first book in 1808: *Cases of Diabetes, Consumption etc. with Observations on the History and Treatment of Disease in General*. Prior to this, in 1806, he helped to found the Paisley Medical Society whose main purpose was to prevent the undercutting of fees; minimum rates were laid down and for many years every new practitioner in Paisley had to sign his agreement to them. In 1807 he became a full Member of the Faculty, being now apparently sufficiently affluent to pay the greatly increased fee. Indeed he was noted to be now visiting his patients in a phaeton while his competitors ambled along on horseback. This may have been sheer ostentation, but Watt claimed declining health and in 1809 left his practice to his partner and went on a tour of England. He had furnished himself with letters of recommendation to many eminent medical men and reached London after a circuitous journey. There he became a member of the London Medical and Chirurgical Society, but there is no record of his other visits. Nevertheless, it must have been during these travels that he made the contacts in University and other libraries without which his *Bibliotheca* would have been impossible to complete.

When he returned to Paisley he found his practice almost gone, since his patients believed, or had been led to believe, that he had gone job-hunting in England. So being now a full Member of the Faculty, he bought in 1810 a large house in Queen Street in Glasgow and the degree of MD from Aberdeen University. The practice of obtaining MD's without examination from Aberdeen and St Andrews at this time has been noted elsewhere, and it is said that Watt's MD 'caused some sneering at the time amongst his medical contemporaries'. It is also fascinating that it was during Watt's Presidency of the Faculty in 1815 that the Faculty raised action against four MD's practising in Glasgow and claimed that two of them had never been examined by their Universities!

He began to teach the Principles and Practice of Medicine partly with the College Street School group but mostly in his own home. By this time he had amassed a respectable library and with a view to attracting more students he published a list of his books in 1812. It is entitled *Catalogue of Medical Books for the Use of Students Attending Lectures on the Principles and Practice of Medicine; with an address to medical students on the best method of prosecuting their studies*. It contains 1,066 entries, nearly all of which are arranged alphabetically by authors. It is exceedingly rare but so important historically as the start of the great *Bibliotheca* that a facsimile was published in New York by Cordasco in 1950.

Even if the *Bibliotheca* had been neither conceived nor achieved, Watt's biography would still be notable. He was assiduous in his attendance at Faculty Meetings, was elected Boxmaster in 1811, joined the Library Committee and was a member of several other committees before becoming President in 1814. He was a founder member and first President of the Glasgow Medical Society in 1814, the same year in which he was elected physician to the Glasgow Royal Infirmary. In 1816 he became President of the Glasgow Philosophical Society.

# TREATISE

ON THE

HISTORY, NATURE, AND TREATMENT

OF

# CHINCOUGH:

INCLUDING

A VARIETY OF CASES AND DISSECTIONS.

TO WHICH IS SUBJOINED,

## AN INQUIRY

INTO THE RELATIVE MORTALITY OF THE PRINCIPAL

DISEASES OF CHILDREN,

AND THE

NUMBERS WHO HAVE DIED UNDER TEN YEARS OF AGE, IN GLASGOW, DURING THE LAST THIRTY YEARS.

---

BY ROBERT WATT, M.D.

MEMBER OF THE FACULTY OF PHYSICIANS AND SURGEONS OF GLASGOW, MEMBER OF THE LONDON MEDICAL AND CHIRURGICAL SOCIETY, &C. AND LECTURER ON THE THEORY AND ON THE PRACTICE OF MEDICINE IN GLASGOW.

---

——— *quæque ipse miserrima vidi,*
*Et quorum pars magna fui.* VIRG.

---

GLASGOW:

PRINTED FOR JOHN SMITH & SON,
AND FOR
LONGMAN, HURST, REES, ORME AND BROWN,
LONDON.

1813.

*The frontispiece of Watt's book on the chincough or whooping cough published in 1813.*

## Total Deaths in the Registers, 1671.

| Months. | Small Pox. | Measles. | Chincough. | Stopping. | W. in Head. | Teething. | Bowelhives. | Still-born. | Fevers. | Under Two. | Under Five. | Under Ten. |
|---|---|---|---|---|---|---|---|---|---|---|---|---|
| Jan. | 5 | 15 | 14 | 14 | 5 | 6 | 8 | 11 | 9 | 66 | 17 | 11 |
| Feb. | 1 | 18 | 10 | 15 | 3 | 5 | 14 | 6 | 13 | 56 | 23 | 8 |
| Mar. | 1 | 10 | 11 | 15 | 7 | 3 | 8 | 8 | 11 | 42 | 19 | 8 |
| Apr. | 2 | 14 | 4 | 9 | 4 | 5 | 11 | 11 | 7 | 52 | 18 | 10 |
| May | 0 | 4 | 6 | 7 | 7 | 3 | 6 | 6 | 7 | 34 | 17 | 5 |
| June | 0 | 1 | 6 | 7 | 5 | 0 | 6 | 4 | 10 | 24 | 15 | 13 |
| July | 3 | 1 | 4 | 8 | 1 | 2 | 5 | 4 | 1 | 36 | 7 | 5 |
| Aug. | 5 | 1 | 6 | 7 | 3 | 3 | 17 | 8 | 7 | 45 | 10 | 3 |
| Sep. | 4 | 3 | 7 | 7 | 2 | 0 | 20 | 5 | 10 | 50 | 5 | 5 |
| Oct. | 11 | 8 | 6 | 6 | 2 | 5 | 10 | 14 | 12 | 57 | 9 | 5 |
| Nov. | 17 | 8 | 24 | 6 | 0 | 4 | 14 | 14 | 14 | 83 | 19 | 2 |
| Dec. | 7 | 7 | 31 | 11 | 4 | 1 | 6 | 13 | 15 | 71 | 29 | 5 |
| Tot. | 56 | 90 | 129 | 112 | 43 | 37 | 125 | 104 | 116 | 616 | 188 | 80 |

*One of the statistical tables from the* Chincough *which showed that while the mortality from smallpox in children had decreased, the overall mortality was unchanged.*

In 1813 he published a book on the *Chincough* or whooping cough in which two of the fatal cases described were Watt's own children, both of whom were examined post-mortem. But it was the second part of the book which was to cause controversy for many years and remains one of the most important early works on epidemiology: the 'Inquiry into the Relative Mortality of the Principal Diseases of Children'. Vaccination had begun in the Faculty in 1801 and Watt compared the mortality of children under the age of ten before and after its introduction. The only source of statistics was the burial registers and after laboriously wading through these, Watt found that although the deaths from smallpox had fallen steeply, the total mortality of young children remained about the same; measles and other diseases had carried off the weaklings saved from smallpox.

He retired from medical practice in 1817 to devote his time to the *Bibliotheca* and died in 1819 having lived just long enough to see it largely completed, in the end directing from his sick bed his amanuenses who included his two sons, William Motherwell the poet and Alexander Whitelaw. The *Bibliotheca* was a monumental work and undoubtedly the greatest bibliography ever made by a single man. To appreciate the Gargantuan nature of the task Watt set himself, go and see the 69 volumes of the manuscripts which are housed in Paisley Public Library; and even these are incomplete. The 'authors' entries are all written longhand and, as these came from the presses, a scissors-and-paste technique with copious additions and deletions was used for the 'subjects'.

It started with his catalogue of 1812 which was just an 'authors' index, and from which he drew out a 'subjects' index. It was first enlarged to include all the medical works in the British Dominions, next books on law and divinity, articles from journals as well as books, and lastly foreign publications. The final manuscript bore the title:

*The*
*Bibliotheca Britannica*
*or*
*A General Index*
*to the*
*Literature of Great Britain and Ireland*
*Ancient and Modern*
*including*
*Such Foreign Works*
*as have been translated into English or printed*
*In the British Dominions*
*As also a copious Selection from the Writings of the most distinguished*
*Authors of all Ages and Nations*

It appeared at first in parts and finally in four volumes, two each of authors and subjects. It was years in advance of any similar compilation and librarians still use it today.

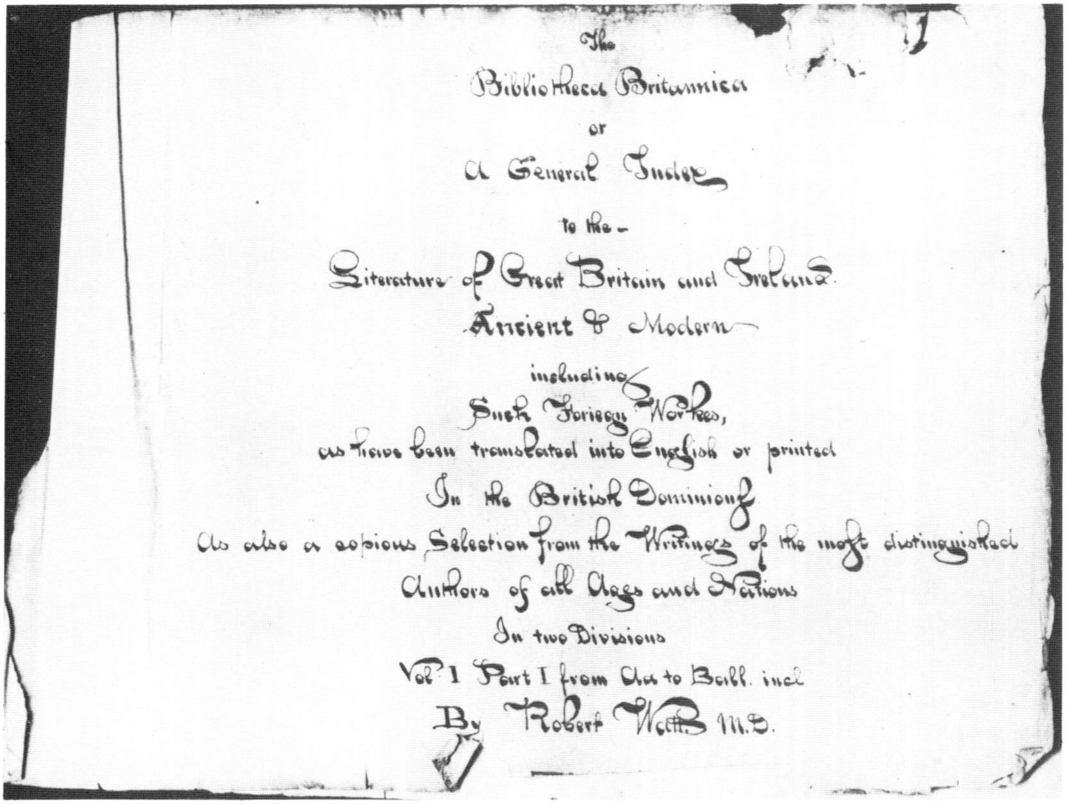

The
Bibliotheca Britannica
or
A General Index
to the
Literature of Great Britain and Ireland
Ancient & Modern
including
Such Foreign Works,
as have been translated into English or printed
In the British Dominions
As also a copious Selection from the Writings of the most distinguished
Authors of all Ages and Nations
In two Divisions
Vol. I Part I from Aa to Ball. incl
By Robert Watt M.D.

*The frontispiece of the manuscript of the* Bibliotheca *preserved in the Mitchell Library.*

## *The tragic end of Robert Watt and his family*

When Watt died he had been forgotten as a medical teacher and practitioner and had yet to be known as a bibliographer. Only a simple notice of his death appeared in the local press, there were no obituaries, and he lies in an unnamed grave in the Cathedral Churchyard. This was but the first of many misfortunes which were to plague the Watt family. In brief:

> His house was plundered and Mrs Watt's rings wrenched from her fingers soon after his death, by Irish ruffians, four of whom were caught, convicted and 'thrown off together by Thomas Young the hangman' in 1820;
>
> The firm of Constable, who were publishing the *Bibliotheca*, went bankrupt and Mrs Watt received not a penny of the £2,000 she had been promised;
>
> Both surviving sons died within a few years of their father, and Mrs Watt was

left with only her daughter Mary and her pension from the Faculty's Widows' Fund;

Mary was engaged to a Fellow of the Faculty but he died from typhus, and soon afterwards she became insane and was confined in Govan Lunatic Asylum. Robert Watt was now famous, public sympathy was aroused and a petition to the Government for an annuity for Mary, signed by such literary figures as Tennyson and Ruskin, was finally granted in 1864; but Mary had died some days before.

Among Mary's effects were several sacks full of slips of paper which proved to be her father's manuscripts. They were purchased for Paisley by Thomas Coats of thread mill fame and in the Library there sorted, bound and housed, a fitting memorial to a very great man.

Robert Watt was President of the Faculty of Physicians and Surgeons of Glasgow from 1814 to 1816.

*Note:* Dr James Finlayson wrote a small book *An account of the life and works of Dr. Robert Watt* which was published by Smith, Elder of London in 1897. See also Goodall, A. L. and Gibson, T. (1963) 'Robert Watt: Physician and Bibliographer'. *Journal of the History of Medicine and Allied Sciences*, 18, p. 36.

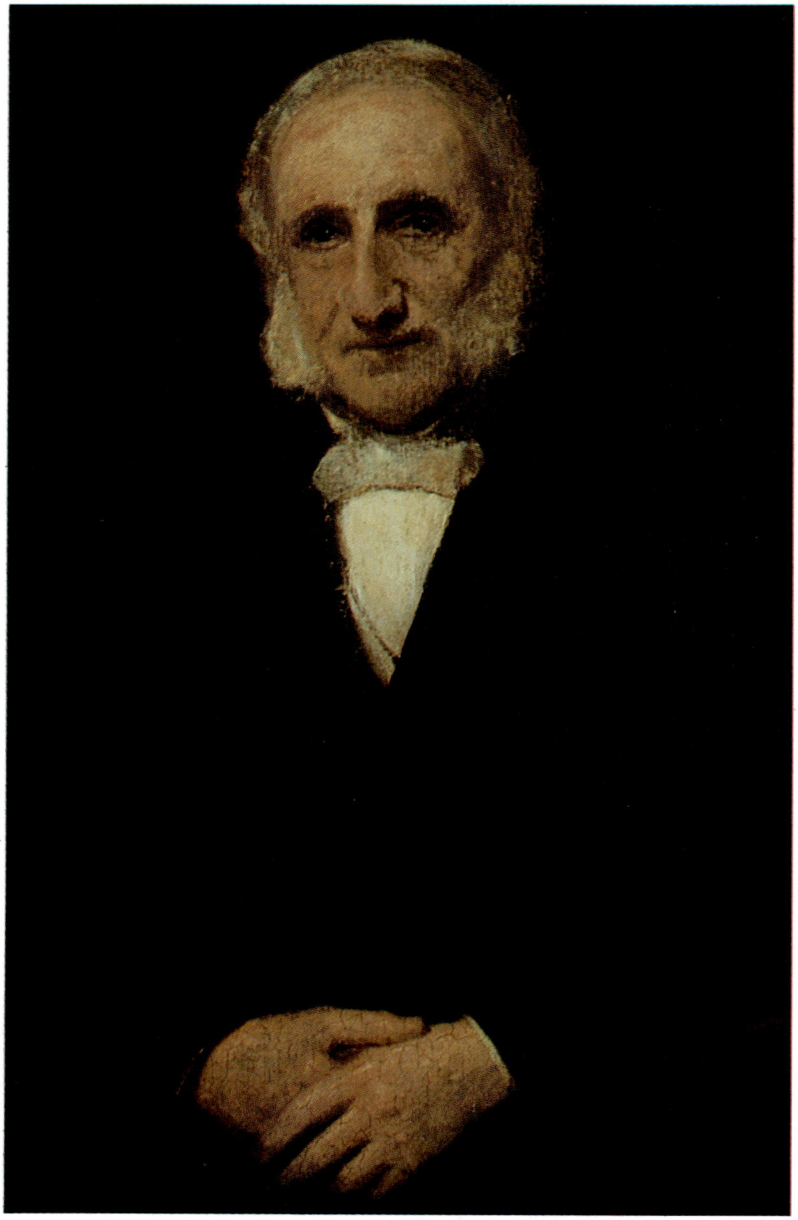

*William Weir (1794 to 1876) made a great contribution to the Faculty's history when he extracted the most relevant details of the Minutes and presented them with his comments to the Library in 1869. The portrait is by Graham-Gilbert. He was President from 1847 to 1849.*

# WILLIAM WEIR

1794 to 1876

*The portrait is by Graham-Gilbert. When found stored away in the College in 1981 it was in poor condition, but as much as possible was cleaned and preserved at that time.*

William Weir was born in Glasgow, the son of John Weir who was a teacher of music and the precentor in St George's Church. William went to Glasgow Grammar School, studied medicine in the University and became a member of the Faculty in 1816. At first he practised in Lochwinnoch but then settled in Glasgow where he graduated MD in 1829.

It will be recalled that only 'pure' physicians could hold the post of physician in Glasgow Royal Infirmary until 1830. So we find Weir, who was by inclination much more physician than surgeon, taking a junior surgical appointment there in 1829, and then in 1840 when a suitable vacancy arose, applying for and obtaining an appointment as a physician.

William Weir was secretary to the Portland Street School and there he was also Lecturer in Medicine from 1830 to 1842. At this time there was great interest in phrenology and we find Weir as Lecturer in Phrenology in the Andersonian University. This 'branch of diagnostic medicine' had been introduced to Scotland in the 1820s by Andrew Combe, an Edinburgh physician, and was soon so popular that by the mid-1830s there were some 36 societies of phrenology in Britain and several 'scientific' journals devoted to it. As an illustration, it may be recalled that when the burial vault of Robert Burns in Dumfries had to be opened in 1834, nearly 40 years after his death in 1796, to receive the remains of Jean Armour, his widow, a group of eminent citizens temporarily removed his skull at dead of night and made a plaster cast of it. The phrenologists, after much study, asserted that it vindicated all their claims; the well-known characteristics of the great poet fitted exactly, or nearly so, the evidence of his cranial contours.

The *Glasgow Medical Journal* started as a quarterly journal in 1828, and Weir was one of the original promoters of this pioneering venture which was the first provincial medical journal to appear in Britain. William Mackenzie was the first editor and after two years was succeeded by William Weir. The *Journal* had a chequered career. It collapsed in 1832 but a second series was started in 1833 with Weir and James A. Lawrie as editors; it only lasted for one year but, undeterred, Weir some 12 years later began editing a third series which ran to 13 volumes. There were subsequent series and eventually it amalgamated with the *Edinburgh Medical Journal* to form the *Scottish Medical Journal*. It was William Weir who saw it through its inception and its first most difficult decades.

The office of 'Treasurer and Collector of the Widows' Fund' in the 1830s and 1840s was probably the most arduous of all the Faculty posts at this time and Weir wrought long and hard at it for many years. The Faculty minutes of these years are full of Widows' Fund business and the wrangles direct and indirect which arose from it. The Act of 1850 which freed the contribution to the Widows' Fund from the Faculty entrance fee and led to the winding up of the Fund was a great relief to all who were connected with it.

William Weir was the first historian of the Faculty. For some years he read in detail all the extant minutes and in 1864 published an address he had given on the 'Origin and Early History of the Faculty'. It was the painstaking work behind this which gave Alexander Duncan the basis on which to write his *Memorials*, the definitive history of the Faculty from 1599 to 1850. Here are Duncan's own words: 'In 1869 Dr. William Weir handed over to the Faculty a MS of considerable size consisting of copious extracts from the Minute Books of the Faculty connected by a thread of comments and reflections of his own. It had not been written with any view to publication and indeed in the letter presenting it he expressly stated that "printing of such a large mass is out of the question". The document was however fitted to serve a useful purpose as a key to the Minute Books rendering their contents more available for reference and also as a kind of annotated digest of their contents'. For many years seekers after information of the early Faculty days have been referred to Weir, as his extracts afforded much readier access than the old minutes with their often crabbed handwriting. Weir himself wrote a fair hand but his 'Extracts' have now been typewritten.

William Weir was President of the Faculty of Physicians and Surgeons of Glasgow from 1847 to 1849.

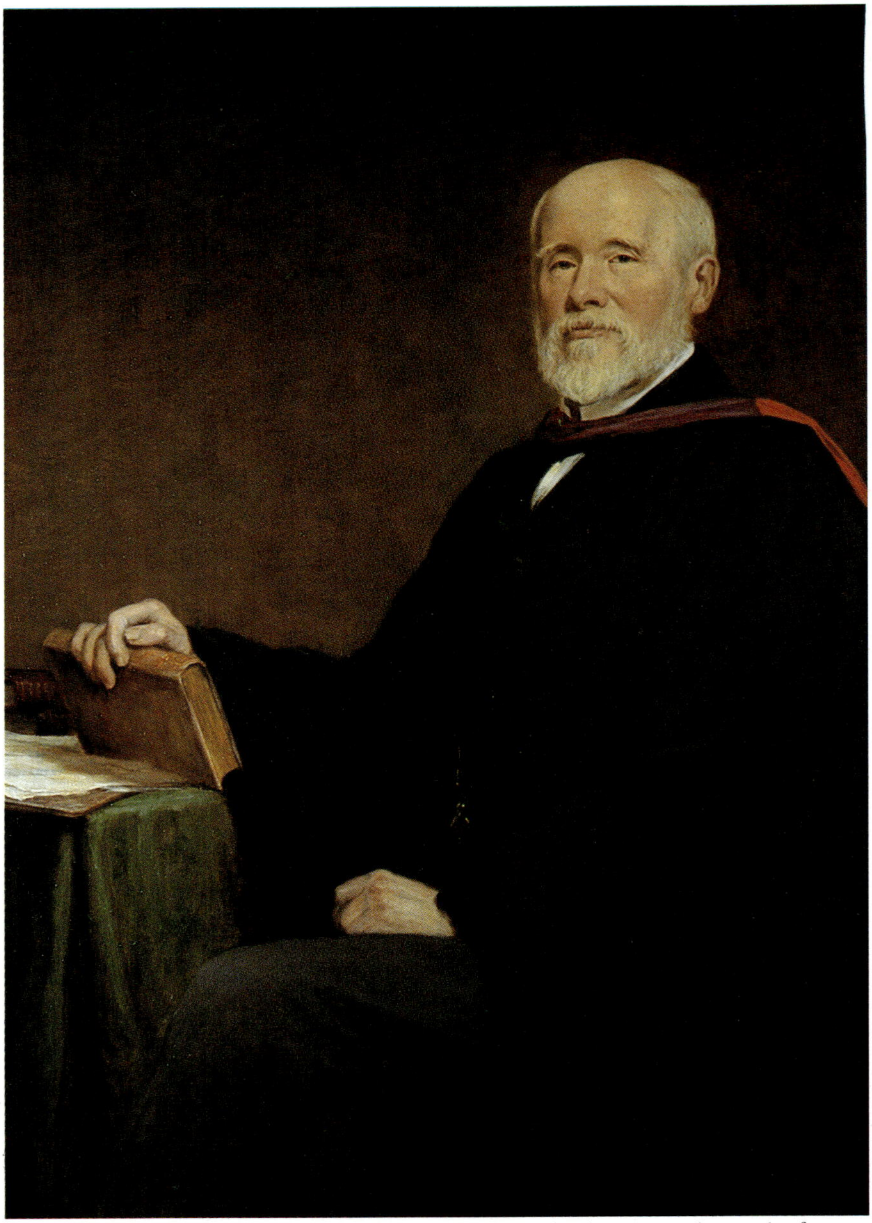

*Alexander Duncan (1833 to 1921) was Secretary and Librarian to the Faculty for 55 years and his major contributions were his* Memorials, *the history of the Faculty until 1850, and his two catalogues of the Library of 1885 and 1901.*
*The portrait is by Joseph Henderson.*

# ALEXANDER DUNCAN

1833 to 1921

*The portrait was commissioned by a group of subscribing Fellows presided over by Dr Lindsay Steven. It was painted by Mr Joseph Henderson of Glasgow and presented formally to the Faculty at their Annual Dinner in 1902. In addition to the larger work there is a smaller replica of the head and shoulders.*

Dr J. Gibson Fleming has already been quoted as saying that his greatest contribution to the Faculty, which occurred during his presidency in 1865, was the appointment as Secretary and Librarian of Alexander Duncan who served the Faculty faithfully and devotedly for more than half a century.

Alexander Duncan was born in Dollar and graduated BA in London University with a view to teaching as a career, and at the time of his appointment to the Faculty he was employed in a school in Kirkintilloch. But he was more suited to the painstaking and often solitary work of a Librarian and Secretary than the daily distractions and disturbances of a dominie, and his achievements for the Faculty went far beyond the routine work for which he was paid. These were, firstly, the Library catalogue of 1885 and its supplement of 1901 and, secondly, the *Memorials*, his history of the Faculty until 1850. At first he was a man feeling his way, a university graduate to be sure, but now working intimately with other graduates of an entirely different discipline with their own language, tradition, foibles and personalities, but his tact and perseverance won him widespread respect in the end.

There had been earlier printed catalogues, as noted above, but they suffered like the rest of their kind in becoming more and more out of date. In 1880 it was resolved to prepare and print a new catalogue, but Duncan found this going rapidly out of date as it was being written because James Finlayson (*q.v.*), the Honorary Librarian, had been surveying the shelves and had found many omissions in all branches of medical literature. Before the catalogue should appear, Duncan tried to fill as many of these as he could, visiting secondhand bookshops in Glasgow, London and Paris and exchanging duplicates with other medical libraries.

For the first time, the books were arranged on the library shelves according to a rough subject classification. This by itself took two or three years but when it was complete it was the beginning of a catalogue of subjects. Further delay occurred when the printing was held up for a time to enter the William Mackenzie collection in 1885, but the catalogue finally appeared later the same year. The 242 pages of subject index are numbered i to ccxlii. Each entry gives the author's name and the date of the publication. To find the full reference one turns to the author index which runs to just over 700 pages. Then there are sections on Periodicals, Reports and Transactions, and a supplement of additions made while the rest was printing. It all adds up to a three-inch thick volume of 1,082 pages which indexes about 25,000 volumes.

Writing in 1896, Duncan said there were now approximately 40,000 volumes. 'The great aim of the successive library committees of the Faculty within the last generation has been to make it a good medical library *all round*, not to pamper one department at the cost of the atrophy of the other'. This great increase in the size of the library of some 15,000 books required another catalogue and it was planned to publish it at the time of the Tercentenary in 1899, but Duncan had other pressures of work including his *Memorials* which appeared in 1896, and it was 1901 before *Catalogue of the Library of the Faculty of Physicians and Surgeons of Glasgow Volume II* was published. This indexes the acquisitions from 1885 to 1900, is of similar design to Volume I, but is only two inches thick and 700 pages long!

There will never be another printed catalogue of the College Library or any similar medical library. The Surgeon General's Library, now the National Library of Washington, tried to continue one; its first catalogue filled 16 volumes from 1872 to 1896, a second and third series were completed, but the fourth came to a complete stop in 1955 with a volume which only went from MH to MN. Current lists, card index catalogues and computerisation have replaced definitive printed catalogues, which could never keep up with the exponential increase of medical literature. But to the interested explorer of medical history in almost any of its branches, Duncan's *Catalogues* are a rich source of information and most of the books he lists are still available from the Library shelves.

Duncan's second great contribution to the Faculty was his *Memorials*, an almost inexhaustible reference for the history of the Faculty before 1850. Its full title is *Memorials of the Faculty of Physicians and Surgeons of Glasgow 1599-1850 with a Sketch of the Rise and Progress of the Glasgow Medical School and of the Medical Profession in the West of Scotland.*

Its beginning, as already noted, was William Weir's extracts from, and comments on, the early Minutes which he handed into the Faculty Library in 1869. But the early Minutes were laconic at best, the second minute book with all the data from 1681 to 1733 had been destroyed by fire, and many other sources, some already in the Faculty Library, some in the University Library, some in the Records of the City authorities, had to be consulted to build up a composite picture of the first 250 years of the corporation and its background. At the time when it was being written, James

Finlayson, the Honorary Librarian, was preparing his *Account of the Life and Works of Maister Peter Lowe*, and this too was of help to Duncan. Indeed, on Duncan's suggestion, Finlayson, Dr John Glaister and Dr Lindsay Steven were nominated by the Faculty to act as a committee of consultation during the preparation of the book for publication. Although it purports to be a history only to 1850 it was not published until 1896, and some aspects are followed into the second half of the century. But 1850 is the cut-off point for the chronological list of the members of the Faculty and their basic known biographical data.

In the preface, Duncan admits to being at some disadvantage in writing the memorials of the 'calling of the healing art' without being a member of it. However, 'he saw no likelihood of the task being undertaken by any of the present Fellows' whom he divides into two categories: those with much professional work to do and those with little. 'The former have rarely adequate time to devote to work of this kind; the latter, who are often juniors, have seldom much taste for it'.

It is impossible to overstress the value of Duncan's work. It is above all accurate, and if there seems to be occasionally too little detail and occasionally too much, the former is readily remedied from other sources he gives and the latter seldom goes amiss.

In 1898 Glasgow University conferred on him the honorary degree of LLD.

Alexander Duncan continued to work in the Royal Faculty until he died in his 89th year in 1921. For some time he had been helped by Mr Walter Hurst as acting Secretary and Librarian, and Hurst succeeded him.

In 1915, when Duncan had served the Faculty for 50 years, the Fellows placed on record their appreciation of his services. What was then said is similar to what the President, Dr Freeland Fergus, said about him when he announced at the March meeting in 1921 that 'Dr. Duncan who had served the Faculty faithfully for fifty-five years had passed away. No one had rendered more distinguished services to the literary side of Medicine in the West of Scotland than Dr. Duncan. He had a wide knowledge of the Literature of Medicine and a knowledge of Modern Languages which gave him great advantages in his extensive researches'. After eulogising the *Catalogues* and the *Memorials* he concluded, 'in all matters which affected the Faculty, its welfare or its honour, he took a deep interest and was a wise and trusted adviser. His relations with the Fellows and all connected with the Faculty were of the most harmonious character and with all his learning and ability he was one of the most modest and retiring of men'.

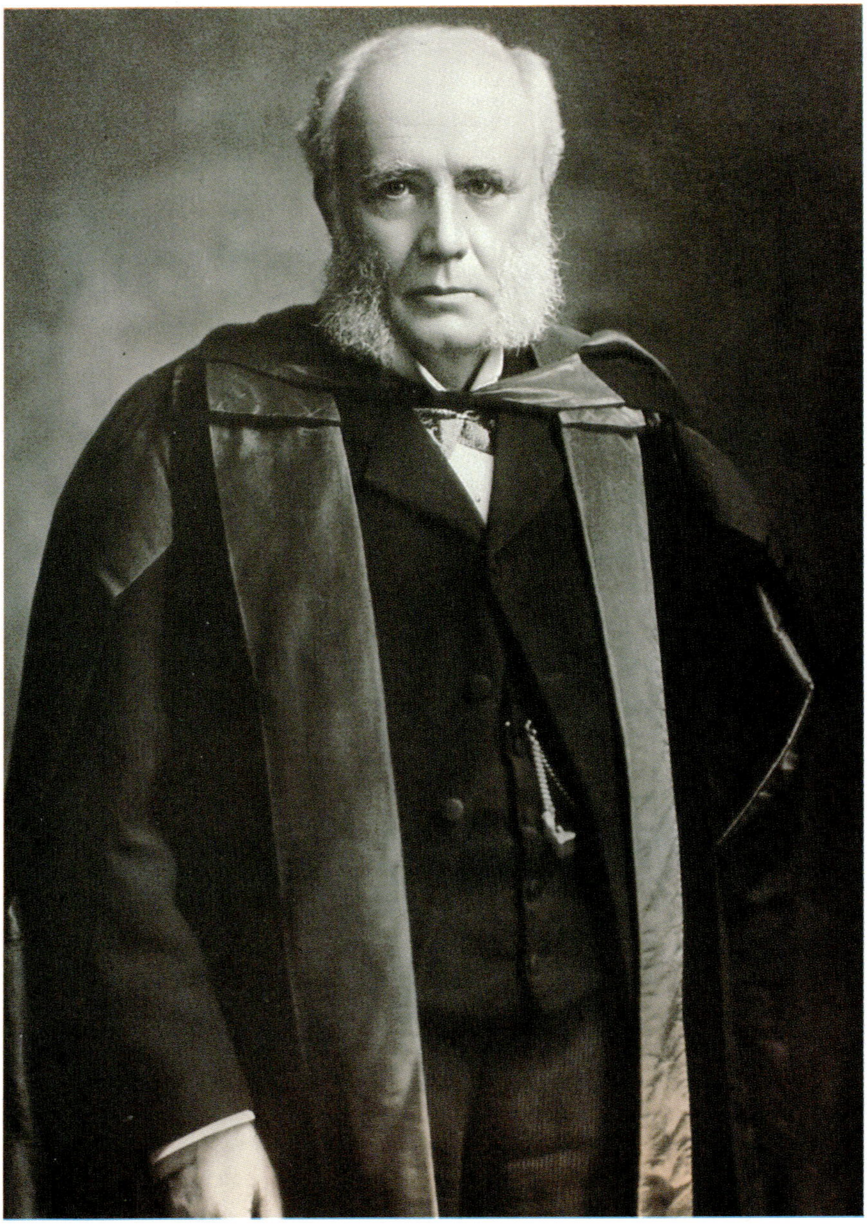

*James Finlayson (1840 to 1906) was known to thousands of medical students and young doctors for his* Clinical Manual *and was also a great medical historian. Together, Duncan and he filled most of the gaps on the Library shelves and his monograph on Peter Lowe is the definitive work. The portrait is an enlargement of a photograph by Annan. He was President from 1900 to 1903.*

# JAMES FINLAYSON

1840 to 1906

*The portrait is a framed enlarged photograph which for many years hung in the original reading room of the Royal Faculty. When the Fraser Reading Room was constructed from the attic rooms in 1963, the original L-shaped reading room was divided into the limbs of the L, the larger with most of its original gallery remaining as part of the Library, the smaller being converted into a lecture room. Even then Finlayson's portrait still hung from the gallery but following the more recent upheaval it has disappeared, or, at least, cannot be located. Fortunately, another photograph by Annan is extant.*

*A bust of James Finlayson was presented to the Royal Faculty in 1929 by relatives of his sister, Miss G. T. Finlayson, who had just died. This bust, like all others in the College, with the exception of Benno Schotz's head of T. J. Honeyman, has vanished during the recent alterations. The high price of bronze must have been attractive to one of the many strangers who invaded the building at that time.*

James Finlayson went first to Glasgow High School and then to Glasgow University where he studied Arts in the 1856-1857 session. He spent the next five years in business; his father was one of the partners of the manufacturing firm, McLean and Finlayson. Determined on medicine as a career, he started in Anderson's College in 1862 and then went to Glasgow University in 1863 and graduated with 'honours' MB,CM in 1867. He seems to have been a clever lad and two years later, the earliest date which the regulations permitted, he received his MD. His earliest hospital appointments were in the Children's Hospital in Manchester, but he came back to Glasgow as assistant to Sir William Tennant Gairdner, the Regius Professor of Medicine, in 1871, and in 1875 was appointed Physician to the Glasgow Western Infirmary, a clinical teaching post which he held until his death. His early interest in paediatrics led to his appointment as Physician to the Glasgow Royal Hospital for Sick Children when it opened in 1883 and this connection, too, he maintained until his death. For many years he was the medical adviser to the Scottish Amicable Life Insurance Company and in later years this claimed much of his time.

These are the basic data of his life, and that he was a good physician to whom even his colleagues turned for advice, there can be no doubt. But Finlayson was so much more. His literary output was phenomenal: his contributions to the medical press at home and overseas numbered about 150, and about 60 of these appeared in the *Glasgow Medical Journal*. Two aspects of his literary work are outstandingly notable:

*Finlayson the clinical teacher.* Countless thousands of medical students, house physicians and junior hospital doctors have known and respected the name of Finlayson. His textbook *Clinical Manual for the Study of Medical Cases* was first published in 1878 and proved so popular that second and third editions appeared in 1886 and 1891. In the United States, editions entitled *Clinical Diagnosis* appeared in 1878 and 1886, and for many years the book was used extensively throughout the English-speaking world. The final edition appeared in 1926, long after Finlayson's death, and was edited by C. H. Browning, Professor of Bacteriology, E. P. Cathcart, Professor of Physiology and Leonard Finlay, Professor of Medical Paediatrics, all in the University of Glasgow. That three such eminent men should keep 'Finlayson' alive in this way speaks for itself. Quite apart from his book, however, he seems to have been a greatly admired teacher. One of his obituarists wrote, 'In many a doctor's home—from Highland glen to London square, from African veldt to Australian bush—the news of his death will be sadly received by hundreds of Glasgow graduates who, in many years gone by, sat at the feet of James Finlayson'.

*Finlayson the Librarian and Medical Historian.* In 1871, on his return to Glasgow, Finlayson became a Fellow of the Faculty. In 1877 the Faculty elected him Honorary Librarian and he held this post for 25 years. He and Duncan together probably did more for the Library than any librarians before or since, and each pays tribute in his work to the other. Here is Duncan in the preface to the *Catalogue* of 1885: 'A careful survey of the library made by Dr. Finlayson, Honorary Librarian, disclosed many omissions in all departments of medical literature, which it seemed important to have filled up'. Together they worked hard to do so until by the turn of the century they had achieved a library which was adequately represented in all branches of medicine and surgery and more than adequately in some, such as ophthalmology, the history of medicine and books on Glasgow and the West of Scotland.

His contemporaries described him as a medical 'archaeologist'. He gave several extremely popular 'bibliographical demonstrations' of the early medical works in the Faculty Library and a number of these were published: 'Hippocrates'; 'Galen'; 'Celsus'; 'Ancient Egyptian Medicine'; 'Herophilus and Erasistratus'; 'The Care of Infants and young children according to the Bible and the Talmud'.

He was equally interested in the history of more recent times and two of his books are classics: *Account of the life and works of Maister Peter Lowe; with portrait* was published in 1889. It is a scholarly attempt to obtain and record as much information as was available about our surgeon founder and little new has been added since, apart from the discovery of Lowe's will which Finlayson recorded in 1898. Duncan based his section on Lowe on Finlayson's work; so did the present writer.

His second historical book was the *Account of the life and works of Dr. Robert Watt; with portrait* which appeared in 1897. More recent research has established a few more details, but Finlayson's *Account* remains the standard work on which the biographical sketch above was largely based.

James Finlayson was a fine physician and a great scholar. He was President of the Faculty of Physicians and Surgeons of Glasgow from 1900 to 1903.

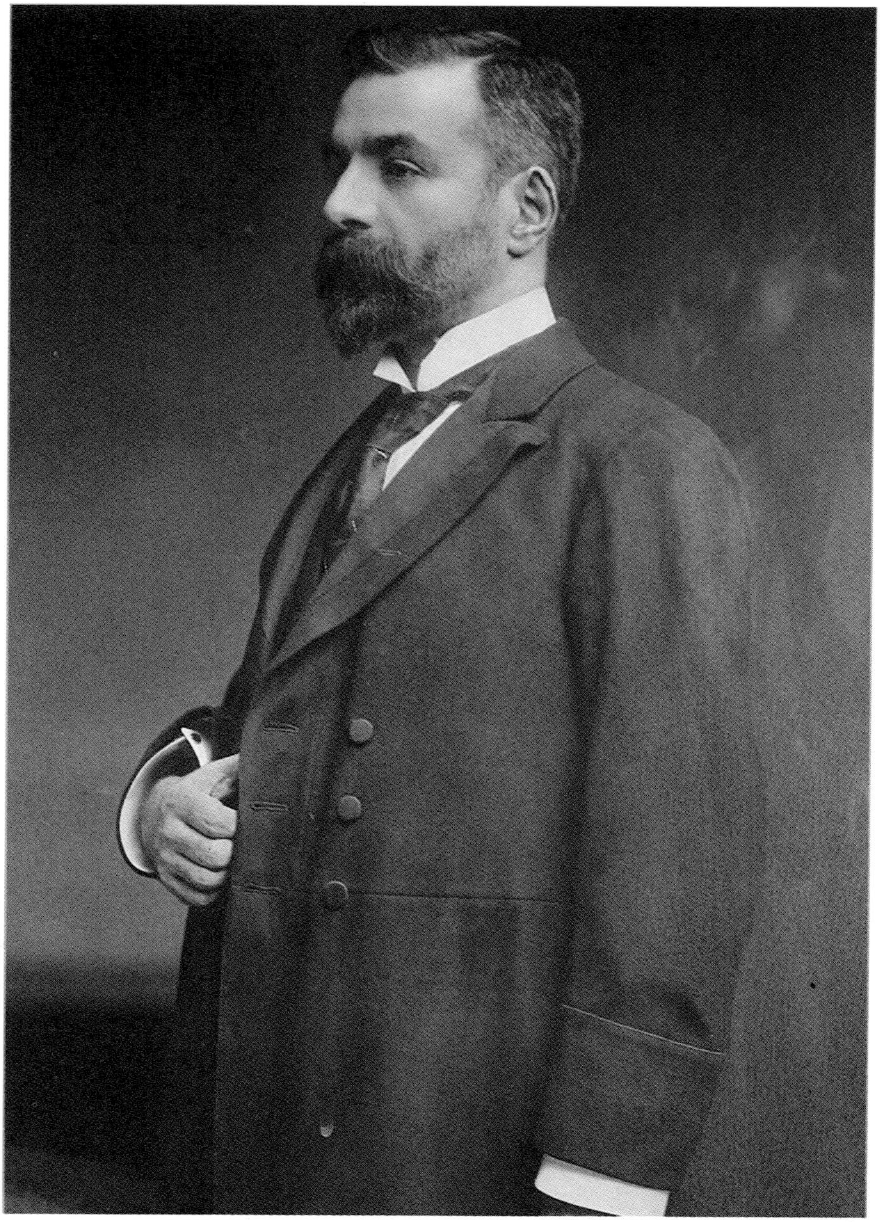

*John Lindsay Steven (1858 to 1909) conducted original research in the blood supply of the heart and fibroid degeneration of the heart muscle. As Honorary Librarian from 1901 to 1909 he continued the progressive improvement in the Library which had been achieved by Duncan and Finlayson.*

*The portrait is a photograph by Annan.*

# JOHN LINDSAY STEVEN

1858 to 1909

*The framed photograph is by Annan and was taken in 1906.*

Lindsay Steven went to school at Glasgow Academy and proceeded to Glasgow University where, in 1880, he graduated MB,CM and was awarded the Brunton Memorial Prize as the most distinguished graduate in medicine of his year.

When he completed his house jobs, he was fortunate in obtaining posts in the two disciplines which he was to combine so successfully throughout his career: pathology and clinical medicine. He became assistant to the Professor of Clinical Medicine (Sir T. McCall Anderson) in 1881 and a year later received the additional appointment of Pathological Chemist, each in Glasgow Western Infirmary. His distinction in both fields was apparent by 1884 when he obtained his MD degree with 'High Commendation' for a thesis entitled 'The Pathology of Suppurative Inflammation of the Kidney'; his classification remained for many years the accepted basis for later works. In 1890 he was appointed Pathologist to Glasgow Royal Infirmary and Professor of Pathology in St Mungo's College there, but he was also appointed Assistant Physician and continued teaching clinical medicine. In 1906 he returned to the Western Infirmary as Visiting Physician and held this post until his death three years later.

He published a textbook of *Practical Pathology* in 1887 and a volume of *Lectures on Clinical Medicine* in 1900, but his total contributions to medical literature numbered over 100 and covered many aspects of clinical medicine and pathology. Probably the most important are those which dealt with cardiac fibrosis and ischaemia and their association with coronary artery disease, and which were published between 1885 and 1898 and were much in advance of current thought.

The following appraisal of this work is by Dr J. H. Wright who was of great help in preparing this short biography.

> 'In the *Lancet* article of 1887, "Lectures on Fibrous Degeneration and Allied Lesions of the Heart and their Association with Diseases of the Coronary Arteries", Lindsay Steven described perfusion experiments which would appear to confute Cohnheim's statement that coronary arteries are end arteries without significant anastomoses. He also stated clearly the relationship between coronary artery occlusion and cardiac infarction and described minor infarcts occurring as the result of occlusion of small vessels.
>
> 'Acute softening of the myocardium is almost invariably caused by complete or sudden occlusion of the arterial branch supplying the affected area of the heart wall. . . . The size of the area and the liability to subsequent rupture are directly dependent upon the size of the obstructed branch. . . . As a general rule cases of infarction leading to rupture are associated with extensive disease of coronary arteries where, in addition to chronic deterioration of the nutrient supply, a sudden obliteration of the arterial trunk has occurred by thrombosis or embolism.
>
> 'But besides this very serious form of infarction there is also a variety of the affection in which the occluded vessels are small.
>
> 'The possibility of diagnosing fibroid degeneration and infarction of the heart should always be kept in sight and by carefully passing in review the whole symptomatology and pathology of cardiac disease a correct opinion in this regard may probably be arrived at.'!

'Lindsay Steven', writes Dr Wright, 'is an excellent example of what happens when the sand is not yet ready to respond to footprints. He was unfortunate to be ahead of his times'.

Apart from pathology and clinical medicine Steven had an absorbing interest in literature and medical history. He had a fine command of English and edited the *Glasgow Medical Journal* for 11 years. As a postgraduate he visited medical centres in Leipzig, Berlin and Paris and had a sound knowledge of French and German. His Presidential Address to the Glasgow Medico-Chirurgical Society was entitled 'Morgagni to Virchow: an Epoch in the History of Medicine'.

He became a Fellow of the Faculty of Physicians and Surgeons of Glasgow in 1889 and a member of the Council in 1895, and his interest in medical education is illustrated by his appointment as Faculty representative on the General Medical Council in 1903 which he continued to hold until his death and on which he was most active. In 1904 he proposed that the Committee on Examinations and Education 'consider the manner in which the fifth year of the curriculum was being swallowed up by the preliminary scientific studies and suggested alternative methods for dealing with this "undoubted evil".' *Plus ca change. . . .* His paper on 'The Evolution of the Medical Curriculum' of 1907 should also be compulsory reading for all interested in medical education.

He will be most remembered by the Faculty, however, by his occupancy of the post of Honorary Librarian when James Finlayson retired from it in 1901. At that period the writer of his obituary says, 'Dr. Lindsay Steven occupied in Glasgow if not in the whole of Scotland, an almost unique position as a student of the history of medicine'.

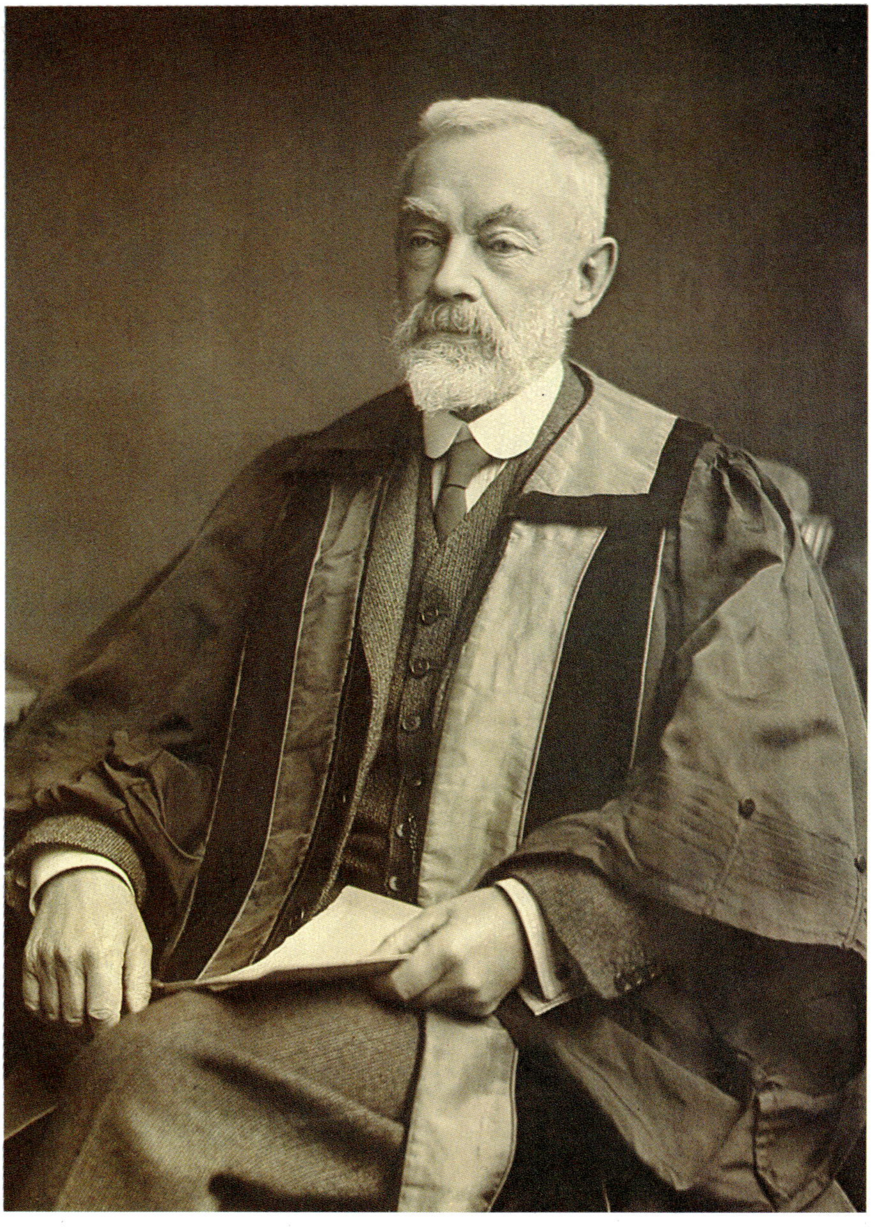

*Ebenezer Henry Lawrence Oliphant (1860 to 1934) was an obstetrician who was also Honorary Librarian of the Royal Faculty from 1919 to 1933 in that period of depression between the Wars when few advances were made.*

# EBENEZER HENRY LAWRENCE OLIPHANT

1860 to 1934

*The portrait is an enlarged framed photograph. In the Royal Faculty minutes of 5th March 1934 (about three months before Oliphant died) it is recorded 'that the Council had pleasure in submitting to the Faculty an enlarged photographic portrait of Dr. E. H. L. Oliphant. This portrait was obtained as a means of thanking Dr. Oliphant for his long and valued services as Honorary Librarian. The Faculty expressed its warm approval and the portrait was instructed to be hung on the walls'. Maybe it was; but by 1979 it was becoming mildewed and tarnished in the basement cellar.*

Dickens in his *Christmas Carol* probably destroyed the name Ebenezer for all time; certainly Oliphant was always known as Lawrence and signed himself E. H. Lawrence Oliphant. He was born in 1860 in Pau on the French slopes of the Pyrenees and spent his early years in France. All his life he continued this French connection, becoming a member of the Rabelais Society in Paris; indeed in 1932 he was invited to give the Watson Lectures and for these he took as his subject 'Rabelais: Physician and Humanist'.

His main education, however, was in Clifton College where one of his contemporaries became Field-Marshal Earl Haig. From Clifton he went to Edinburgh and graduated MB,CM in 1882 and MD in 1886, having spent some time at the medical schools of Paris and Vienna. He came to Glasgow about 1885 as house physician to Samson Gemmell, but already he seems to have been interested in obstetrics as a career and with the help of Dr W. Loudon Reid (*q.v.*), with whom he was closely associated for many years, he obtained a staff appointment at the Royal Maternity Hospital. His promotion there was rapid and he became first an Assistant Obstetric Physician and then a full Obstetric Physician. When he retired from the latter post he became for the rest of his life Honorary Consultant Obstetric Physician to the Hospital. He was Dispensary Physician for Diseases of Women at the Western Infirmary and during the 1914-18 War worked on the staff of the Woodside Red Cross Hospital and acted on the Pensions Board.

Lawrence Oliphant was bilingual, much travelled and an excellent host and companion. He was apparently comfortably well off and little interested in the financial aspects of his work so long as he could maintain a quiet, cultured life style.

He was Honorary Librarian of the Royal Faculty of Physicians and Surgeons of Glasgow from 1919 to 1933. These inter-war years were, for the Faculty, a period of marking time and, in some respects, slow decay. Oliphant wrote a short article in the *Glasgow Medical Journal* in 1928 on the Royal Faculty of Physicians and Surgeons of Glasgow. It is couched in tactful terms but is really meant to show how the Universities, and that of Glasgow in particular, had taken to themselves more and more of undergraduate medical teaching. It begins with the litigation between the Faculty and the University in the early years of the 19th century and comments on the decision of the House of Lords in favour of the Faculty in 1840: 'So ended the second round, but the triumph of the Faculty was short-lived; it had won the war but the Universities won the peace'. At the time of writing, this was becoming increasingly true although the death knell of the Royal Faculty's part in undergraduate education did not come until 1947 after the Goodenough Report was published, and the extra-mural schools were abolished. It may well be true that the Universities have the statutory powers to take over all the functions of the Royal Colleges, but this has not happened. The vast expansion in all branches of medicine, and the need for increasing specialised postgraduate education, has not only infused new vitality into the old Colleges but created new.

Lawrence Oliphant retired about ten years before his death. He devoted himself to his wife during her prolonged illness and when she died never resumed active practice.

# 14

## THE TWENTIETH CENTURY: UP TO AND BETWEEN THE WORLD WARS

George Stevenson Middleton (1853 to 1928)
James Hogarth Pringle (1863 to 1941)
John Freeland Fergus (1865 to 1943)
Archibald Young (1873 to 1939)

By the turn of the 20th century, the Faculty was a strong sturdy pillar of the Victorian professions: a stable teaching and licensing medical institution. Glasgow now had two thriving extra-mural medical schools most of whose students took the 'Triple' qualification, a joint diploma between the Faculty and the Royal Colleges of Surgeons and Physicians of Edinburgh. This brought in revenue not only to the Faculty but to the examiners appointed by the Faculty all of whom were, of course, Fellows. With the aid of Duncan, Weir, Finlayson and others, the Faculty now had one of the best medical libraries in the country. The Tercentenary celebrations of 1899 had been a great success and the then President, Hector Cameron, had been knighted by Queen Victoria.

The Faculty, under the Presidency of Dr John Glaister, petitioned King Edward VII for the privilege of adding the adjective 'Royal' to the Faculty's title, and a special meeting was called on 20th December 1909 to announce that the King had granted this boon, and the Fellows loyally drank his health. Thus encouraged, they had their Armorial Bearings, which they had adopted in 1863, 'matriculated' by the Lord Lyon King of Arms. Dr James Walker Downie arranged for a mace similar to that of the House of Commons to be made by Frank Lutiger of London and presented it to the Royal Faculty.

These tokens of success were celebrated in a Grand Conversazione held on 28th October 1910. It was a great occasion for the Fellows and their ladies and representatives from the Sister Corporations in Edinburgh, and in all 620 people attended an evening of vocal and instrumental music, scientific demonstrations, and the presentation of the new mace by Dr Walker Downie.

This was the zenith of the Faculty as an institution for undergraduate medical teaching. So far, apart from its library developments, it had played little part in postgraduate work; indeed there was little demand for such. But already its old enemy the University was taking from it more and more of its medical students. Paradoxically, the reason was the action of perhaps the greatest of all Scottish educational philanthropists, Andrew Carnegie. Born in Dunfermline in 1835, emigrating to America in 1848, he made a vast fortune there in the expanding steel industries and gave back much of his wealth to Scotland. Two million pounds were handed over in 1901 to trustees who were prepared, virtually on request, to pay the fees of Scottish students at Scottish Universities; so the University flourished at the expense of the extra-mural schools which were not so endowed. In paying their University fees, the Carnegie Trust expected but did not demand that the fees would be repaid after the supported graduate became adequately affluent. It came as a disagreeable surprise that this was not a common facet of the 'sturdy

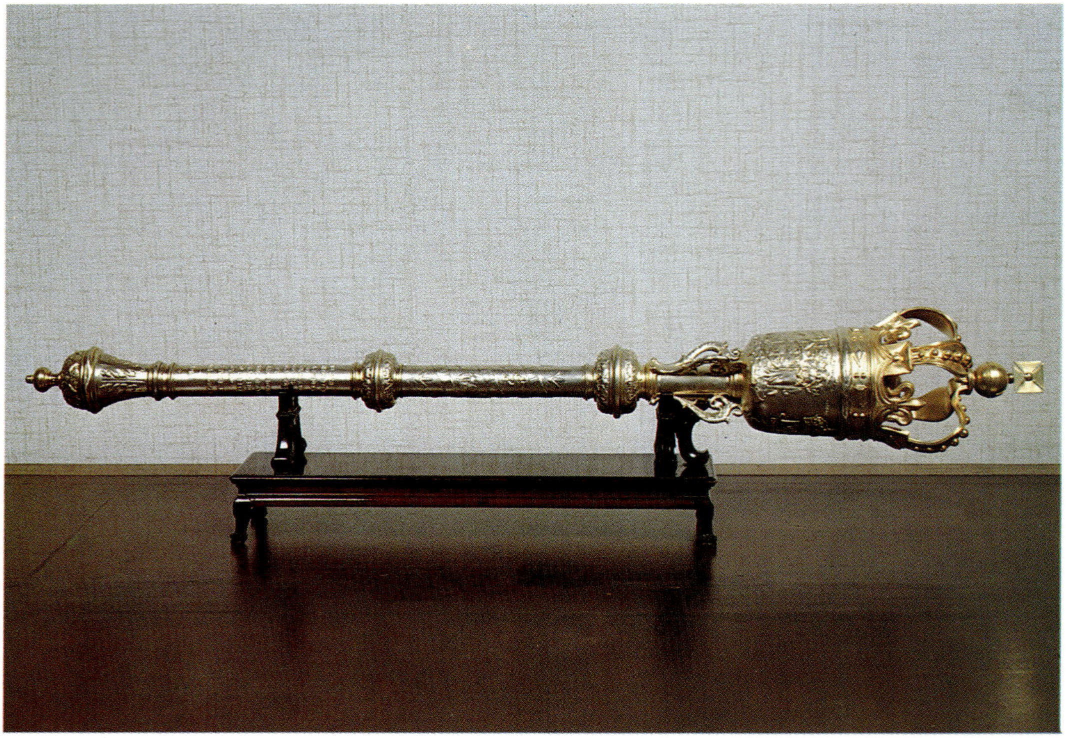

*The Mace laid on the table when the College is in session was made by Frank Lutiger and presented in 1910 by Dr James Walker Downie. It is similar in size, shape and general design to that in the House of Commons.*

independence' of the Scottish student, but there was still enough cash to pay a significant part of student University fees for the next forty years or so.

The students attending the extra-mural schools were now those who, for one reason or another, could not obtain entry into University medical schools and so both quantity and quality declined. More subtly, the status of the Triple Qualification declined; it still allowed its holder to practise medicine but, in open competition for a post, the candidate with the University degree was usually preferred.

Simultaneously the status of the Fellowship of the Faculty was considered to be much lower than that of the Royal Colleges of Physicians or Surgeons. A Fellow of the Faculty, even the 'Royal' Faculty, seemed to be neither a specialist surgeon nor a specialist physician; it was not until 1939 that the General Medical Council permitted the addition of the '(S)' or '(P)' after the letters of their degree to signify their qualification *qua* surgeon or *qua* physician. Meanwhile there are four subjects of our portraits of this era who, if they did not altogether halt the downwards slide of the Royal Faculty's place in medical education, kept up the standards of the Glasgow Medical School.

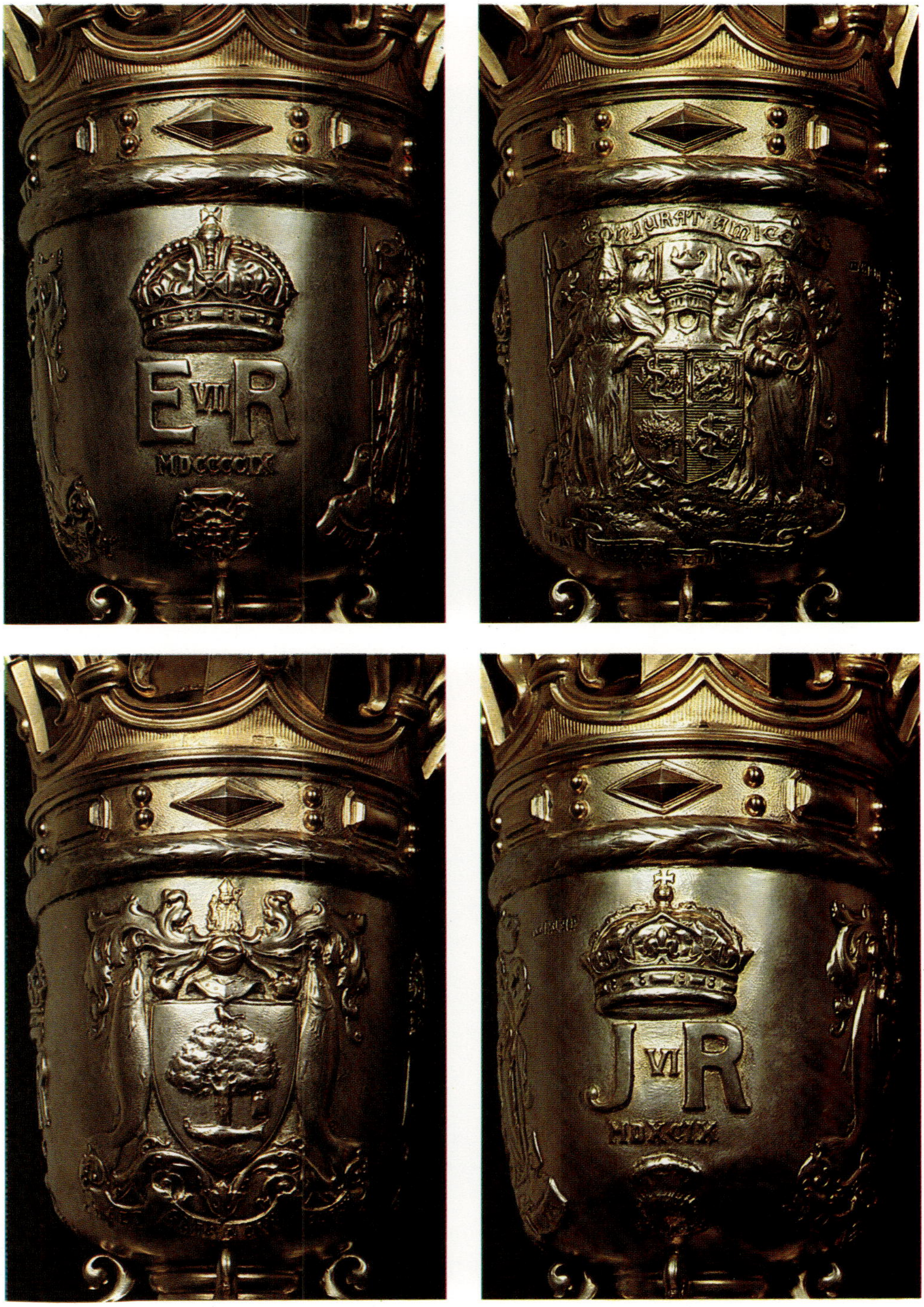


*The four faces of the Mace to show the various emblems.*

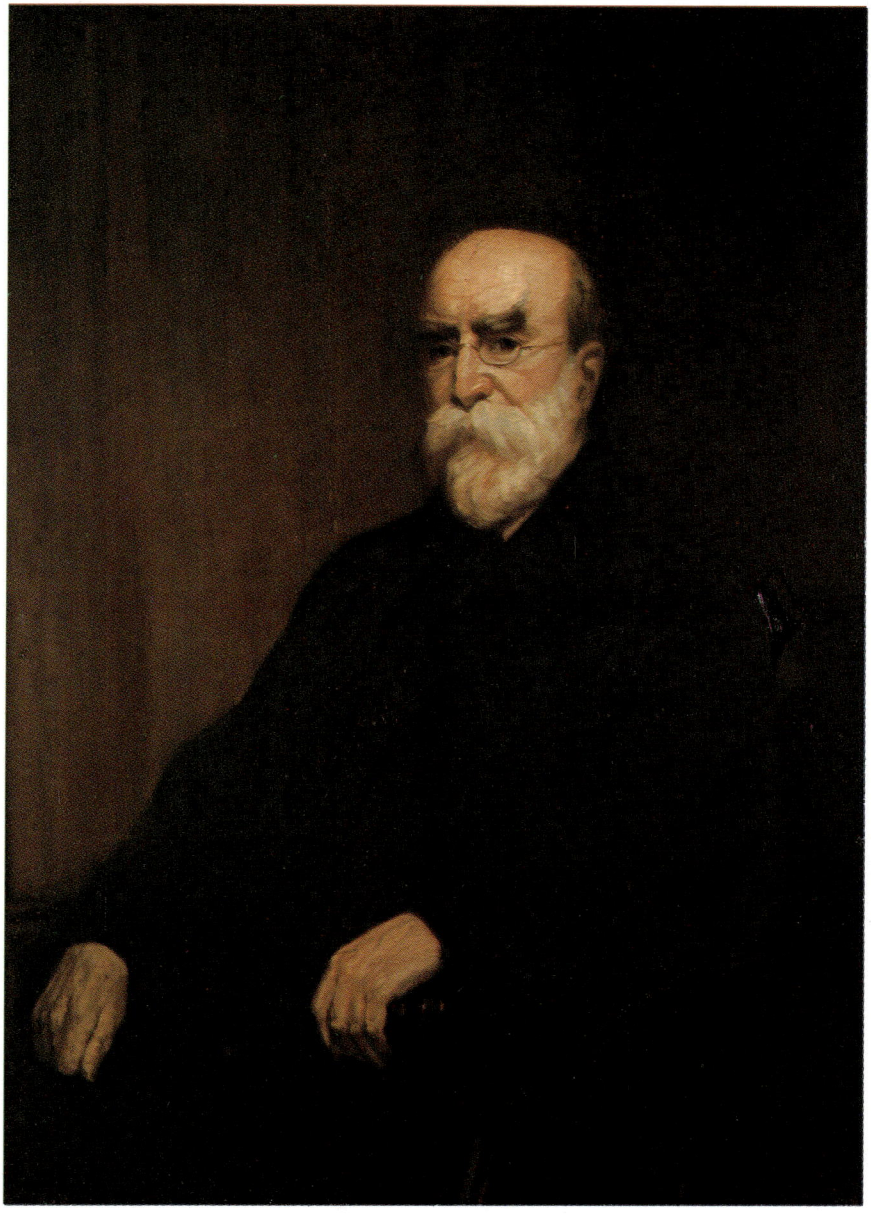

*George Stevenson Middleton (1853 to 1928) was a physician and noted clinical teacher in Glasgow Royal Infirmary. The portrait is by J. Raeburn Middleton. The Royal Faculty made him an Honorary Fellow in 1926.*

# GEORGE STEVENSON MIDDLETON

1853 to 1928

*The following extract is taken from the minutes of the Royal Faculty of 8th April 1929.*

132 West Regent Street
Glasgow C.2. 25th March 1929.

The President,
Royal Faculty of Physicians and Surgeons,
Glasgow.

Dear Sir,

I have been requested by a few Fellows of the Faculty who were all intimate friends of the late Dr. George S. Middleton, but desire to remain anonymous to forward for acceptance by the Royal Faculty the accompanying portrait of their distinguished Honorary Fellow which I executed some five years ago and which I have now much pleasure in doing.

Yours faithfully

*(Signed)* J. Raeburn Middleton.

*The Secretary was then instructed to intimate to Mr J. Raeburn Middleton and to ask him to convey to the donors their cordial thanks for this much appreciated addition to the collection of portraits of Fellows of Faculty.*

George Stevenson Middleton was born in Aberdeen and received his schooling in Aberdeen Grammar School. He started in the Arts Faculty in the University there, but then his father died and the rest of his family moved to Glasgow where his elder brother was an engineer. George, however, by dint of his own efforts, such as tutoring in the evenings, managed to continue his Arts Course in Aberdeen and graduated MA with honours in 1873. He then followed his family to Glasgow, decided to take up medicine and graduated MB,CM, again with honours, in 1876.

Like others who have achieved fame in medicine, he showed early promise and within two years of graduation was invited to become University Assistant in Medicine to Professor (later Sir) William Tennant Gairdner; and he worked with Gairdner for 13 years laying the foundation of his later abilities as an outstanding clinical teacher. In 1892 he was appointed Visiting Physician to Glasgow Royal Infirmary and there, until his retirement at the age limit of sixty in 1913, his teaching of clinical medicine was so acceptable to successive generations of students, that those who had later qualified and were in practice locally persuaded him to conduct a teaching ward round on Sunday mornings. One of his obituarists states: 'it was this class which inaugurated post-graduate teaching in Glasgow'.

He did not write much. His thesis for the MD degree which he obtained with honours in 1884 was on the pathology of pseudo-hypertrophic muscular paralysis, and his interest in pathology is also evident in a paper on 'Vascular Lesions in Hydrophobia' which appeared in the *Journal of Anatomy* in 1880. He had an aversion to premature publication; otherwise he might be known as the discoverer of rat-bite fever. In 1895 a little girl with a history of having been bitten by a rat came under his care with a fever recurring every five to seven days. Since nothing else was found to account for it, Middleton spoke of her case as one of rat-bite fever, but it was some years before the entity was established elsewhere.

In 1906 he succeeded James Finlayson as Visiting Physician to the Royal Hospital for Sick Children. Specialisation was still slow in spreading and the distinction had yet to be drawn between the general and the paediatric physician. Later both he and Sir Hector C. Cameron were to be Vice-Presidents of the Board of the Royal Hospital for Sick Children. In 1914, now 61 years old, he was mobilised with the rank of Lieutenant-Colonel in the RAMC and given charge of medical wards in the 4th Scottish General Hospital at Stobhill where he worked unremittingly until 1919.

'Old George was the hairiest man I ever saw, except for his bald head', wrote O. H. Mavor. 'Hair luxuriated from every other square inch of his face and overhung his steel spectacles. He wore a little black alpaca jacket and carried an old wooden stethoscope. He talked in a high-pitched, testy, old man's voice and kept strictly to the point'. Others speak of his shy and retiring disposition, and it is reported that 'he had his aversions, but though he avoided some of his fellows, he never brawled'. All write of his sympathy and kindness to his friends.

George Middleton became President of the Association of Physicians of Great Britain and Ireland in 1912 when the Association visited Glasgow. He was the representative of the Royal Faculty of Physicians and Surgeons of Glasgow on the Boards of the Royal Technical College and the Royal Samaritan Hospital and, for the last ten years of his life, was an Assessor to Glasgow University Court. The University had previously, in 1915, conferred on him the honorary degree of LLD.

George Stevenson Middleton was made an Honorary Fellow of the Royal Faculty of Physicians and Surgeons of Glasgow in 1926.



o

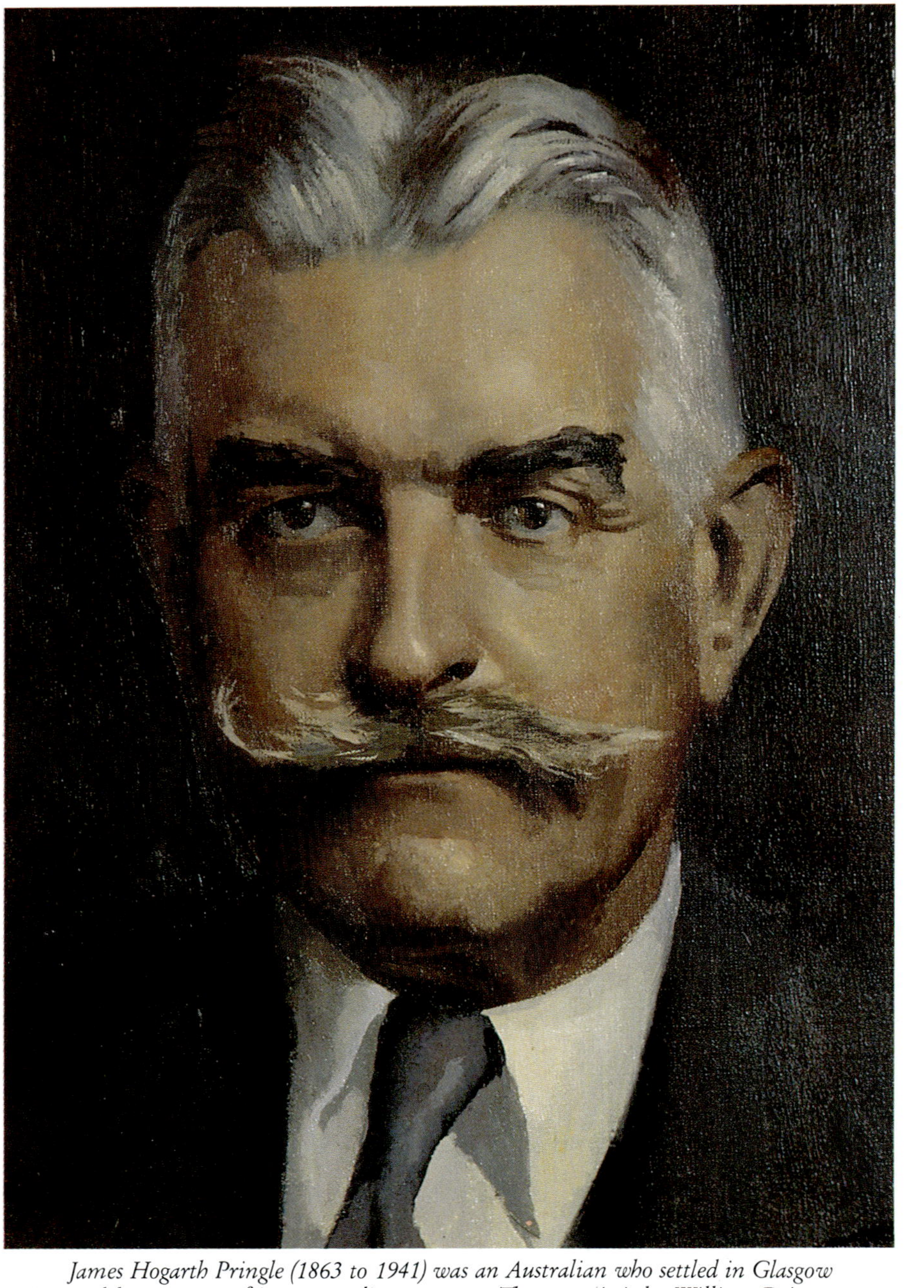

*James Hogarth Pringle (1863 to 1941) was an Australian who settled in Glasgow and became one of its outstanding surgeons. The portrait is by William Dring. He was Visitor from 1923 to 1924.*

# JAMES HOGARTH PRINGLE

## 1863 to 1941

*The portrait by William Dring appears to have been painted when Pringle was in his forties. A photograph when much older was published in his obituaries and still shows the asymmetrical twirl of his moustache.*

James Hogarth Pringle was born in Parramatta, New South Wales, the son of a well-known Sydney surgeon, George Hogarth Pringle. The family appears to have been wealthy and James seems never to have wanted for money; even when a successful surgeon he spent most of his days in his wards and was little interested in private practice. He was sent first to Sedbergh for his schooling and then to Edinburgh University where he graduated in Medicine in 1885. After house surgeon posts in Edinburgh, Glasgow and London he made a European Grand Tour and studied further in Berlin, Vienna and Heidelberg. He was back in Glasgow by 1888 assisting William Macewen with his pathological studies and his surgical work. In the same year he took his Membership of the Royal College of Surgeons of England and became a Fellow there in 1892. In 1896 he was appointed Surgeon to Glasgow Royal Infirmary, a post which he held until his retirement in 1923. In 1899, the year of its Tercentenary, he became a Fellow of the Faculty of Physicians and Surgeons of Glasgow.

Pringle's whole life revolved around surgery. He was an original member of the British Association of Surgeons, and a co-member of the Chirurgical Club with Moynihan, Robert Jones and Stiles. He was a dexterous operator and, as his writings show, made a point of following up his patients for many years after most surgeons would have dismissed them.

His writings ranged over a wide spectrum of surgery: vein grafts to bridge arterial aneurysms and maintain limb circulation; animal urethral grafts to replace strictures; percussion as an aid to diagnosis of skull fractures; the radical cure of hernia. His paper in the *Annals of Surgery* of 1908, on the arrest of haemorrhage from an injured liver, is mainly concerned with deep sutures to close the wound, but it also includes what has

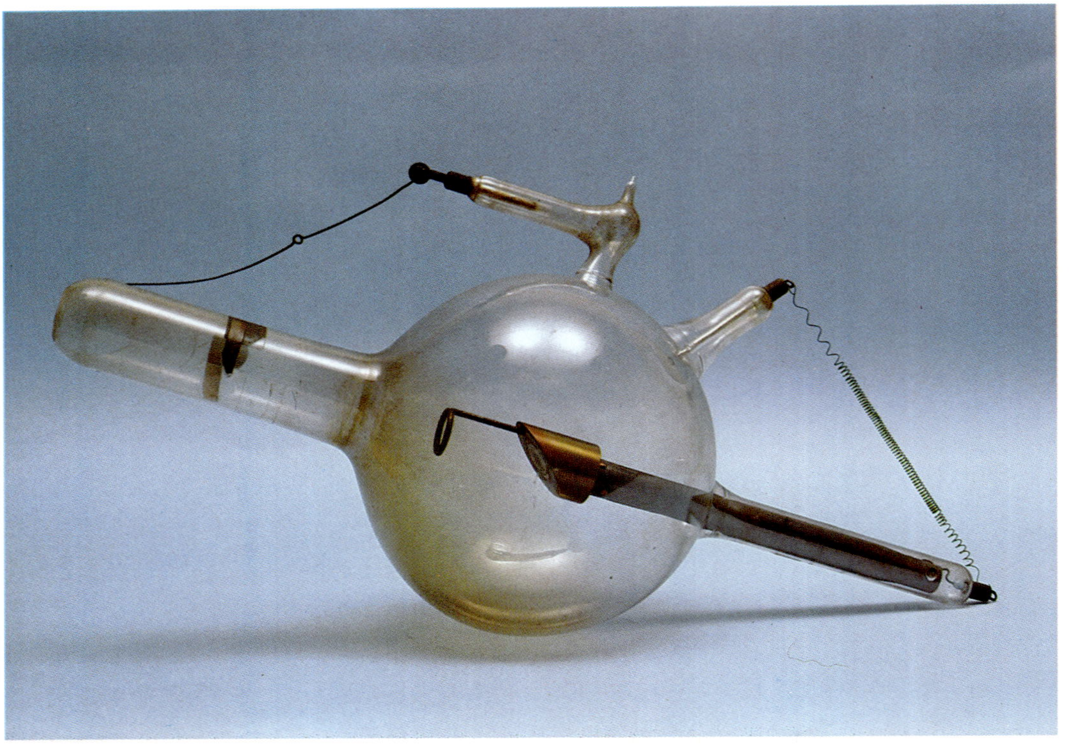

*One of the earliest x-ray tubes. The very first were blown by the investigators themselves and have been broken long since. This probably dates from around the turn of the 19th/20th centuries and enabled accurate reduction of fractures to be carried out for the first time.*

come to be called 'Pringle's manoeuvre': stopping bleeding from the liver by compressing the hepatic artery and the portal vein by a finger and thumb around the foramen of Winslow.

Two other publications are particularly memorable: his textbook on fractures and his extraordinary experiences with malignant melanomas.

His *Fractures and their Treatment* appeared in 1910. It will be recalled that Röntgen discovered x-rays in 1895, but it was some time before reliable routine films of fractures were available. Pringle's book was one of the first to be based on treatment with radiological control and was also notable because Pringle treated his fractures himself; elsewhere they were usually left to the house surgeon. A proportion of the medical profession always resists any change, and so it was with fractures and x-rays. A reviewer writes about the 'conflict of opinion that still rages furiously as to the indispensability of exact existing mechanical form for perfect service of mechanical requirements in the skeleton'. But the 384 pages of his book are full of commonsense and did much to place the treatment of fractures on a sound basis.

His paper on melanoma which he gave to the Glasgow Medico-Chirurgical Society in 1937 was so astounding that it coloured surgical thought on the subject for some years.

In his whole career he says: 'I only saw 3 patients with melanoma'. The first was an old man with a primary near the elbow, large axillary metastases, and many satellite tumours along the lymphatics leading from the primary; the lesion was inoperable and the patient died. The next was a girl with a similarly situated lesion in the flexure of her elbow and enlarged axillary nodes. Pringle excised the primary with a wide strip of lymphatic bearing subcutaneous tissue up to the axilla and the axillary nodes. The patient went to Canada but was still sending him Christmas cards to say she was alive and well 38 years later. His third patient was equally remarkable. A man aged thirty had a primary just above the medial condyle of the left femur and enlarged nodes in Scarpa's triangle and the left iliac fossa. Pringle excised a 'good margin of skin' with the primary and a strip of subcutaneous tissue, deep fascia and muscle fascia 2½ inches wide between the primary and the metastases which he cleared out as far as the iliac bifurcation. At the Medico-Chirurgical Society meeting he was able to produce not only the specimen which had been stored in the Pathology Museum of the Glasgow Royal Infirmary, but the patient himself alive and free of recurrence 30 years after the excision.

This method of Pringle became routine treatment for some time. The wide undermining of the skin to remove the lymphatic-carrying subcutaneous strip led inevitably to skin necrosis, and the cases were referred to plastic surgeons for excision of a strip of subcutaneous tissue with the overlying skin and immediate skin grafting. The increasing use of lymphangiography, however, showed that the lymphatic drainage was not so simple as Pringle had envisaged and for this and other reasons the method was later given up.

James Hogarth Pringle was Visitor of the Royal Faculty of Physicians and Surgeons of Glasgow from 1923 to 1924, when he resigned because of a wish to travel to his native land of Australia. For this reason he never became President.

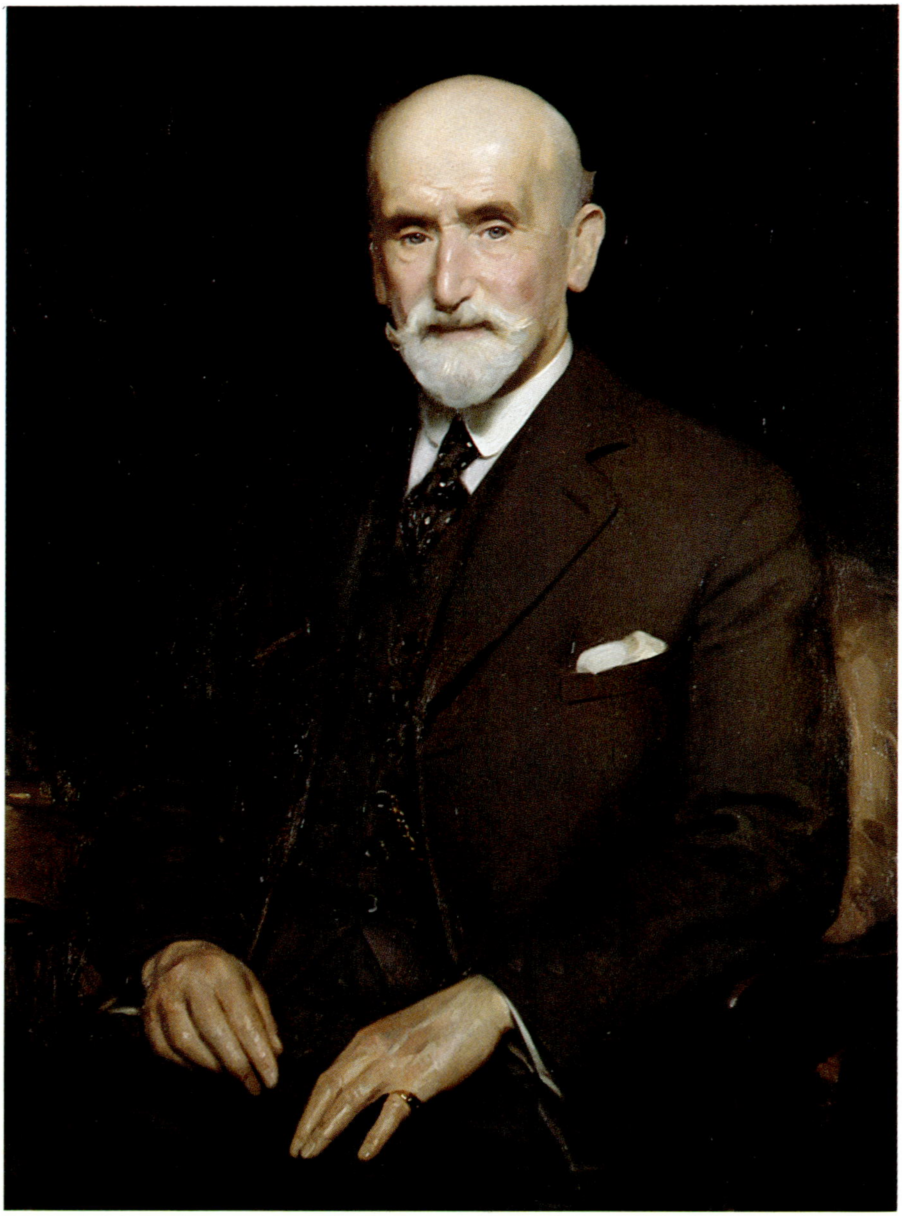

*John Freeland Fergus (1865 to 1943) was a respected clinical teacher in medicine in Glasgow Royal Infirmary, a medical historian, and a poet. His portrait is by Andrew Law.*

*He was President from 1929 to 1931.*

# JOHN FREELAND FERGUS

1865 to 1943

*The portrait is by Andrew Law and was presented to the Royal Faculty by Dr Fergus' widow in 1946.*

The father of John F. Fergus was Andrew Fergus who was President from 1883 to 1886, while John's elder brother, also Andrew (*q.v.*), was President from 1918 to 1921. Both Andrew and John had the middle name Freeland, which Andrew always used in full to distinguish himself from his father, while John either omitted it or abbreviated it to a simple 'F'.

John Fergus was born in Glasgow and was educated at the High School and Glasgow University where he graduated MA in 1883, MB,CM in 1888 and MD in 1897. After graduating he studied in Jena and Vienna and thereafter his professional life was spent in practice as a physician attached latterly to Glasgow Royal Infirmary. He became a much loved family physician, and was a competent clinical teacher, and is remembered mostly on three counts: as a good committee man, as a medical historian and as a poet.

Throughout his professional life he played an active part in medical affairs. He represented the Royal Faculty on the boards of several institutions; he was a Manager of the Royal Infirmary and for several years Convener of its Medical Committee; he was also a member of the Board of the Royal Technical College and a number of smaller institutions such as the Broomhill Home for Incurables. He was particularly proud of his appointment as Assessor to Glasgow University Court, which he continued to hold until he was 74 years old.

His medical historical writings include *Short Sketch of the History of Early Medicine*, *Some medicines of our Ancestors*, *The Medical School of Salerno* and *The Glasgow Hospitals of a Century Ago*, and these prose writings reflect the sensuous feeling for words which is found in his poetry. Some of his poems were written for after-dinner speeches or similar occasions, and are little more than kindly humorous versifications, but others show great depth of feeling.

To one who spent some of his early boyhood in a box bed in a kitchen, lulled to sleep by a dying fire, there is a rich nostalgia about:

THE LUM
*(A wean's night thoughts)*

Bogles come
Doon the lum.
Santa Claus
Brings geegaws
Doon the lum.
The wind howls,
Growls, prowls
Roon' the lum.
The fire roars,
Snores, pours
Up the lum.
The reek swirls,
Dirls, twirls
Up the lum.
The sparks flee
Past the swee,
Faur on hie,
Up the lum.

The cauld mune
Faur abune,
Keeks, sneaks
Doon the lum.
A wee staur,
Awa' faur,
Blinks, jinks,
Doon the lum.
Will the De'il
Wi' a squeal
Come for me,
Sma' and wee
When I dee,
Doon the lum?
Or will I flee
Wi' God to be,
Faur on hie
Up the lum?

For an amateur poet he was fortunate in having most of his verses published in *Fancies of a Physician* (Glasgow; Brown, Son & Ferguson, 1938). Some are in English, some in Scots and his interest in medical history spills over into some of his poems. Two of the longer are addressed to Maister Peter Lowe; then there is 'The Auld Parish Doctor', 'The Gold-heided Cane' and several others. The book is still readily available and it is a continuing pleasure to dip into its contents.

John Fergus was President of the Royal Faculty of Physicians and Surgeons of Glasgow from 1929 to 1931 and the last poem in his book will serve as epitaph.

Carry me forth and let me lie
With my dying face to a northern sky
Where the scent of the heather, the sound of the bees,
The falling of water, the rustle of trees,
The whisper of winds, blowing soft on the bent,
The fragrance of pine trees and bog myrtle's scent,
The mavis's song and the whaup's plaintive cry
Shall be lullaby, incense and dirge as I die.

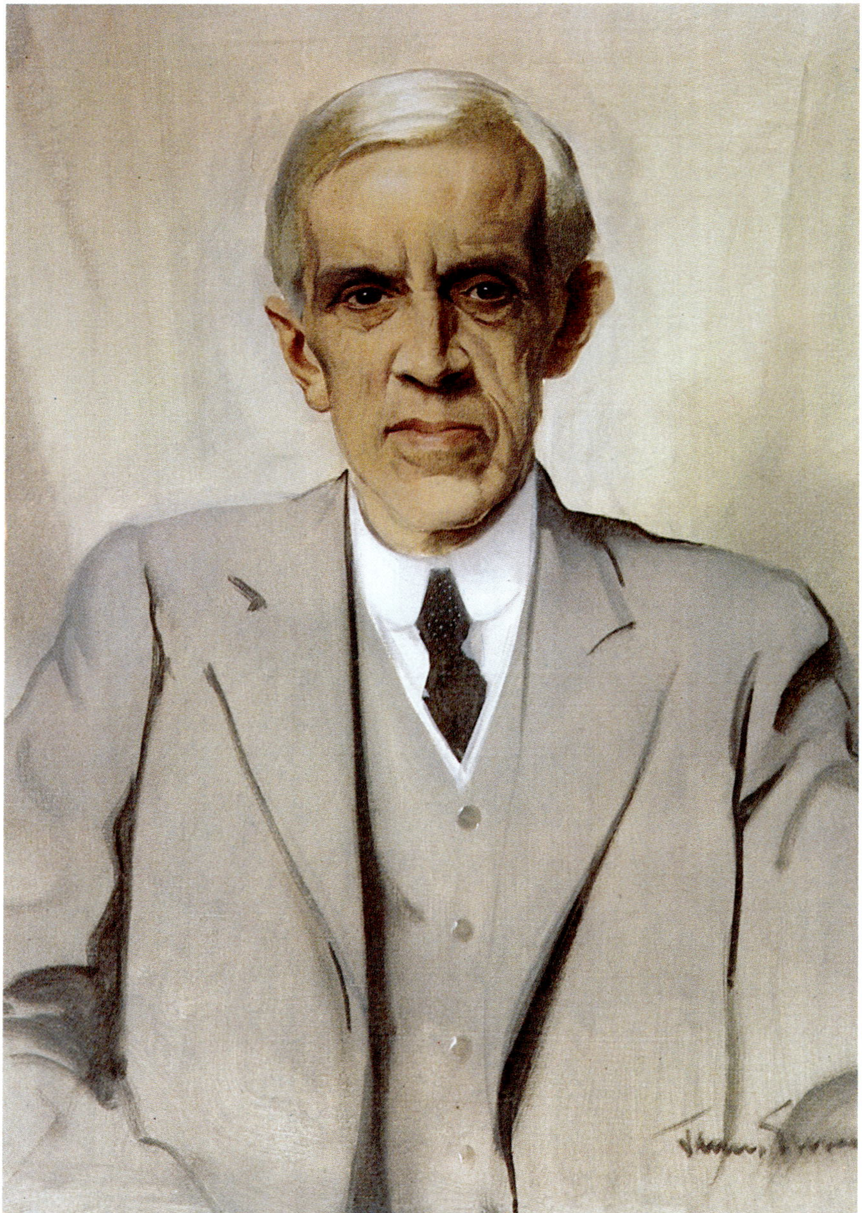

*Archibald Young (1873 to 1939) succeeded Sir William Macewen in the Regius Chair of Surgery in 1924 and added much to the renown of that Chair. The portrait is by James Gunn.*

*He was President from 1935 to 1937.*

# ARCHIBALD YOUNG

1873 to 1939

*Commissioned by, and subscribed to, by many friends and colleagues, a portrait of Archibald Young by James Gunn was presented to him at a Ceremony in Glasgow University only six days before he died in July 1939. That portrait hangs in the Hunter Hall in Glasgow University. A second portrait for Professor Young's family was undertaken by James Gunn from sketches he had made when preparing the first version. After the death of Professor Young's widow in 1966, his sons Archibald and Stuart, both Fellows of the Royal College, presented this second portrait to the College.*

Archie Young was born in Glasgow, educated at its High School and University, and qualified BSc in 1893 and MB,CM with high commendation in 1895. With surgery much in mind he continued his studies in Berlin, Breslau and Heidelberg, and returned to Glasgow to assistantships with Joseph Coats in Pathology, and Sir William Macewen in Surgery in 1898. Thereafter his career developed in the Western Infirmary from the lowliest surgical post to the highest:

1903 Extra Dispensary Surgeon;
1905 Dispensary Surgeon;
1912 Assistant Surgeon;
1913 Fellow of the Royal Faculty of Physicians and Surgeons of Glasgow;
1913 Professor of Surgery at the Anderson College of Medicine;
1917 Visiting Surgeon to the Western Infirmary, The Broadstone Jubilee Hospital in Port Glasgow and the Govan Parish Council Hospitals;
1924 Regius Professor of Surgery of Glasgow University.

He served in two wars. In the Boer War he acted as Civil Surgeon to No. 3 General Hospital at Kroonstad and was recognised there for his work on peripheral nerve injuries. Because of this he served with the rank of Major as a neurological expert in cases suffering from such injuries at No. 4 Scottish General Hospital during the 1914-1918 War.

He wrote much. His experiences with peripheral nerve injuries were published in the official surgical report of the War and read to the International Congress of Surgery in 1923. He was an exponent of the open reduction and fixation of fractures and the use of full thickness skin grafts even on granulating wounds. His pioneering work on the surgery of the autonomic nervous system was well known, particularly in the treatment of causalgia, and this interest culminated in his last publication in 1939, the translation of the book by his great friend Rene Leriche of Strasbourg, *The Surgery of Pain*.

He received wide recognition and many honours at home and abroad. He was invited to the United States in 1926 to deliver the Murphy Oration and chose as his subject 'Sir William Macewen and the Glasgow School of Surgery'. While in the States he received honorary fellowships from the American College of Surgeons, the American Surgical Association and the Academy of Surgery of Philadelphia. In Europe he was elected a Member of the Royal Academy of Physicians in Rome, an Honorary Member of the French Academy of Surgery and an MD of Strasbourg University. At home the City of Glasgow created him a Deputy Lieutenant and a Justice of the Peace. He was President of the Association of Surgeons of Great Britain and Ireland when their annual meeting was held in Glasgow in 1927.

The present writer was an intensive student with Professor Young, and his house surgeon at the time of his death. Although he was often absent from ill health, the memory remains of the firm but kindly man in the grey suit with its cut-away coat, of his dexterity as an operator although his hands were damaged by early over-exposure to irradiation, of his late evening visits to see the patients he had operated on that morning, and of the sound basis of his surgical teaching.

Archibald Young was President of the Royal Faculty of Physicians and Surgeons of Glasgow from 1935 to 1937.

# 15

## THE TURN OF THE EBB

Roy Frew Young (1879 to 1948)
Archibald Lamont Goodall (1915 to 1963)

During the first forty years or so of the 20th century, the Faculty's influence in medical training slowly decreased. The impact on the extra-mural schools of Andrew Carnegie's beneficence in paying the fees of Scottish students at Scottish Universities has already been referred to. The number of students attending the extra-mural schools was further diminished as medical schools opened in such new Universities as Birmingham, Bristol, Leeds, Liverpool, Manchester, Sheffield and Wales.

The 1914-1918 War took its toll of Fellows, and the post-war years with their economic depression and industrial and social unrest did little to encourage even an inclination for expansion and forward thinking in the Royal Faculty's affairs. Immediately after the War the standard of the entrance examination had been lowered, and although this was later tightened, the Faculty began to acquire the reputation of being an institution inferior to any of the Royal Colleges. It became known locally as 'The Chum Club' and nationally was slightingly referred to as the 'Photographic Society' from its initials. The main incentive to becoming a Fellow seemed to be the possibility of becoming an examiner and earning some fees from the few students still presenting themselves for the 'Triple' or the Fellowship. In these days before the salaried Health Service, every little counted.

By the late 1930s, the Fellowship of the Faculty was regarded, even in the Glasgow area, as barely adequate qualification for a hospital appointment, and young graduates wishing to specialise either took an MD or ChM degree, or went to Edinburgh or London for a Royal College Membership or Fellowship; outside of Glasgow such a degree was a *sine qua non* for a hospital appointment.

The subjects of the next two portraits did much to turn the tide. Roy Young recognised and defined the problem of the lowered status of the Fellowship and began the long struggle to give it equal standing with those of the Royal Colleges. Archie Goodall helped in many different ways to set the Royal Faculty on the road to its present status as a Royal College with a reputation second to none and in some respects unique.

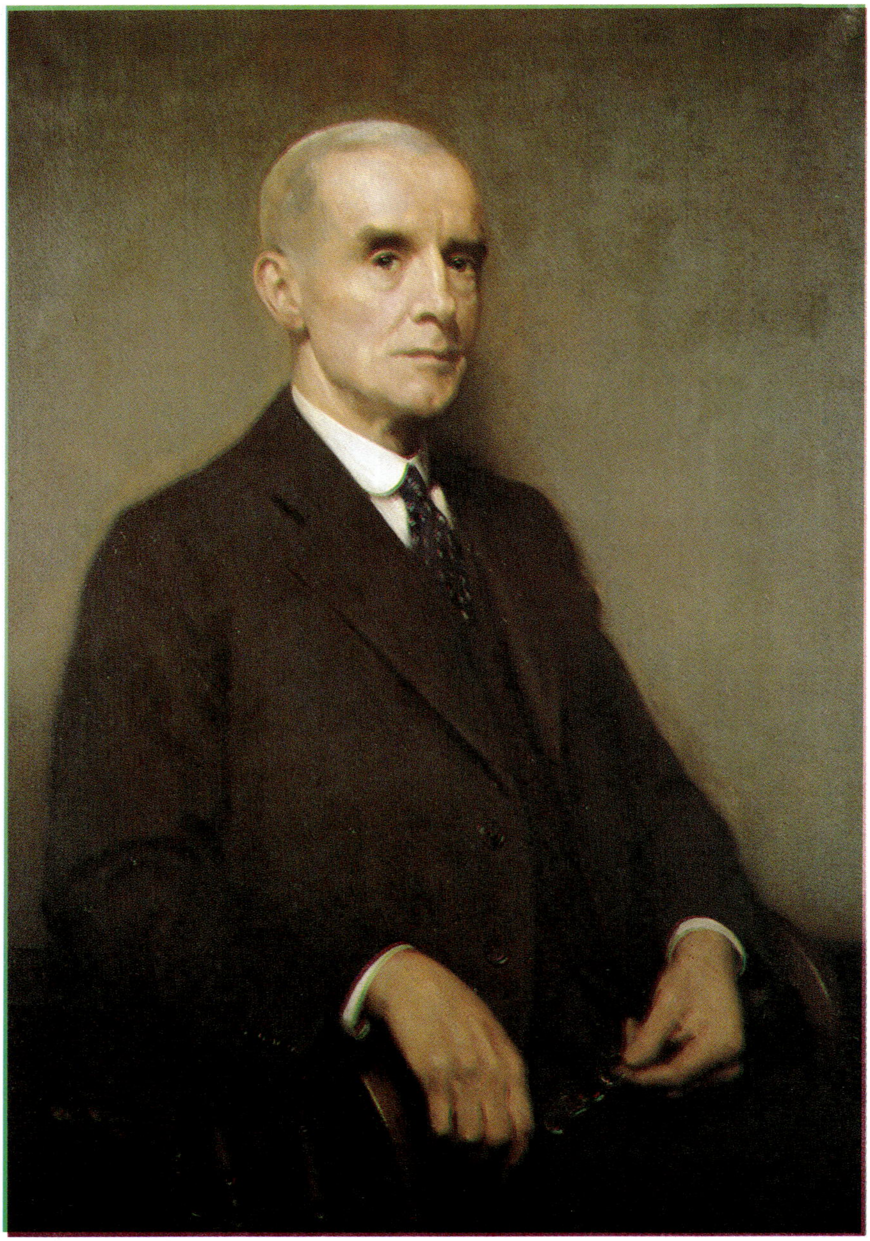

*Roy Frew Young (1879 to 1948) was a general surgeon in Glasgow Western Infirmary where he was widely respected as a clinical teacher. During his presidency he began the rise in status of the Fellowship examinations. The portrait is by Andrew Law.*

*He was President from 1940 to 1942.*

# ROY FREW YOUNG

1879 to 1948

*Following Roy Young's death, Geoffrey Jefferson, who had been his great friend since the days of World War I, wrote an appreciation in the* Glasgow Medical Journal. Inter alia, *he wrote: 'The two events which gave him the greatest pleasure that he ever experienced came towards the end of his life—his honorary degree* and the presentation of his portrait. He told me how the approach for the latter had to be made through his wife (whose death affected him so much) because his admirers feared that he would have kicked them downstairs if they had come to him direct. "I probably would have done", he added. And yet once the ice was broken he was, as everyone knew he would be, immensely grateful for this very considerable mark not only of respect but of gratitude'.*

*The portrait by Andrew Law was commissioned by those who had been his house surgeons and assistants and was bequeathed to the Royal Faculty in Roy Young's will.*

Roy Young was educated at Glasgow Academy and Sedbergh and then took the medical course combined at Cambridge and Glasgow University, graduating BA and MB,BCh in 1909. He was set on surgery as a career and, apart from the 1914 to 1918 War years, spent his professional life in Glasgow Western Infirmary. Soon after graduating he became an extra-dispensary surgeon and then, in turn, dispensary surgeon, assistant surgeon, visiting surgeon and finally, when he retired at age 65, honorary consulting surgeon. He was also associated as a consultant surgeon with the Vale of Leven Hospital, Bellahouston Hospital and the Royal Alexandra Infirmary in Paisley.

* LLD, Glasgow University.

During the 1914 to 1918 War he served with the RAMC in France, latterly as a surgical specialist with No. 14 General Hospital, and he was awarded the MC and was twice mentioned in dispatches. On his return to civilian life he quickly became known as an excellent clinical teacher, a surgeon intensely interested in his patients whose operation to him was but a part of their overall treatment, and a man who was beloved and respected not only by his patients but by his medical and nursing colleagues. He served on many committees and is particularly remembered for his work on the Boards of Management of the Western Infirmary and the Royal Cancer Hospital.

Roy Young became President of the Royal Faculty of Physicians and Surgeons of Glasgow in November 1940 and during his two years in office there occurred three most important events in the institution's history:

> The Royal Faculty realised how low the status of its Fellowship had become and started to raise it;
>
> The death throes of the extra-mural schools began;
>
> The importance of the Royal Faculty as a post-graduate rather than an undergraduate teaching centre began to be realised.

In his *Memorials of the Faculty*, Duncan noted how seldom was there any mention in the minutes of what was happening in the outside world. Roy Young was President during two of the darkest war years but when the war is mentioned at all in the Faculty minutes, it is nearly always in the phrase 'after the war'. There was never the slightest implication that anything other than complete victory would ultimately be achieved and plans were being made for it.

*The Fellowship.* There had of course been previous disquiet about the Royal Faculty's Fellowship but Roy Young took early action and already by the College Meeting of 3rd March 1941, a Memorandum which had been prepared by the Council was submitted to the Faculty with the proposal to send it to the Chairman and Secretaries of the 11 biggest hospitals in Glasgow. It created much discussion and was sent back to Council for further consideration and amendment. A final version, however, was approved by the Faculty on 5th May 1941 and sent to the hospitals. Here is most of it:

> 'At the present time when there is taking place considerable discussion regarding the future of hospital practice the Council of the Royal Faculty of Physicians and Surgeons of Glasgow has been considering the relations of the Faculty with the hospitals of the West of Scotland.
>
> 'In England and elsewhere it is an established rule that any candidate for a senior appointment to the medical or surgical staff of any of the teaching or other large hospitals must hold the Higher Qualification of one of the Royal Colleges of Physicians or Surgeons.
>
> 'In Glasgow prior to 1914 few senior appointments in our teaching infirmaries

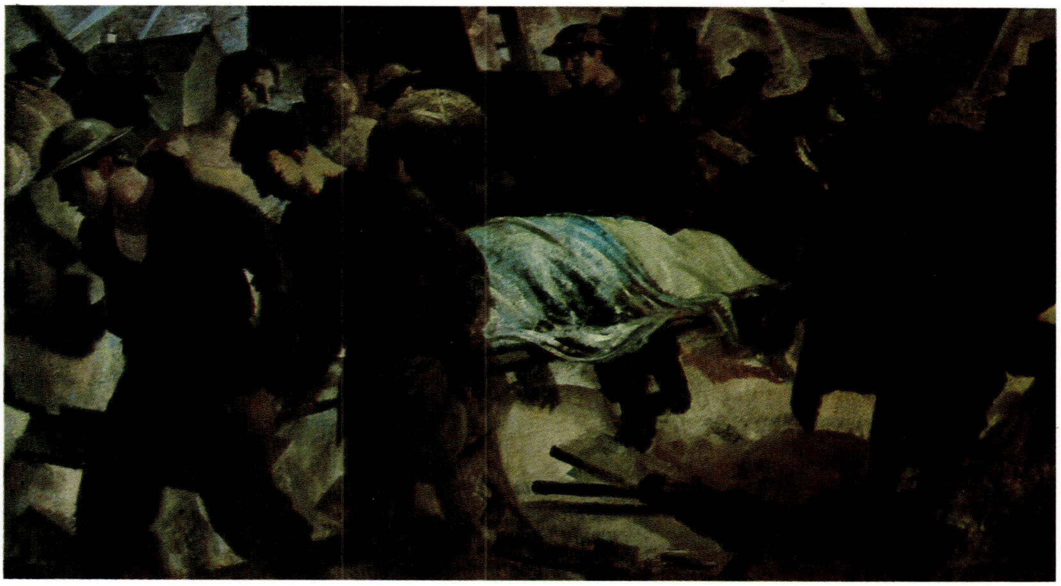

'STRETCHER-BEARERS, CLYDEBANK, 1941'
*by Hugh Adam Crawford RSA (1898 to 1982)*

*The 'blitz' on Clydebank was the worst bombardment suffered in the Glasgow area. This painting, made there at that time, was exhibited in the Royal Academy in 1942, and acclaimed by critics 'the picture of the year'.*

were held except by those who were Fellows of the Royal Faculty of Physicians and Surgeons of Glasgow which for nearly three hundred and fifty years has been closely associated with the development of the voluntary hospitals. Since the last war, this policy, for various reasons, has been allowed to lapse.

'It is of obvious advantage to our infirmaries that the senior medical and surgical posts should be held by men who, in taking a Higher Qualification, have proved both their interest and ability in medicine or surgery. This would also be of great benefit to the younger men in encouraging them to reach a higher standard of work in preparing for the Fellowship Examination. Such a procedure then would be of material benefit to our infirmaries and their medical staffs.

'In view of these considerations it is suggested that for the posts of assistant physician and assistant surgeon or for equivalent appointments special attention should be paid by Selection Boards to the possession by the candidates of the Fellowship of the Royal Faculty of Physicians and Surgeons of Glasgow'.

On the motion of the President, seconded by the Visitor, the Report by the Council was approved—Mr James Russell dissenting—and it was remitted to the Council to deal with the matter.

Although there were dissenters, particularly those who were in favour of the higher

University qualifications of MD and ChM rather than the Fellowship, the President reported at the Annual General Meeting in November 1941:

> 'The Fellowship has been almost continuously the subject of anxious consideration of the Council during the past year. There was a good deal of severe criticism, especially from Fellows resident in England, about the neglect of the Faculty to insist upon the importance of the Fellowship for appointments, particularly in Glasgow. The fact that the possession of the Fellowship was not an essential condition of Hospital appointments and especially of the Visiting Surgeons and Physicians in the Glasgow Hospitals was severely animadverted upon as giving rise to the belief outside Glasgow that the Fellowship must be an inferior qualification. Whatever grounds there may have been at one time for such an impression have long disappeared. The Examination for the Fellowship is a really stiff one and those who do not attain a high standard do not receive it. The qualifications of those who receive the Fellowship without examination have to be of an unquestionably high character. A memorandum stressing the importance of candidates for posts as physician or surgeon, or assistant physician or assistant surgeon in the teaching hospitals in Glasgow holding the Fellowship or other higher qualification was addressed to the various hospitals concerned. The replies received from the Governors of the Hospitals indicated that the representations of the Faculty will receive due consideration.'

One year later when he demitted office at the Annual General Meeting in November 1942, he was able to report, 'We have now had assurances from practically all the hospitals that the possession of the Glasgow Fellowship in Medicine or in Surgery will be expected of all those who hold the more senior appointments'.

The struggle to obtain national recognition of the equivalent status of the Fellowships of the Royal Faculty and those of the Royal Colleges took some years but a good start had been made.

*The Goodenough Committee, the extra-mural schools and post-graduate education.* In June 1942, the Royal Faculty received a letter from the Ministry of Health informing them of the setting up of an 'Inter-departmental Committee on Medical Schools' under the chairmanship of Mr W. M. Goodenough, DL, JP, and asking for the Faculty's cooperation in giving evidence to the Committee 'for the future development of medical education and the health services of the country and of the need for the Government to be in a position to take action as soon as the war is over'.

The Goodenough Committee had wide terms of reference and its report was the basis for much of the Acts of 1946 and 1947. Only two items concern us here:

*A.* 'The desirability or otherwise of all medical students being required to obtain a University degree as the sole or as one of the qualifications for registration. (The Committee would be glad if in the consideration of this question regard could be made to the effect on the Scottish Triple Qualification and the extra-mural medical schools in Scotland)'.

The Royal Faculty resisted, but the extra-mural schools had little future and closed in 1947. At the same time the 'Triple' was retained as a registrable medical qualification and is still in use today, particularly for overseas graduates wishing to settle in practice in Britain.

*B.* 'The training of physicians and surgeons of consultant status likely to be needed after the war'.

This matter of postgraduate training was closely linked with that of the Fellowship examinations and the regulations for these differed markedly. It was only in 1939 for example that the General Medical Council allowed the Glasgow Fellowship in Surgery or Medicine to be registered other than plain FRCPS Glasg. by permitting '(S)' or '(P)' as appropriate to appear at the end. The College of Physicians of Edinburgh had examinations which could be taken in special subjects, that of England insisted on a wider spectrum of knowledge. Both created Members; to become a Fellow required later election by the College concerned. The English College of Surgeons insisted on a primary examination in basic science, while the Edinburgh College did not introduce this until 1943.

Each College and the Faculty had its own traditions and its own economic needs, but a surprising degree of agreement was eventually reached. The matter is still not fully resolved and will be alluded to again. The following extract from the minutes of 9th April 1945 is, however, valid to show how deeply Roy Young was thought of in the long negotiations which accompanied the Goodenough Committee's investigations into postgraduate education.

> 'Letters of date 28th ult. and 7th inst. from the Secretary of the Royal College of Surgeons of England were submitted inviting the Faculty to appoint someone who can speak in a representative capacity on behalf of the Faculty at a Conference to discuss the question of a common curriculum for the different Fellowships in Surgery (otherwise the co-ordination of Fellowship Regulations) to be held in London on 3rd May at 10 a.m. in the premises of the Royal College of Surgeons of England in Lincoln's Inn Fields.
>
> 'On the motion of the President the Faculty agreed to accept the invitation and appointed Mr. Roy F. Young as their representative'.

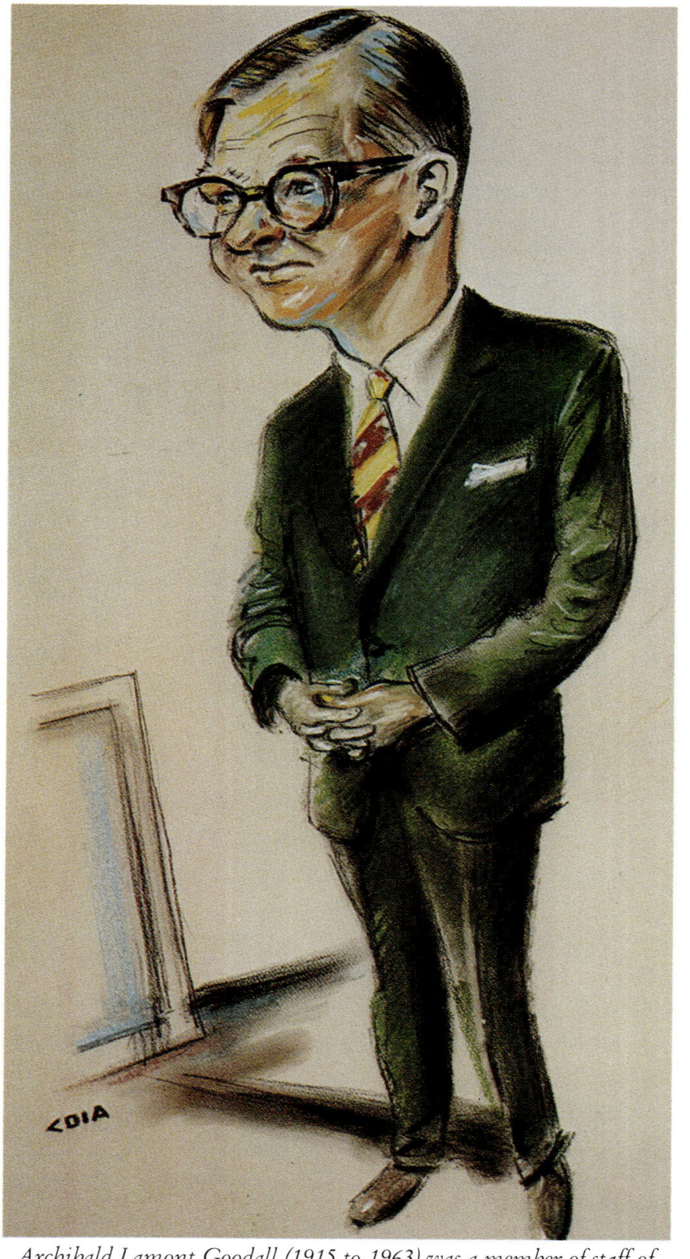


*Archibald Lamont Goodall (1915 to 1963) was a member of staff of the University Department of Surgery in Glasgow Royal Infirmary and a scholarly bibliophile and historian. He was Honorary Librarian from 1946 to 1963 and as a member of Council during these years worked tirelessly to improve the standing of the Royal Faculty. The cartoon is by Emilio Coia.*

# ARCHIBALD LAMONT GOODALL

1915 to 1963

*The portrait is a caricature by Emilio Coia painted in 1962 and presented to the College by his widow after Dr Goodall's death.*

Archibald Goodall was born in Glasgow and in later years was proud of his 'Burgess Ticket'; i.e. he was of the third generation of his family who were members of one of the Guilds of the Glasgow Trades House. He graduated MB,ChB with commendation in Glasgow in 1937 and went on to take the Diploma in Public Health in 1939. His first intention was to be a physician, and indeed he became a Fellow of the Royal Faculty of Physicians and Surgeons of Glasgow in 1940 *qua* physician, the obligatory special subject in which he was examined being 'Specific Fevers'. But he became attached shortly afterwards to the University Department of Surgery in Glasgow Royal Infirmary and remained there for the rest of his life, at first with Professor Burton and then with Professor Mackey. He graduated MD with commendation in 1944, took the Fellowship of the Royal College of Surgeons of Edinburgh in 1946 and, when the National Health Service began in 1948, was given the rank of Consultant Surgeon and held an Honorary Lectureship in Surgery in the University.

He was a severe diabetic. Many who knew him quite intimately were unaware of this since he tried in every way to live an outwardly normal life. At dinners he would eat everything, calculating in some magic way the exact amount of insulin to cope with the meal. But he had no illusions about the progression of his condition. Having sprained an ankle when he was still under thirty years of age, an x-ray was taken which showed no fracture but calcification in the posterior tibial artery. He knew that his span of life would be short and this showed firstly in a desire to do and see as much as he could while he could, and, secondly, in an urgency about everything he undertook to complete it before it might be too late.

He had an encyclopaedic knowledge of his specialty and wrote a number of clinical papers, but it was as an under- and post-graduate teacher of surgery that he excelled. He tried to stimulate the student to think for himself and not just 'swot up the books'. He was passionately fond of professional meetings, with their free interchange of ideas, and was a member of the Association of Surgeons of Great Britain and the International Society of Surgery; on two occasions he attended meetings of the American College of Surgeons. During the war years, he began the Glasgow Royal Infirmary Surgical Club and for many years organised their fortnightly meetings. He was vice-convener of the Postgraduate Medical Committee for a number of years and played a large part in inaugurating and administering not only courses for postgraduates preparing for higher degrees, but the popular twice-yearly symposia in the Royal Faculty.

He loved books, whether new or old, and was a member of the Glasgow Bibliographical Society. From books came his associated love of history, particularly that of Scotland, Glasgow and the Royal Faculty, and he was a founder member and later President of the Scottish Society for the History of Medicine.

When the office of Honorary Librarian in the Royal Faculty fell vacant in 1946, Archie Goodall was the obvious choice for successor and he held the office until his death. At that time the Honorary Librarian had automatically a seat on the Council and for 17 years he exerted a profound influence on the development of the Royal Faculty, as every President under whom he served would testify.

This appointment as Honorary Librarian when he was only 31 years old recognised the status which he already held as scholarly bibliophile and historian. He established this reputation indelibly when he gave the Finlayson Memorial Lecture in November 1949. To be invited to do so was in itself a great honour. The Lectureship had been set up by public subscription in 1909 in memory of James Finlayson (*q.v.*) and was given every three to five years. It was regarded as one of the Royal Faculty's most important occasions and of the 11 lecturers before Goodall, seven were Knights and only one was a local man.

Archie decided as his subject 'The History of the Royal Faculty of Physicians and Surgeons of Glasgow', partly because of the ignorance and lack of interest of his contemporaries and partly because of the lowly status which the institution had reached between the wars. Although there is, by definition, nothing new in history, Archie worked hard to present original material. He set out to solve two of the mysteries of the Faculty: what meant the word 'Arellian' that Peter Lowe added to his name, and where was the original Charter of James VI.

The term 'Arellian' has been variously interpreted as meaning either 'of Orléans', where Lowe could have been a graduate at the College of Medicine, or implying a place of birth, and Ayr, Errol and Airlie have all been suggested. Finlayson in his life of Lowe is rather in favour of Orléans, mainly because of a dogmatic letter to him from Dr A. Dureau of the Bibliotheque de l'Académie de Médicine in Paris. '*Arellian veut dire Orléanais*', he writes, and says that he has seen Lowe's name in several registers of 1596. But when Archie wrote to find out if he could see the registers, he learned that they had been destroyed by bombing in 1940, and the Archivist in Orléans thought that 'Arellian' was more likely from a place name in Scotland! So Archie wrote to the Minister at Errol, he visited the Bibliotheque Nationale in Paris, he wrote to the Curator of Historical Records in the Register House in Edinburgh, to the Librarian and Keeper of the Records of the Church of Scotland, to C. J. Fordyce, Professor of Humanity in Glasgow University and to others. But the trail was cold and he had no success; the replies to his letters are still extant, however, and should be consulted by any who wish to try again.

He had as little success in finding the Charter. It seemed likely that it would have had to be produced during the litigation with the University in the first half of the 19th century, but the lawyers of that time had been taken over and their successors taken over in turn, and nobody knew what had happened to the Charter. Perhaps it was taken to the House of Lords when the University appealed to them in 1838 and lies there with countless others gathering dust in an ancient cupboard.

Although he failed in the aims which he had set himself, he learned a great deal of history, made many friends, and his Finlayson Lecture was a memorable success. The War was over, the last of the mobilised doctors had come back to civilian life, the outlook was still bleak, but young and new and promising. Archie's lecture to a full audience revealed to them what they either didn't know or knew but vaguely, that Glasgow had a medical corporation of which they could and should be proud, and which had the potential for development into an organisation as good as, if not superior to, anything similar in the world.

It would be facile to say that the lecture was a turning-point in the Faculty's history; turning-points like U-turns are sudden events, and the fortunes of the Faculty had already begun to turn some years before when Roy Young had drawn attention to the low reputation of the Fellowship. Dr Joe Wright has likened Archie Goodall to an enzyme, and this analogy is good because there was at hand the perfect substrate on which to initiate the series of reactions needed to forge ahead. But Archie was also a constantly pricking conscience; his sense of urgency has already been alluded to and was a useful goad if the pace of change seemed to be slackening.

Archibald Goodall would certainly have become President had he lived, but he saw many of the changes he had planned and worked for come about and envisaged others which have now taken place or soon will do so. The change of name from Royal Faculty to Royal College in 1962 gave him great pleasure and satisfaction.

# 16

## SINCE 1948

Hector James Wright Hetherington
*(1888 to 1965)*
H.R.H. Princess Alexandra of Kent
*(Honorary Fellow 1960)*
Stanley Alstead
*(President 1956 to 1958)*
Joseph Houston Wright
*(President 1960 to 1962)*
Charles Frederick William Illingworth
*(President 1962 to 1964)*
Archibald Brown Kerr
*(President 1964 to 1966)*
James Holmes Hutchison
*(President 1966 to 1968)*
Robert Brash Wright
*(President 1968 to 1970)*
Edward McCombie McGirr
*(President 1970 to 1972)*
Andrew Watt Kay
*(President 1972 to 1974)*
William Ferguson Anderson
*(President 1974 to 1976)*
Thomas Gibson
*(President 1976 to 1978)*
Gavin Brown Shaw
*(President 1978 to 1980)*
Douglas Henderson Clark
*(President 1980 to 1982)*
Thomas James Thomson
*(President 1982)*

Although Alexander Duncan entitled his work *Memorials of the Faculty of Physicians and Surgeons of Glasgow, 1599-1850*, he did not publish it until 1896.

> 'The question of the date to which these Memorials should be brought down was not settled without some hesitation. In fixing the middle of the present century as the line, the dominant consideration was, that it was obviously very undesirable to extend the limit down to a period in which men now living would to any extent figure as the actors in the transactions recorded'.

This latter argument is still extremely valid, but the Royal College has portraits of subjects up to the present day and somehow these must be included in this account; but how to prevent them figuring, in Duncan's words, 'as the actors in the transactions recorded'? No matter how it be done, there might arise resentment at items omitted or wrongly accredited. The fact that during the Presidency of X, item Y occurred or was brought to fruition does not necessarily mean that President X was the prime mover or the effective agent of Y. Previous Presidents, other office-bearers, members of Council and individual Fellows and Members of the College may have done as much as, if not more than, the President of the time.

After many years it may be possible to assess fairly the contributions of the subjects of the more recent portraits to the College and its development. Meanwhile the following compromise seems least likely to offend either the subjects themselves or others of the College who have lived through and remember these exciting years of expansion, locally, nationally and internationally.

Firstly, the 'biographical sketches' of each surviving ex-President are the basic facts of his career and nothing more. They were taken from his entries in the *Medical Directory* and *Who's Who*, paraphrased into more or less readable sentences, and sent to each who either agreed to, amended or rewrote his entry; what appears therefore is his own. There is no allusion to the work of the College and its development, but the sketches are arranged chronologically so far as their presidential term is concerned.

Secondly, only an outline history of these years has been given. So much has happened that anything more would be impossible here.

The first General Election at the end of the War in 1945 saw a wide swing towards socialism, and one of the greatest effects of this was the creation of the National Health Service by the Acts of 1946 and 1947. The Beveridge Report, the wranglings in the Royal Faculty, the Royal Colleges and the British Medical Association and its branches up and down the country, and the work of Aneurin Bevan who did more than any other to create, depending on one's point of view, either the best health service in the world or the worst: these are matters about which full histories have still to be written and are still fresh in the older memories; they need not concern us in detail here.

The major effect of the implementation of the Acts in 1948 on the Royal Faculty was the radical change from hospitals supported essentially by charity or local rates, and staffed by virtually unpaid 'voluntary' surgeons and physicians who made their living from private practice and teaching, to hospitals paid for by the state and staffed with consultants, thoroughly trained in their specialty, who were either fully salaried or partly so with permission to indulge in limited private practice. No longer were the hospitals outside the major cities staffed by general practitioners with a leaning towards medicine or surgery. Consultants with the same qualifications as those in teaching hospitals were appointed, and such hospitals were raised to the same standard as those of the main teaching hospitals; indeed, many became 'teaching' hospitals. The change was of course eased and indeed foreshadowed by war-time practice; doctors in the armed forces were fully salaried and the Emergency Medical Services hospitals built to treat the casualties of war were staffed with salaried medical personnel.

The National Health Service Acts gave to the Royal Faculty the same rights as the Royal Colleges of supervising postgraduate training and examining candidates for specialist qualifications. But changing semantics had degraded the term 'Faculty'; it now signified to many a branch of an academic body and it had become the odd man out among similar institutions. FRFPS(S) or FRFPS(P) still sounded inferior to FRCS, MRCP or FRCP. It was essential therefore that the Royal Faculty became a Royal College and that it should be able to grant such registrable higher degrees as FRCS, MRCP and FRCP. This took time, diplomacy and much friendly intercourse with the Royal Colleges at a high personal level; such a change could hardly take place without their willing cooperation.

Meanwhile the Royal Faculty forged ahead with postgraduate projects. A joint Postgraduate Medical Committee composed of equal numbers of the Royal Faculty and the University Medical Faculty came into being. Symposia on topics which would, wherever possible, interest equally surgeons and physicians, were organised at least twice a year, while courses in basic science and on specialist topics were arranged for the trainee specialists. The Principal of Glasgow University who was particularly concerned with the Faculty/University cooperation at this time is the subject of our next portrait.

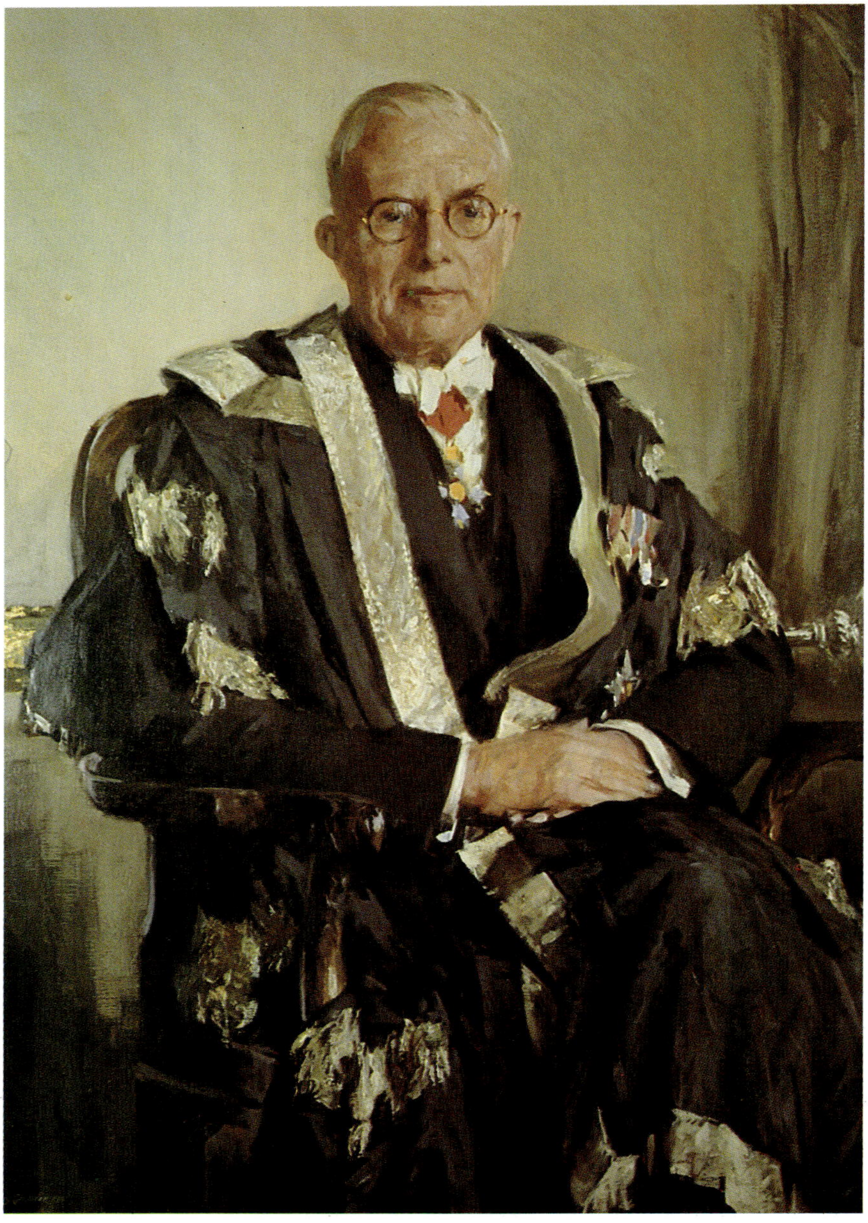

*Sir Hector Hetherington (1888 to 1965) was Principal and Vice-Chancellor of Glasgow University from 1936 to 1961.*

# HECTOR (JAMES WRIGHT) HETHERINGTON

GBE, Kt, MA, LLD, LittD, Hon.ARIBA, Hon.FRCPS, FKS, Hon.FEIS
(1888 to 1965)

*The portrait was commissioned by the Royal Faculty, painted by the Queen's Limner, Sir Stanley Cursiter, and presented at a ceremony in the Royal Faculty in 1961.*

Hector Hetherington was born in Cowdenbeath and when his family moved shortly afterwards to Tillicoultry he went to primary school there and had his secondary school education at Dollar Academy. In 1905 he matriculated at Glasgow University and graduated MA with honours in 1910. Although he had, initially, thoughts of Divinity as his career, he became assistant to the Professor of Moral Philosophy in Glasgow for four years. In 1914 he was appointed to a Lectureship in Philosophy in Sheffield University but moved on to Cardiff a year later as Professor of Logic and Philosophy. In 1920 he became Principal of University College, Exeter where he also held the Chair of Philosophy. Although he now seemed set on a course of University administration, he returned to Glasgow in 1924 as Professor of Moral Philosophy. In 1927 he returned once more to University government when he accepted the post of Vice-Chancellor of the University of Liverpool. He held this post with great distinction for nine years, and when Sir Donald MacAlister, the Principal and Vice-Chancellor of Glasgow University, retired in 1936, Hetherington was the obvious choice as successor. He held this post until he retired for reasons of health in 1961 when he was 73 years of age.

Sir Charles Illingworth has written a biography of Hetherington (*University Statesman*. Perth. Outram and Company Ltd., 1971) and this should be consulted for further details of his life. Hetherington's views on medical education caused much rancour when he first came to Glasgow, because he was firmly opposed to those who held academic appointments indulging in private practice. Illingworth writes that his 'firm action in his early days provoked bitter reactions at the time but are now seen to have been a necessary catharsis'. Others might still dissent.

During Hector Hetherington's term as Principal, the Postgraduate Medical Committee was set up.

He was made an Honorary Fellow of the Royal Faculty of Physicians and Surgeons of Glasgow at the 350th Anniversary in 1949.

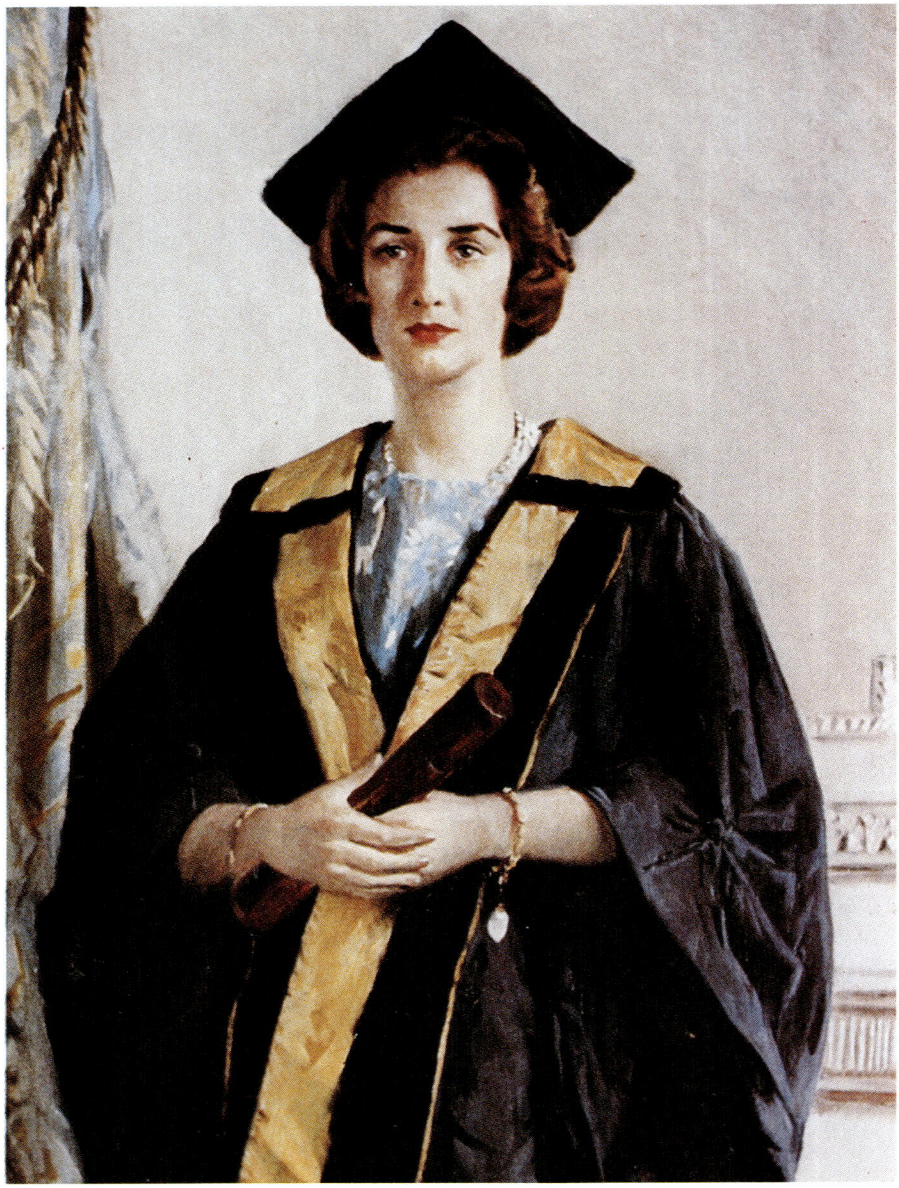

*HRH Princess Alexandra graciously accepted the Honorary Fellowship of the Royal Faculty in 1960 and her portrait by Sir Stanley Cursiter was unveiled the following year.*

The increasing number of courses and lectures required more space than the Faculty Hall could provide, and so, with the aid of a grant of £20,000 from Sir Maurice Bloch, a large lecture room taking up much of the old garden between the Royal Faculty building and St Vincent Lane at the rear, was conceived, built and opened in 1959. It has excellent acoustics, every possible visual teaching aid and a tendency to chill the feet of those in the first two rows, a fault which many improvisations have helped but failed radically to cure.

Furthermore, appeals had been made to industrial and charitable organisations and funds had been raised which put the Royal Faculty on a sounder financial footing than it had been for many years.

## HRH PRINCESS ALEXANDRA OF KENT

(1936- )

In 1959, HRH Princess Alexandra agreed to become an Honorary Fellow of the Royal Faculty and was duly elected at a ceremony on 1st June 1960. She has since visited the Royal College on a number of occasions. Her portrait was commissioned by the Royal Faculty and painted by the Queen's Limner, Sir Stanley Cursiter; it was unveiled on 28th April 1961. Unfortunately the portrait was vandalised to an irreparable degree in July 1979. It is hoped that there will soon become available a replacement portrait of this, our most important, Honorary Fellow.

Biographical details of Her Royal Highness are so widely available as to be unnecessary here.

On 30th November 1961 the then President, Dr J. H. Wright, received from Sir Hugh Fraser a letter to say that the Hugh Fraser Foundation would contribute £22,500 towards the rehousing of the Library.

Previously the main reading room of the Royal Faculty was L-shaped and included the present Lock Room, while the short limb of the L was later incorporated into a new lecture room and is now a seminar room. Many of the books were stored on the floor above in a series of attic rooms radiating out from a central aperture through which light from a cupola in the roof filtered to the floor below. From this floor the new spacious reading room was created. The central aperture was covered over and now accommodates the librarian on duty and all reference books and indexes. On the reading room shelves are the bound volumes of the journals taken by the library which remain there for at least ten years. The new reading room was formally handed over by Sir Hugh Fraser on 1st May 1963 and the architect, Mr W. N. W. Ramsay, presented Sir Hugh with a blotter.

The years thereafter were the heyday of the reading room; the Library staff was increased, and while it had always been traditional that the Library remained open on Friday evenings, it now became possible to open the Library from 9.30 a.m. to 9.00 p.m. each weekday and on Saturday mornings. But physical presences in the Library decreased progressively after photocopying was introduced and became more and more popular. The Medlar system of computerisation of the indexes and photocopies of selected papers made the old personal 'search of the literature' virtually obsolete; and yet, when one learned how to do it, the search through the indexes, the Catalogues of the Surgeon-General's Library, Callisen, Hirsch and all the rest brought its own rewards.

The position of the Library in the College has changed. It is still by far its greatest asset and its books are of incalculable value; 'incalculable' because their exact worth can only become known if they should ever be put up for auction; but certainly at today's prices its worth is many millions of pounds. It is, however, no longer the only source of medical literature in the West of Scotland apart from the University. Inter-library loan schemes are so thoroughly organised that virtually any article in any medical journal from any part of the world can be obtained in photocopy form. Books may be borrowed from libraries not just in the UK but internationally. The Library still continues to take the most important journals in nearly all medical specialties and sufficient textbooks to keep up-to-date information on these specialties ready to hand. It remains one of the most magnificent of historical medical libraries, although its treasures are too seldom appreciated and too rarely tapped.

The acceptance by Princess Alexandra in 1959 of the Honorary Fellowship of the Royal Faculty may well have been a straw in the wind that the negotiations to change 'Faculty' to 'College' were not without approval in high places. Only two out of 400 Fellows who had voted for or against the change of name had voted 'against', the other Colleges raised no objections and, indeed, encouraged the change; the General Medical Council, having tidied up some loose ends, gave its blessing and Her Majesty agreed that if the title were changed, the 'Royal' adjective would still be appropriate. It all took time, but finally the required Act of Parliament, after passing through the House of Lords, received the Royal Assent on 6th December 1962.

The Royal College of Physicians and Surgeons of Glasgow has two important attributes. Firstly, it is the only joint College of Physicians and Surgeons in the United Kingdom, and secondly, it is a Royal College both in Scotland and in the UK, and it is to be remembered that different medical acts cover the practice in England and Wales and in Scotland. In a sense, therefore, although one or two of the others might dispute it, the Glasgow College is involved in twice as much activity as the Colleges of Edinburgh and four times as much as those of England and Ireland. It is not merely a Royal College of Physicians and Surgeons; it is a Royal College of Physicians *and* a Royal College of Surgeons, and each entity has the same powers and privileges as the single Colleges of Edinburgh, England and Ireland.

Higher qualifications in Medicine and Surgery are granted which are not only of the same standing and quality as those of the other Royal Colleges but are registrable with the same initials. The higher surgical qualification FRCS is followed by the abbreviation 'Glasg.' to distinguish it from that of Eng. or Edin. or Irel., but the labelling of the MRCP is more complex. The standardisation of a higher qualification in medicine is one of the outstanding results of post-war inter-collegiate discussion and negotiation. That there should be quite different examination routines leading to the same higher qualification was recognised, and it was seen as ridiculous that budding young physicians were taking the MRCP examinations in Glasgow, Edinburgh and London, to be quite sure of having the right one, a course which wasted years of their lives and came to be known as 'multiple diplomatosis'. Common Part 1 and Part 2 examinations were finally agreed upon which would be exactly the same in all the Colleges and would lead to the degree of MRCP(UK). Thereafter, depending on where the graduates should settle and the corporate advantages they might desire, they could become 'collegiate' members of Glasg., Edin., or Eng. While much logistic detail has to be observed in the simultaneous sitting of the examination in widely separate sites, and in spite of some lingering nostalgia on the part of the traditionalists, the system seems to work well and gives coherence to the Colleges of Physicians. The Collegiate Member may be elected Fellow in due time and by agreement of his Collegiate peers.

The evolution of a standard Fellowship for the Surgical Colleges has not proceeded so happily. After much negotiation, and particularly after the introduction of the Multiple Choice Questions type of examination, 'reciprocity' of the Primary Surgical Fellowship examination was achieved; i.e. the candidate could sit his Primary in any Surgical College and, having passed, was then eligible to sit the Final Fellowship in the same or any of the other Colleges. The English College, however, was concerned at the lack of an 'essay' question in the reciprocal primary and recently withdrew from the scheme; at the time of writing the Colleges are still some distance from the introduction of a standard British Surgical Fellowship similar to that of the Colleges of Physicians.

The FRCS and the MRCP examinations are searching, and expect from the candidate a wide range of knowledge in surgery or medicine; the pass rate rarely exceeds 30 per cent. But in spite of the many hours of study, of the host of facts memorised, of the tensions imposed, they have proved inadequate as certificates of competence for hospital consultancies. Specialisation has expanded exponentially as the advances in all branches of technology have made possible more and more new methods of patient treatment and care, which demand increasing expertise and full time application to branches of medicine and surgery which a few decades ago were regarded as well within the range of the 'general' physician or surgeon.

Some specialties have long felt that the Royal Colleges did not fulfil their needs, and proceeded to form their own Colleges. The Royal College of Obstetricians and Gynaecologists was the first, in 1929, but now there are Royal Colleges of Pathology, General Practice and Psychiatry, and 'Faculties' of the traditional Colleges in Anaesthesia, Radiology and Community Medicine. To pass the examinations of these bodies is adequate for a consultant appointment without a FRCS or M(or F)RCP. At the same time, because all of these new bodies are concentrated in London, there is a continuing demand from their Fellows who practise, for example, in the West of Scotland, and would like corporate facilities there, to seek election as Fellows of the Glasgow College, in the words of the regulations, 'under Chapter II, Paragraph 5', which means in effect without examination.

A 'College' or a 'Faculty' has, of course, more standing than an 'Association' or a 'Society', but is only practicable when the members are numerous enough to finance it; there are other arguments too against a multiplicity of such organisations. One alternative is for Colleges to provide specialist examinations at the end of the training period to qualify the candidate as a specialist in his chosen field. This is common overseas. The American 'Board' examinations are typical examples, and specialist examinations are now provided by the Colleges in Canada, Australia and South Africa and a pass is virtually obligatory to obtain a hospital consultant post in many of the specialties.

In the UK, there has been strong resistance to specialist examinations although one or two of these are now available in the Royal College of Surgeons of Edinburgh, and in the Glasgow College it has been possible for many years to take the Surgical Fellowship in Ophthalmology or Oto-rhino-laryngology. In general, however, the MRCP and the FRCS are not 'exit' examinations; their holder is not to be regarded as a fully qualified physician or surgeon. It is common knowledge, of course, that in many countries overseas, one who has passed his membership or fellowship is indeed recognised as qualified to a standard requiring no further training, but in the UK the Colleges have stressed that these degrees are but 'entrance' examinations and, before full qualification is achieved, several more years of training in a specialty are essential.

Such training years are taken in senior registrar posts, so, in essence, one must become MRCP or FRCS before obtaining a senior registrar post and then remain there for three, four or more years until a signature from the senior consultant in the unit says that training is satisfactorily completed. It sounds inflexible and dependent on the whim of an individual who may not be favourably disposed to the trainee. But in practice the training is so well safe-guarded that it virtually guarantees the qualifications of any specialist in the hospital service in the U.K.; but its rigidity, however fair it may seem to the majority, is still felt by some to hold back the more brilliant trainees at a time when they are most capable of creative work.

The main safeguard to the training period was the setting up of joint supervisory committees of members from the Colleges and from the specialist associations. The first was the 'Joint Committee on Higher Surgical Training', with its subcommittees in the various surgical specialties. Then came the JCHMT in medicine, with even more specialist subcommittees, and finally the JCHDT for dentistry. To begin with the committees were financed by the Colleges and the Specialist Associations. Today they are mostly supported by the National Health Service, but much of their time-consuming, investigative work is carried out voluntarily by the committee members. Every unit which has a senior registrar establishment, or wishes to have one, is inspected by members of the appropriate specialist subcommittee who report either its full approval or its possible approval conditional upon certain improvements in facilities and amenities becoming available. Inspections are repeated every few years or more frequently if recommended changes are to be approved. These visitations by senior respected members of each specialty have ensured that training posts throughout Britain offer to their holders the best possible opportunities for specialist training. The great majority of trainees have, of course, an overwhelming enthusiasm for their specialty and make the most of these opportunities, but there are still those in authority who feel that an 'exit' examination would be the only infallible way to ensure that they did.

There is another complication to the higher qualifications of the Royal Colleges. The majority of those who sit the examinations are graduates of foreign universities and while, in the past, the high standards of many of these were readily acceptable, the political, social and economic upheavals of the last 20 or 30 years have meant that only a few are now recognised. Many overseas candidates for the fellowship and membership wish to work for a spell in British hospitals before taking the examination, and it is obvious that they must be not only professionally competent but able to speak and write good idiomatic English. So they have to sit a preliminary examination to test such proficiency and this is organised by the Royal Colleges in turn. The so-called PLAB (Professional and Linguistics Assessment Board) examination has greatly helped to improve the standards of those applying for junior hospital posts and those sitting the College examinations.

It is a pity that the College does not have a portrait of a Dental Fellow; otherwise more

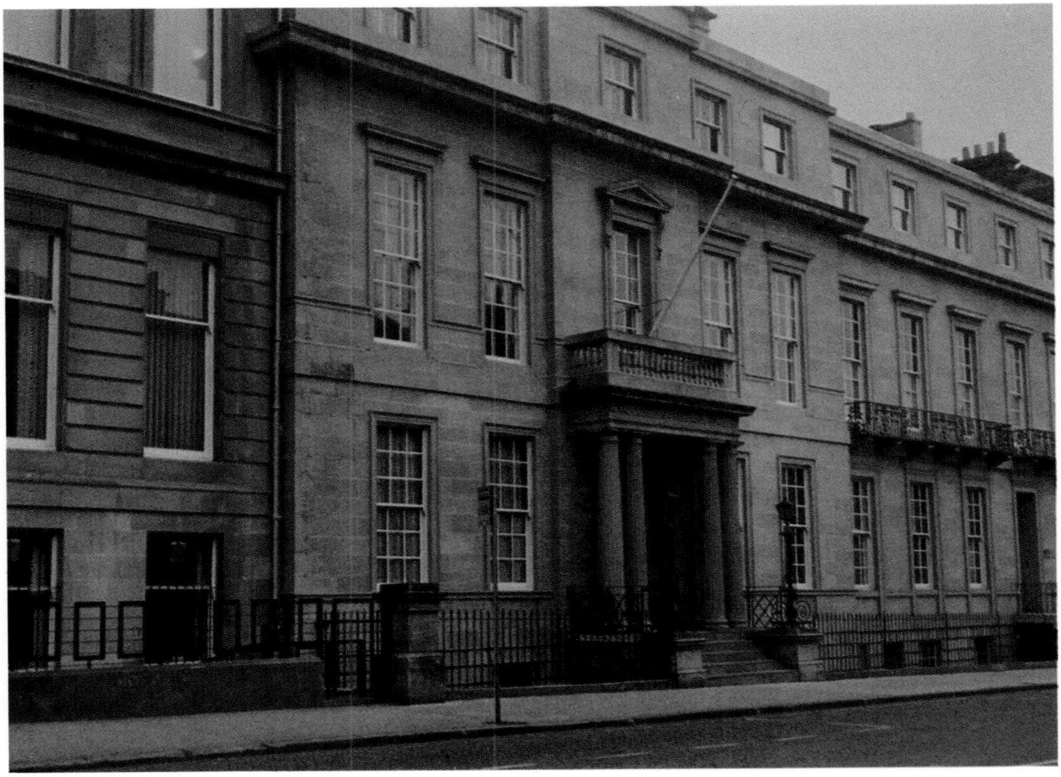

*The Royal College of Physicians and Surgeons of Glasgow today, looking east. The main entrance leads to the initial building, 242 St Vincent Street, purchased in 1862. The adjoining building at 238 was obtained in 1900 and the entrance converted into an office. The latest acquisition is the next building at 234 whose entrance, for security reasons, is that most commonly used. The balcony links 238 and 234.*

might be said of the role of the Faculty in dentistry, particularly since it became a licensing body by the Dental Act of 1868 and is represented on the General Dental Council. As in medicine, the undergraduate training and licensing of dentists has been taken over by the University, but the Royal College still plays an important role in granting higher dental degrees. Its Fellowship in Dental Surgery is now on a par with similar Fellowships in the other Surgical Colleges. The Fellows have their own Council, their convener is ex officio a member of Council of the College, and they now have full rights in the College.

The degree of Diploma in Child Health, begun in 1957, is similar to that given by other Colleges of Physicians and continues to attract about 100 applicants each year. It is intended for those who are concerned with aspects of child care short of those requiring the services of a consultant paediatric physician or surgeon. The MRCP or FRCS are regarded as essential for the latter posts, although it is not uncommon for those who wish to make consultant paediatrics their career to take the DCH at an earlier stage.

As an illustration of the extent of the postgraduate examinations, the following is extracted from the Report of the Honorary Secretary to the Annual General Meeting of the Royal College on 1st November 1982.

Examination activity has continued at a high level as shown by the following figures:

| | *1979-80* Sat | *Passed* | *1980-81* Sat | *Passed* | *1981-82* Sat | *Passed* |
|---|---|---|---|---|---|---|
| Membership (Physicians) Common Part II | 734 | 221 | 729 | 214 | 759 | 210 |
| Primary Fellowship (Surgeons) | 1,584 | 289 | 1,457 | 184 | 1,265 | 248 |
| Final Fellowship (Surgeons) | 533 | 155 | 665 | 186 | 798 | 168 |
| Diploma in Child Health | 111 | 36 | 118 | 42 | 137 | 49 |
| Primary Fellowship (Dental Surgery) | 69 | 16 | 61 | 13 | 62 | 11 |
| Final Fellowship (Dental Surgery) | 70 | 31 | 79 | 22 | 67 | 17 |

In addition to the above examinations the College also participates in the PLAB Examination. The Triple Qualification Examination too continues to be attractive to many people seeking medical qualifications registrable in the U.K.; almost 200 candidates sat in 1982.

The College held its Primary Fellowship Examination in Tripoli for the first time in 1982 and it is hoped to continue these diets in Libya.

The holding of examinations and the granting of qualifications is one aspect of today's work in the College; the other is postgraduate education. For those preparing for examinations there are regular courses in applied basic sciences, higher medicine and higher surgery, and occasional courses in other specialties. In the sphere of continuing education, for those already established as well as those in training, there are several symposia organised each year, monthly invited lectures throughout the winter months, and for the past few years a series of 'supper colloquia' on a wide variety of topics.

Accommodation has been extended by the purchase in 1975 of No. 234 St Vincent Street, 'the building next door', and the successful fund-raising activities needed to finance its purchase, conversion and incorporation in the College took much of the College's time for two or three years. But even the additional accommodation is not always adequate; the numbers sitting some of the examinations are such that space must be hired elsewhere, usually in the University.

Today the Royal College is more active than it has ever been in its almost four centuries of existence, and its steady expansion shows no sign of abating. On the international scene it was host in 1976 to a meeting of the Presidents of all the English-speaking Colleges of Physicians; in 1981 it hosted a similar meeting of Presidents of the Colleges of Surgeons. At home, as already indicated, it is a member of many committees concerned particularly with postgraduate training, but is in a similar position to any of the Royal Colleges in any matter which affects their interests. It has the added power of speaking with the voices of both physicians and surgeons, and nearly always the voices are in complete harmony. *Conjurat amice.*

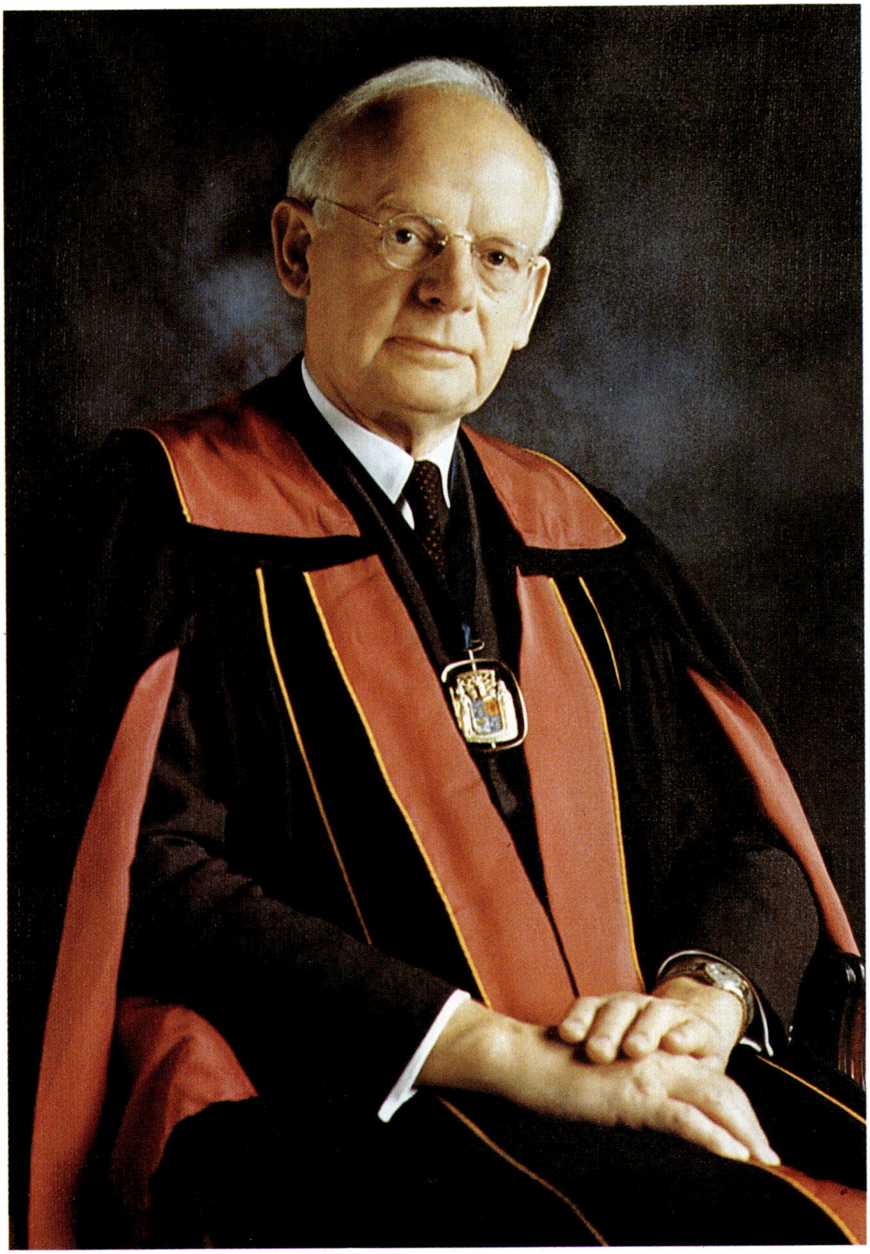

STANLEY ALSTEAD (1905- )
*President, 1956 to 1958.*
*Portrait by Elliot Robertson, 1978.*

# STANLEY ALSTEAD

CBE, MD, Hon.FRCPSGlasg., FRCP(Glasg, Edin, Lond), FRSE
(1905- )

*The portrait/photograph by Elliot Robertson was made in 1978.*

Stanley Alstead was educated at Wigan Grammar School and Liverpool University. After holding junior appointments in Liverpool, Birmingham and Salford, he joined the staff of the University of Glasgow as Pollok Lecturer in Pharmacology in 1932; his interests were mainly in the clinical aspects of the subject and in teaching. At this time he was on the Dispensary (OPD) staff of the Western Infirmary of Glasgow and assisted in the wards.

During the Second World War (1939-45) he served as a Medical Specialist in No. 5 Casualty Clearing Station in Algeria, Tunisia and Sicily, and later as OC Medical Division of 67 General Hospital in Italy and of 63 General Hospital in Egypt. He was mentioned in dispatches. After the War, he was Physician to the Highlands and Islands Medical Service, based in Inverness (1947-48).

In 1948 he was appointed Regius Professor of Materia Medica, a post which carried responsibility for a clinical unit at Stobhill General Hospital, Glasgow. During 1965-66 he was an Honorary Professor in the University of East Africa and an Honorary Physician to the Kenyatta National Hospital in Nairobi. He acted as External Examiner in Clinical Pharmacology and in Medicine in many universities at home and abroad. Later he served on a number of national committees including the British Pharmacopoeia Commission.

He has published a number of papers on the results of original research in clinical pharmacology and was joint editor of a *Textbook of Medical Treatment* (Churchill Livingstone) and editor (later joint editor) of *Clinical Pharmacology* (Dilling) (Bailliere Tindale).

In retirement he joined the Society of Friends of Dunblane Cathedral; he was successively Editor of the Society's journal and joint-chairman of the Society. Over a period of ten years he contributed biographical and religious articles to this journal.

He was President of the Royal College of Physicians and Surgeons of Glasgow from 1956 to 1958.

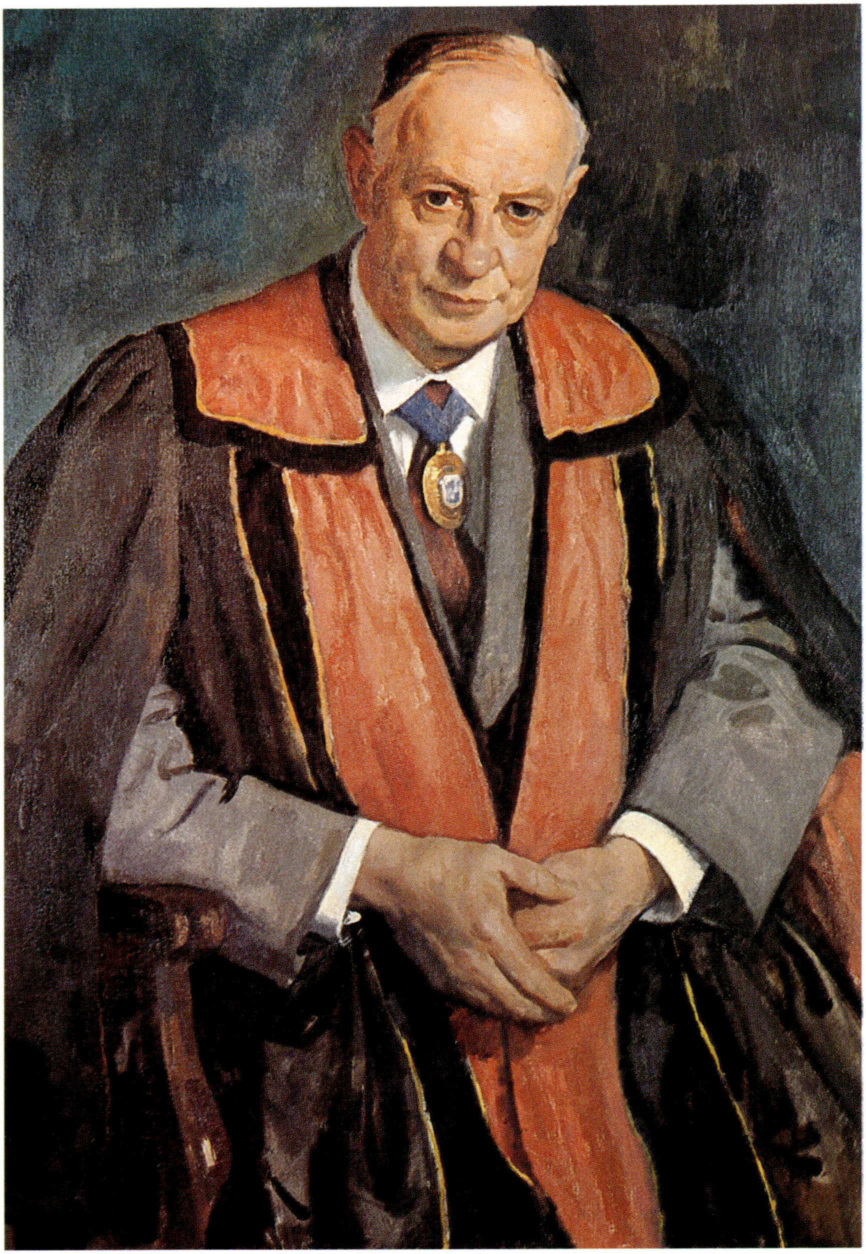

JOSEPH H. WRIGHT (1899- )
*President, 1960 to 1962.*
*Portrait by Alberto Morrocco, 1963.*

# JOSEPH (HOUSTON) WRIGHT

CBE, LLD, JP, MD, FRFPS, FRCPEdin, FRCPLond, Hon.FRCPS
(1899- )

*The portrait was commissioned by the Royal College and painted by Alberto Morrocco in 1963.*

Joseph Wright graduated MB,ChB in Glasgow University in 1922 and was awarded its MD with High Commendation in 1932; in the same year he became a Fellow of the Royal Faculty of Physicians and Surgeons of Glasgow. Fellowships of the Royal Colleges of Edinburgh (1953) and London (1964) followed. Until his retirement from the National Health Service in 1964, he was Senior Consultant Physician in Glasgow Royal Infirmary and for many years a Clinical Lecturer in the University.

Glasgow University has bestowed on him the honorary degree of LLD and he is a Justice of the Peace.

He was President of the Royal Faculty of Physicians and Surgeons of Glasgow from 1960 to 1962 when the Royal Faculty became the Royal College.

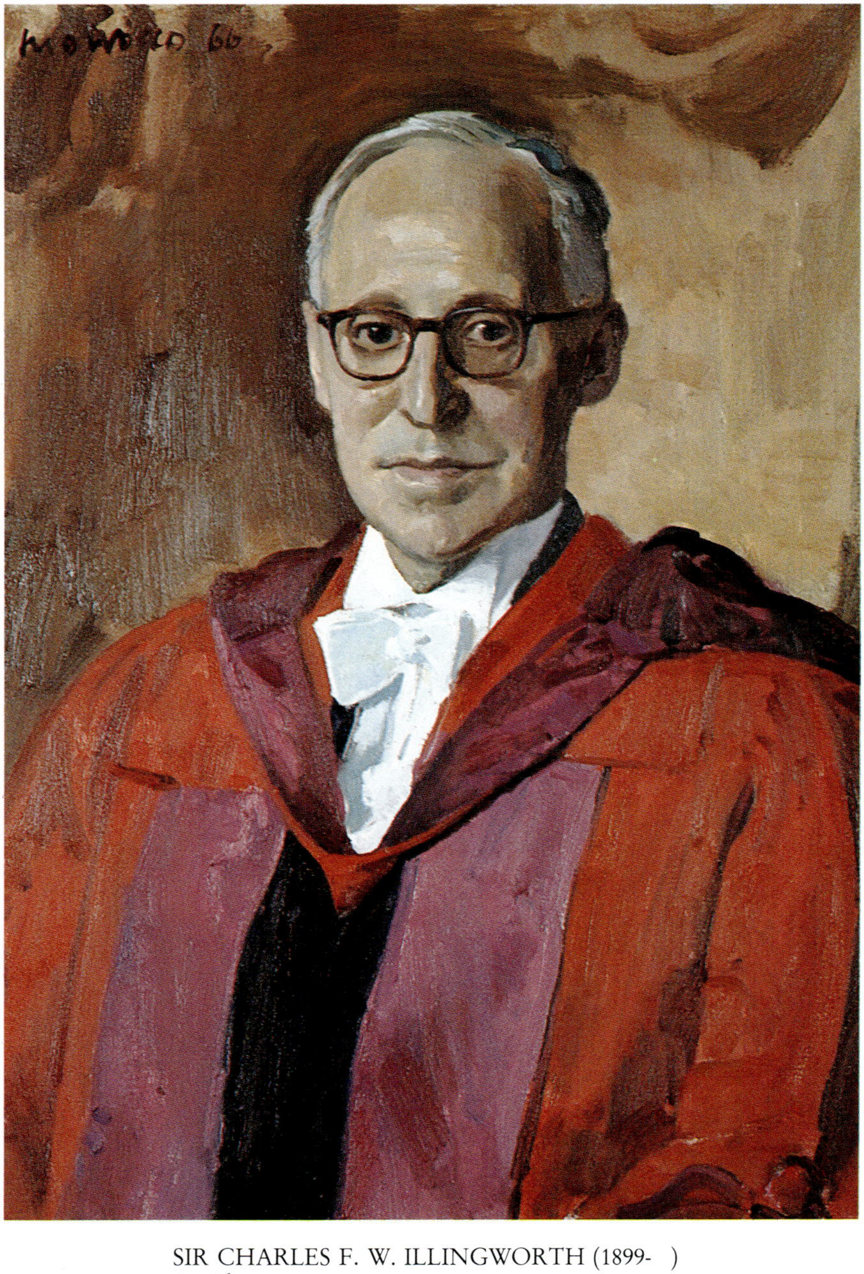


SIR CHARLES F. W. ILLINGWORTH (1899- )
*President, 1962 to 1964.*
*Portrait by Alberto Morrocco, 1964.*

# SIR CHARLES (FREDERICK WILLIAM) ILLINGWORTH

(1899- )

*The portrait is a copy by the artist of that painted for Glasgow University by Alberto Morrocco in 1964.*

Charles Illingworth was educated at Heath Grammar School, Halifax, and Edinburgh University, where he graduated in Medicine in 1922 and later took the degrees of ChM and MD. His education was interrupted by war service as 2nd Lieutenant in the Royal Flying Corps, part of which service he spent as a prisoner of war. He became a Fellow of the Royal College of Surgeons of Edinburgh in 1925 and was soon established as a general surgeon in Edinburgh, interested in gastro-enterology, under- and postgraduate surgical education and surgical research. In 1939 he succeeded the late Archibald Young (*q.v.*) as Regius Professor of Surgery in Glasgow University, which Chair he held until he became Emeritus in 1964.

He has been given many honorary degrees: DSc of Sheffield (1962) and Belfast (1963), LLD of Glasgow (1965) and Leeds (1965), and is an Honorary Fellow of the following surgical Colleges: Glasgow, England, Ireland, America, Canada, and South Africa. He became CBE in 1946 and was knighted in 1961.

Apart from various contributions to surgical literature mainly on digestive disorders, he has published several books. His *Short Textbook of Surgery* has run to nine editions, the last in 1972, while his *Textbook of Surgical Pathology*, which he wrote with the late Mr Bruce Dick, had its 12th edition published in 1979. The *Textbook of Surgical Treatment*, first published in 1943, ran to four editions and has been followed in 1980 by *Surgical Treatment. The Story of William Hunter* appeared in 1967, *The Sanguine Mystery* in 1970, and *University Statesman: Sir Hector Hetherington* in 1971.

His *Monograph on Peptic Ulcer* of 1953 remains the standard work of its time.

He was Honorary Surgeon to the Queen in Scotland from 1961 to 1965 and has been Extra Surgeon to Her Majesty since 1965.

He was President of the Royal College of Physicians and Surgeons of Glasgow from 1962 to 1964 and Honorary Librarian from 1975 to 1980.

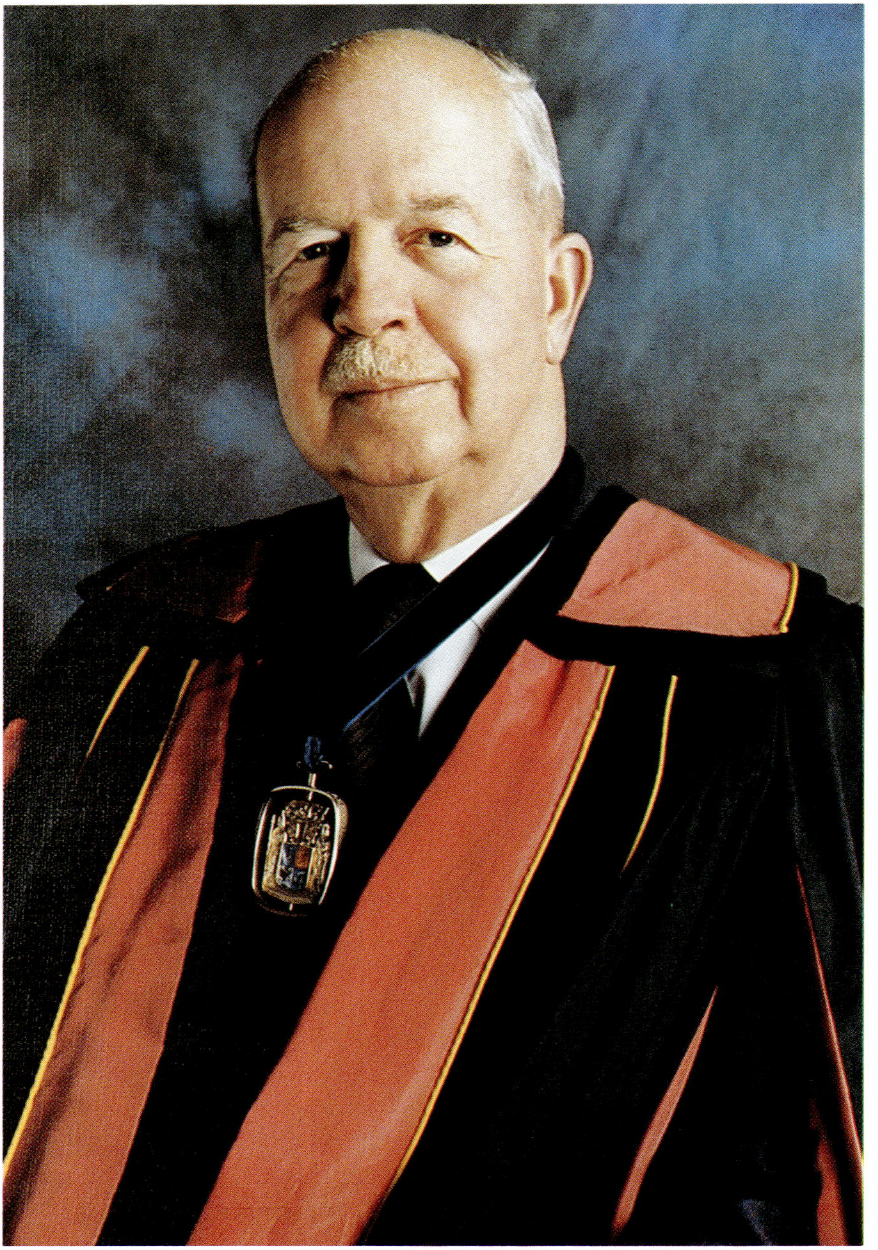

ARCHIBALD B. KERR (1907- )
*President, 1964 to 1966*
*Portrait by Elliot Robertson, 1978.*

# ARCHIBALD (BROWN) KERR

CBE (1968), (OBE, Mil, 1945), TD, BSc, MB,ChB,
FRCSGlasg, FRCSEdin, Hon.LLD(Glasg)
(1907- )

*The portrait/photograph by Elliot Robertson was made in 1978.*

Archibald Kerr was educated at Glasgow High School and Glasgow University where he graduated in Science in 1927 and in Medicine two years later.

He was assistant to Sir Robert Muir, Professor of Pathology in Glasgow University, from 1931 to 1933 and thereafter became a Surgeon to Out-Patients in the Western Infirmary and an assistant to Roy F. Young (*q.v.*) who was subsequently President of the Royal Faculty. He had served in the Infantry Unit of Glasgow University Officer Training Corps for 15 years and on the outbreak of war in 1939 he mobilised with 156 (Lowland) Field Ambulance. He then spent five years in Palestine, France and Germany as Surgical Specialist, Officer in Charge of Surgical Division and Colonel Commanding No. 23 (Scottish) General Hospital.

On his return to civilian life he was appointed Assistant Surgeon to the Western Infirmary, Glasgow, in 1945 and Surgeon to the Royal Alexandra Infirmary, Paisley in 1946. Both these posts he held until 1954 after which he continued as Consultant Surgeon in Charge of Wards in the Western Infirmary until his retirement in 1972. From 1946 to 1972 he was an Honorary Lecturer in Clinical Surgery to the University and it was under his care that Paisley first became accepted as a centre for University clinical classes.

He was, in 1951, President of the Royal Medico-Chirurgical Society of Glasgow which made him an Honorary Member in 1971. He served as a member of the Western Regional Hospital Board and from 1973 has been a member of Court of the University of Glasgow.

His contributions to surgical literature have dealt largely with military and historical subjects and with the surgery of the colon and rectum. He is the author with Loudon MacQueen of *The Western Infirmary 1874-1974: A Century of Service to Glasgow* published in 1974.

He was President of the Royal College of Physicians and Surgeons of Glasgow from 1964 to 1966.

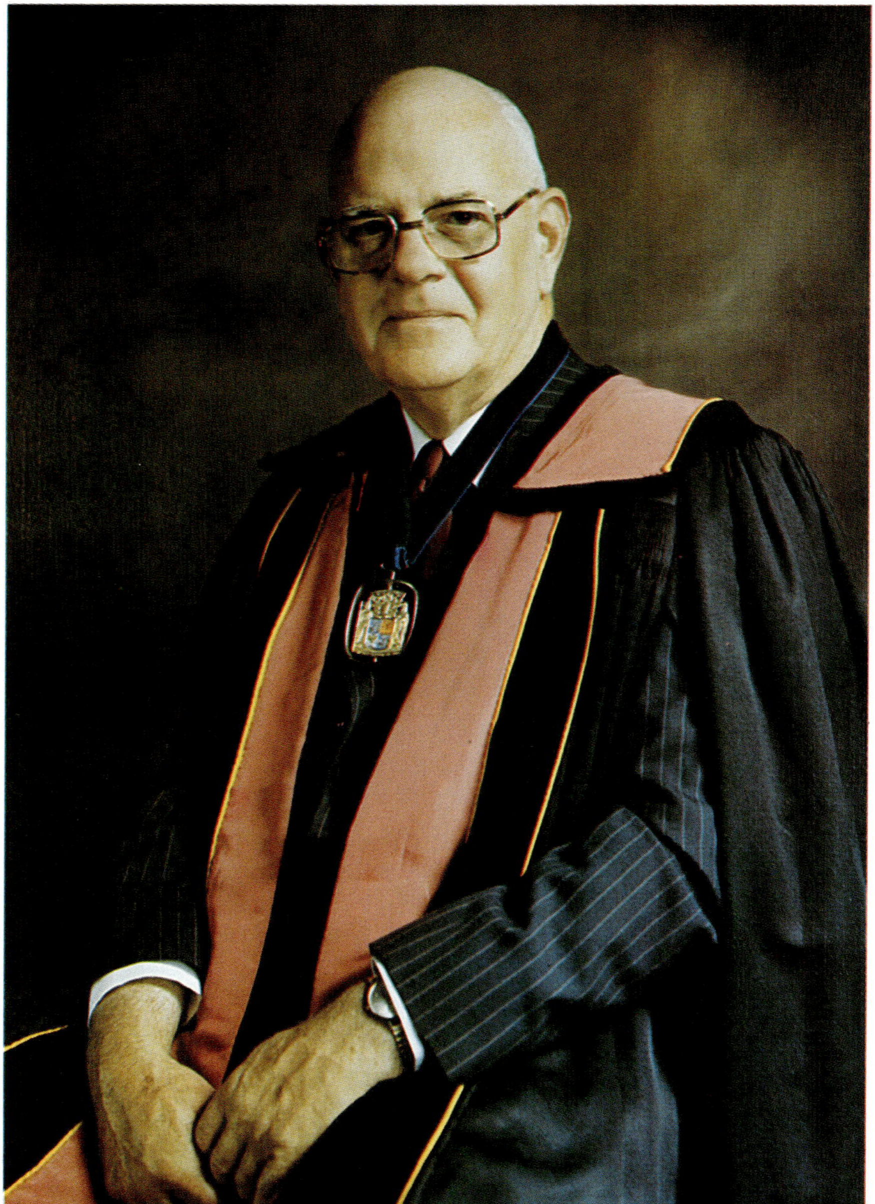

JAMES H. HUTCHISON (1912- )
*President, 1966 to 1968.*
*Portrait by Elliot Robertson, 1978.*

# JAMES (HOLMES) HUTCHISON

CBE, (OBE, 1945), FRCPLond (1947), FRCPEdin (1960), FRCPGlasg (1962), MD (Hons, Glasgow 1938), FRSE (1965)
(1912- )

*The portrait/photograph by Elliot Robertson was made in 1978.*

James Hutchison went to Glasgow High School before proceeding to Glasgow University where he graduated MB,ChB in 1934. After his resident posts he became the McCunn Research Scholar at the Royal Hospital for Sick Children in Glasgow from 1936 to 1938 when he was appointed Assistant Visiting Physician to that hospital. During the Second World War, he served from 1939 to 1945 in the RAMC with the rank of Major and Lieutenant-Colonel and was awarded the OBE (Military) in 1945. After his return to civilian life he became a Physician in charge of wards at Sick Children's Hospital, a Consultant Paediatrician to the Queen Mother's Hospital, Glasgow (Maternity) and the Leonard Gow Lecturer on Medical Diseases of Infancy and Childhood at the University of Glasgow. These posts he held until 1961 when he became the Samson Gemmell Professor of Child Health at the University of Glasgow, in which Chair he continued until his retirement in 1977. Since then he has served for three years as the Professor of Paediatrics in the University of Hong Kong.

He has published many papers on paediatrics and has contributed chapters on various aspects of paediatric medicine to many textbooks, e.g. *British Encyclopaedia of Medical Practice* (2nd edition, 1952), *Paediatrics for the Practitioner* (1953), *Recent Advances in Paediatrics* (1958), *Emergencies in Medical Practice, Textbook of Medical Treatment, Endocrine and Genetic Diseases of Childhood* (1969), *Paediatric Endocrinology* (1969), *Textbook of Paediatrics* (2nd edition, 1978). He is also the author of *Practical Paediatric Problems* (5th edition, 1980).

He has been a member of many Government committees and was Chairman of the Scottish Health Services Council from 1970 to 1974. The British Paediatric Association elected him President from 1969 to 1970 and he was President of the Association of Physicians of Great Britain and Ireland from 1973 to 1974. He was awarded the CBE (Civil) in 1971.

He was President of the Royal College of Physicians and Surgeons of Glasgow from 1966 to 1968.

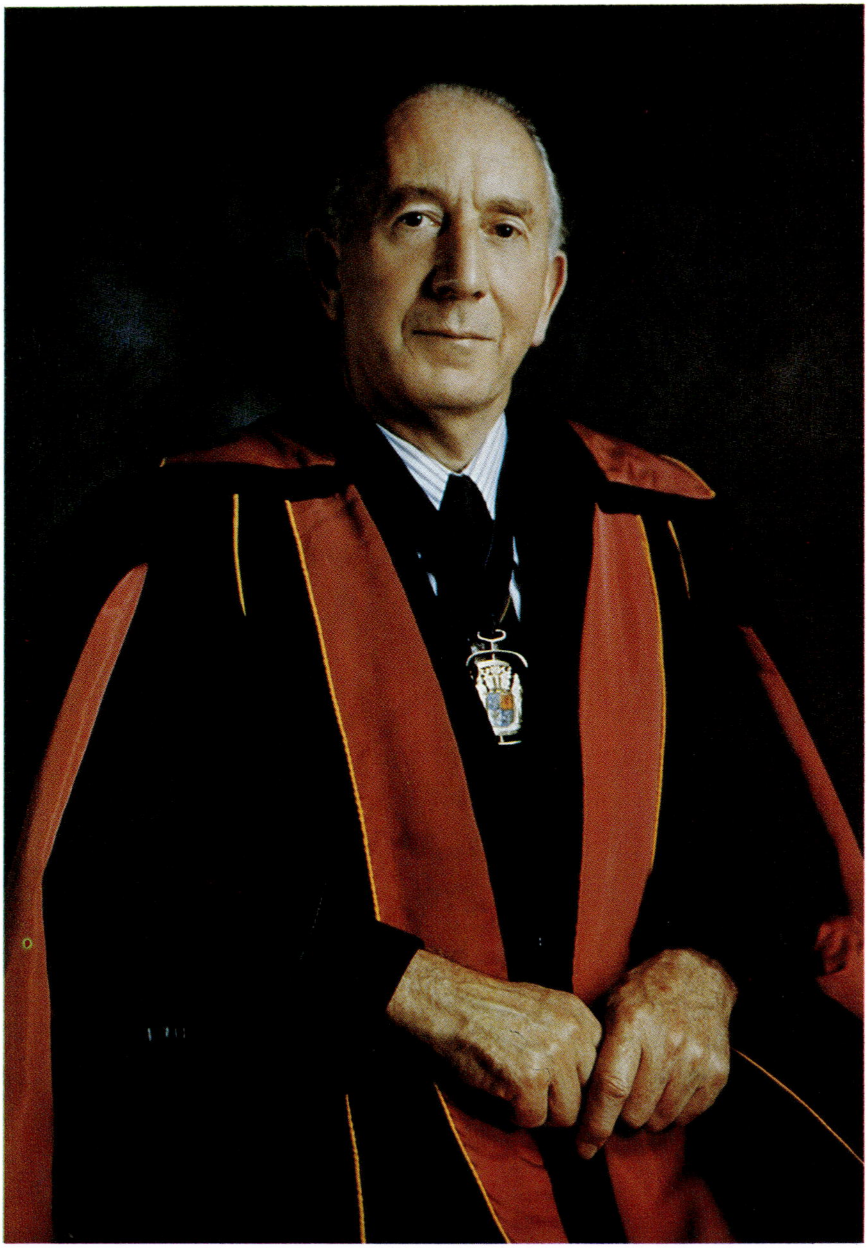

SIR ROBERT B. WRIGHT (1915 to 1981)
*President, 1968 to 1970.*
*Portrait by Elliot Robertson, 1978.*

# SIR ROBERT (BRASH) WRIGHT

1915 to 1981

*The portrait/photograph by Elliot Robertson was made in 1978.*

Robert Wright was educated at Hamilton Academy and Glasgow University where he graduated BSc in 1934, MB,ChB with Honours in 1937, ChM in 1953, and LLD in 1981. He served with distinction in the RAMC from 1939 to 1946 during which he was awarded the OBE (1944) and the DSO (1945). He was an Assistant Surgeon in the Western Infirmary during the post-war years until he was appointed Surgeon in Charge at the Southern General Hospital, Glasgow in 1953, a post which he held until his retirement from the National Health Service in 1980.

He took the Fellowship of the Royal College of Surgeons of Edinburgh in 1947, became a Fellow of the Glasgow College in 1962 and was awarded the Honorary Fellowship of the Royal College of Surgeons of England in 1975 and that of the Australasian College in 1968. He was knighted in 1976.

He was a member of the General Medical Council from 1970, the Chairman of its Disciplinary Committee from 1974 to 1980 and was appointed its President in 1980. He was also a member of the General Dental Council from 1971 to 1980.

He published papers on gastro-enterological topics, vascular disorders and postgraduate education and training.

He was President of the Royal College of Physicians and Surgeons of Glasgow from 1968 to 1970.

*Note:* Sir Robert Wright died on 4th December 1981, not long after he had checked and amended these biographical notes. Obituaries and appreciations of his outstanding career will be found in the *British Medical Journal* of 12th December 1981 and 16th January 1982 and in the *Lancet* of 9th January 1982.

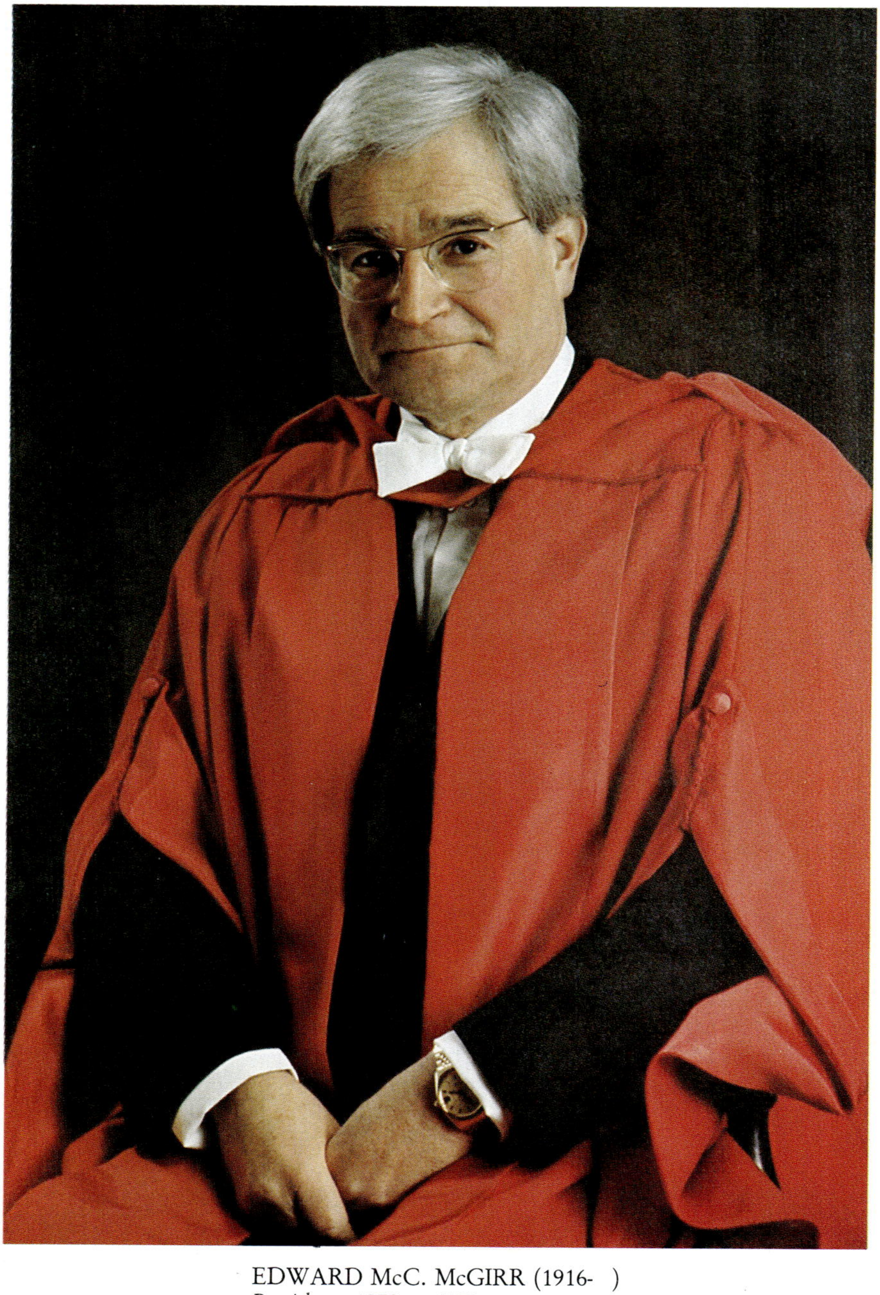

EDWARD McC. McGIRR (1916- )
*President, 1970 to 1972.*
*Portrait by Elliot Robertson, 1978.*

# EDWARD (McCOMBIE) McGIRR

CBE, BSc, MD, FRCPLond, FRCPEdin, FRCPGlasg,
FACP(Hon), FFCM, FRSE
(1916- )

*The portrait/photograph is by Elliot Robertson and was made in 1978.*

Edward McGirr was educated at Hamilton Academy and the University of Glasgow where he graduated BSc in 1937 and MB,ChB (with honours) in 1940. He saw service in the RAMC from 1941 to 1946 in the UK, India, Burma, Siam and Indo-China, latterly as a medical specialist; he was demobilised with the honorary rank of Major. His post-war appointments from 1947 to 1978 were held in the University Department of Medicine, Royal Infirmary, Glasgow where he pursued his clinical interests in general (internal) medicine, endocrinology and nuclear medicine. His main research interest was thyroid disease, particularly dyshormonogenesis. He was appointed to the Muirhead Chair of Medicine in the University of Glasgow in 1961 and was appointed Dean of the Faculty of Medicine in 1974. He resigned from the Muirhead Chair in 1978. From 1978 until his retiral in 1981 he combined the offices of Dean of the Faculty of Medicine and of Administrative Dean. From 1975-1981 he was honorary consultant physician to the army in Scotland.

He has been examiner in medicine in many universities in the UK and overseas and also examiner for the MRCP of the Royal Colleges of Physicians. He delivered the Sir William Gull memorial lecture at Guy's Hospital, London in 1973 and was Harveian Orator of the Harveian Society of Edinburgh in 1979.

His interests in the National Health Service and in postgraduate medical education are reflected in the many committees on which he served and continues to serve, such as Scottish Health Service Planning Council (Chairman 1978- ); Scottish Council for Postgraduate Medical Education (Chairman 1979- ); Greater Glasgow Health Board; General Nursing Council for Scotland; National Board for Scotland for Nursing, Midwifery and Health Visiting; National Radiological Protection Board. Other committees included Scottish Council for the British Medical Association; Joint Consultants Committee and Scottish Joint Consultants Committee; Boards of Management of Glasgow Royal Infirmary and of Glasgow Dental Hospital; Joint

Committee for Higher Medical Training and its specialty advisory committee in endocrinology; West of Scotland Committee for Medical Education; Scottish Committee for Hospital Medical Services; National Medical Consultative Committee; Medical Subcommittee of the University Grants Committee; Medical Advisory Committee of the Vice-Chancellors and Principals; Medical Appeals Tribunal.

He is a member of many learned societies: Association of Physicians of Great Britain and Ireland (member of the editorial panel of the *Quarterly Journal of Medicine*, 1968-1976 and member of Council 1972-1976); Scottish Society of Physicians; Scottish Society for Experimental Medicine (treasurer 1960-66); American Thyroid Association (corresponding member); Medical Research Society (member of Council 1967-69); Royal Medico-Chirurgical Society of Glasgow (President 1965-1966); Harveian Society of Edinburgh (President 1979).

His publications are mainly in the fields of thyroid disease, nuclear medicine and medical education.

He was President of the Royal College of Physicians and Surgeons of Glasgow from 1970 to 1972.

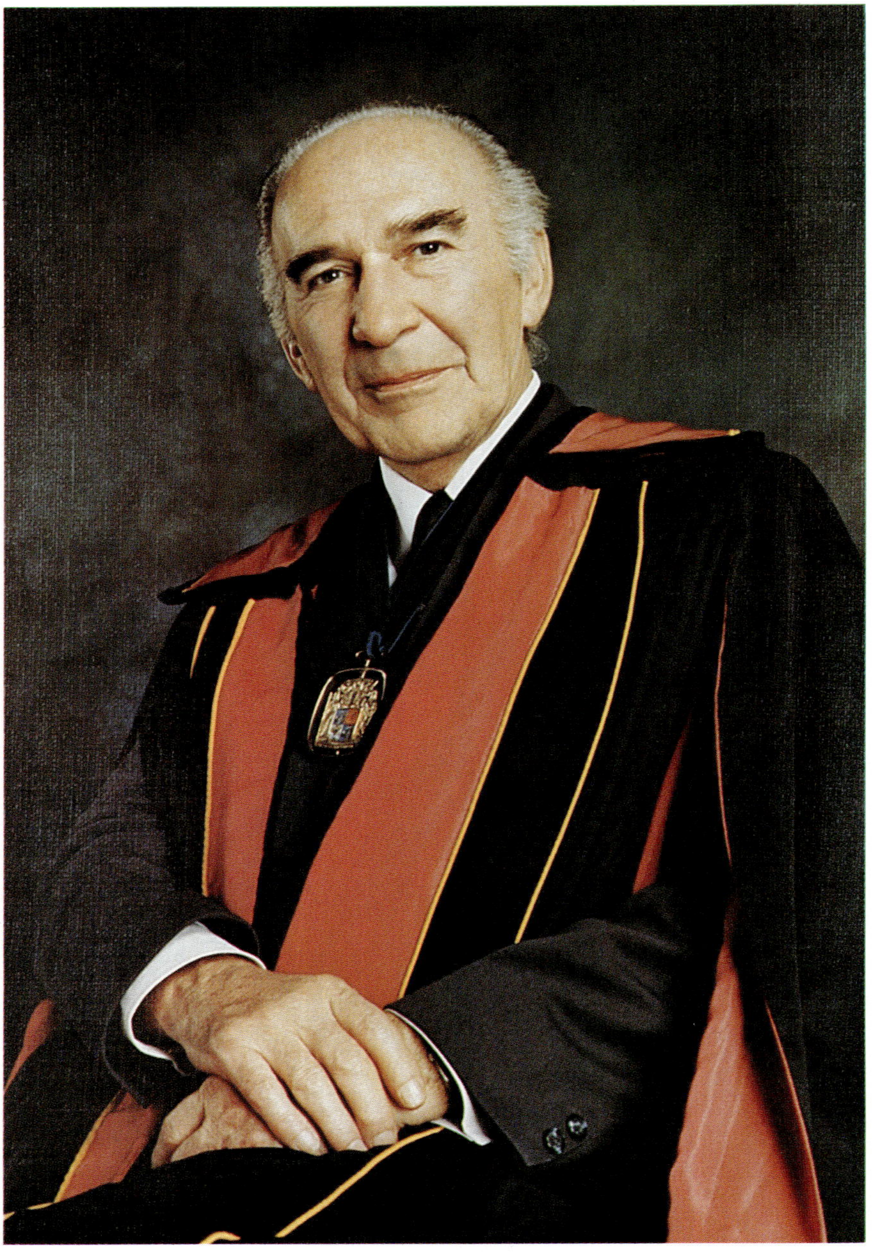

SIR ANDREW WATT KAY (1916- )
*President, 1972 to 1974.*
*Portrait by Elliot Robertson, 1978.*

# SIR ANDREW WATT KAY

(1916- )

*The portrait/photograph by Elliot Robertson was made in 1978.*

Andrew Kay was educated at Ayr Academy and Glasgow University where he graduated MB,ChB with Honours and received the Brunton Memorial Prize in 1939. He was awarded the MD with Honours and the Bellahouston Gold Medal in 1944, and the ChM with Honours in 1949. His assistantship to the Regius Professor of Surgery in Glasgow University from 1942 to 1956 was interrupted by military service; from 1946 to 1948 he was a Major in the RAMC in charge of the Surgical Division of Millbank Military Hospital in London. In 1956 he became Consultant Surgeon in charge of wards in Glasgow Western Infirmary. Two years later he went to Sheffield where he was Professor of Surgery in the University until he succeeded Sir Charles Illingworth (*q.v.*) as the Regius Professor of Surgery in Glasgow University in 1964. Since 1973 he has been part-time Chief Scientist to the Scottish Home and Health Department. He is a Fellow of all the Surgical Colleges in the UK: Edinburgh, 1942; Glasgow, 1956; England, 1960. In addition he is Honorary Fellow of the Australasian College of Surgeons (1970), the Canadian College of Physicians and Surgeons (1972), the College of Surgeons of South Africa and the American College of Surgeons. He has travelled extensively and in 1969 was the Sims Travelling Fellow to Australasia and the following year the McLaughlin Foundation Edward Gallie Visiting Professor in Canada; in addition he is an Honorary Member of the North Pacific Surgical Association, the Belgian Surgical Association and the American Surgical Association. Apart from the prizes noted above, he has been awarded the Cecil Joll Prize of the Royal College of Surgeons of England (1969), the Gordon-Taylor Lectureship and Medal (1970), and has received the honorary degree of DSc from Leicester (1973), Sheffield (1975), Manchester (1981) and Nebraska (1981) Universities. The honorary degree of MD was conferred by the University of Edinburgh in 1981. He was knighted in 1973.

His interests in research and education are illustrated by his presidency of the Surgical Research Society (1969-71) and his membership of the Royal Commission on Medical Education (1965-68) and of the Medical Research Council (1967-71).

He has published several papers on gastro-enterological subjects and is co-author (with R. A. Jamieson) of the *Textbook of Surgical Physiology* (1959, 1964).

He was President of the Royal College of Physicians and Surgeons of Glasgow from 1972 to 1974.

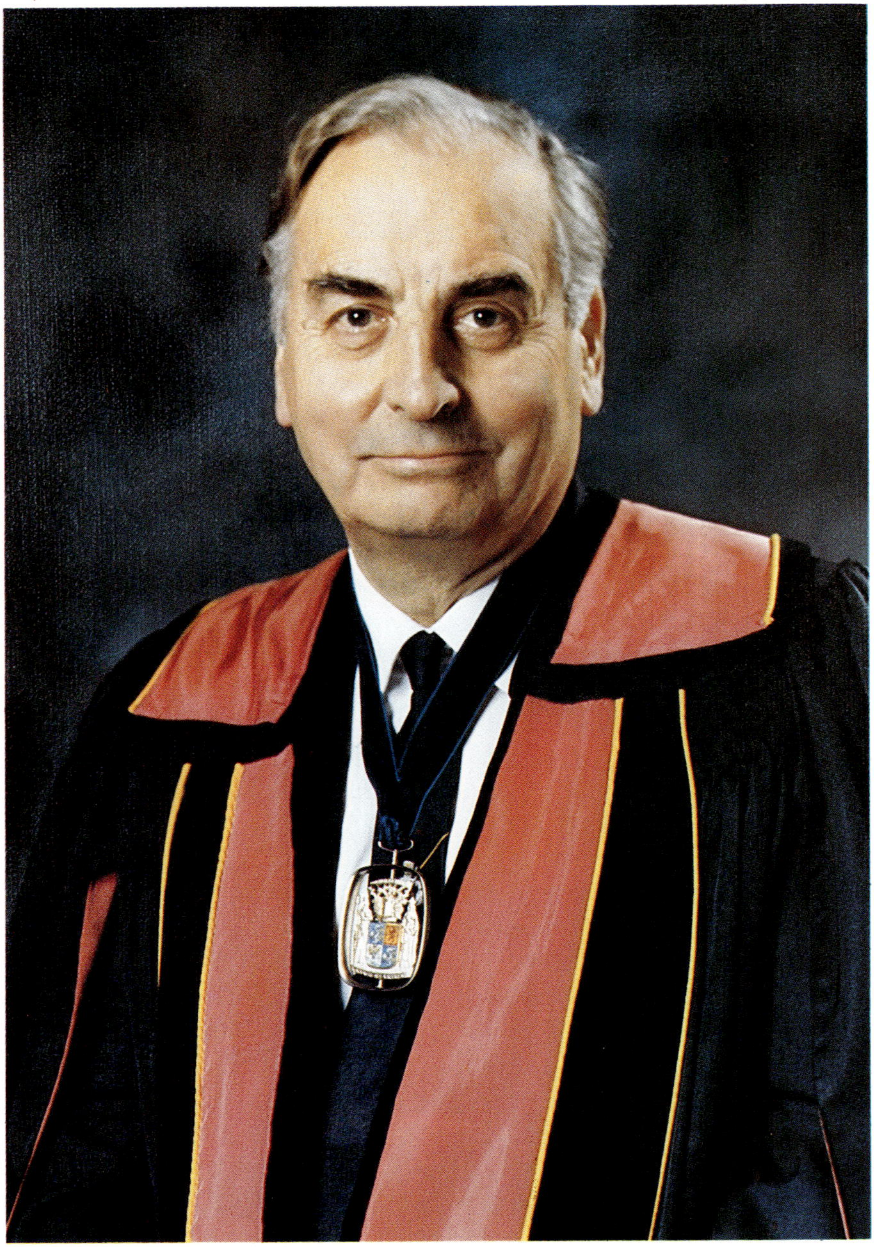

SIR W. FERGUSON ANDERSON (1914- )
*President, 1974 to 1976.*
*Portrait by Elliot Robertson, 1978.*

# SIR (WILLIAM) FERGUSON ANDERSON

(1914- )

*The portrait/photograph by Elliot Robertson was made in 1978.*

Ferguson Anderson spent his schooldays at Merchiston Castle School and Glasgow Academy and graduated MB,ChB with honours at Glasgow University in 1936. He was awarded the MD with honours of Glasgow University in 1942 (with the Bellahouston Gold Medal) and subsequently became a Fellow of all three Colleges of Physicians and an Honorary Fellow of the Irish, Canadian and American Colleges. He was a Medical Specialist in the RAMC with the eventual rank of Major from 1941 to 1946 and on returning to civilian life was appointed Senior Lecturer in the Department of Materia Medica and Therapeutics in the University of Glasgow, and Assistant Physician to the University Medical Clinic in Stobhill Hospital. In 1949 he went to Cardiff for a three-year stay as Senior Lecturer in the Medical Unit and Honorary Consultant Physician to Cardiff Royal Infirmary. On returning to Glasgow in 1952, he became Physician in Geriatric Medicine to Stobhill Hospital and Adviser in Diseases of Old Age and Chronic Sickness to the Western Regional Hospital Board. In 1965 he was appointed the first David Cargill Professor of Geriatric Medicine in Glasgow University, a post which he held until his retirement in 1979.

He did much to improve the lot of the elderly sick: thus, he was Chairman of the Glasgow Retirement Council, Chairman of the Marie Curie Foundation, Strathclyde House, Honorary Chairman of St Mungo's Old Folks Club in Glasgow, and for this and other work he was awarded the St Mungo Prize by the City of Glasgow in 1971.

He has published many papers on Geriatric Medicine and Preventive Aspects of Geriatrics and is the author of *Practical Management of the Elderly*, 2nd Edition (1971) and jointly with B. Isaacs of *Current Achievements in Geriatrics* (1964).

He was awarded the OBE in 1961 and became a Knight of St John in 1974.

He was President of the Royal College of Physicians and Surgeons of Glasgow from 1974 to 1976.

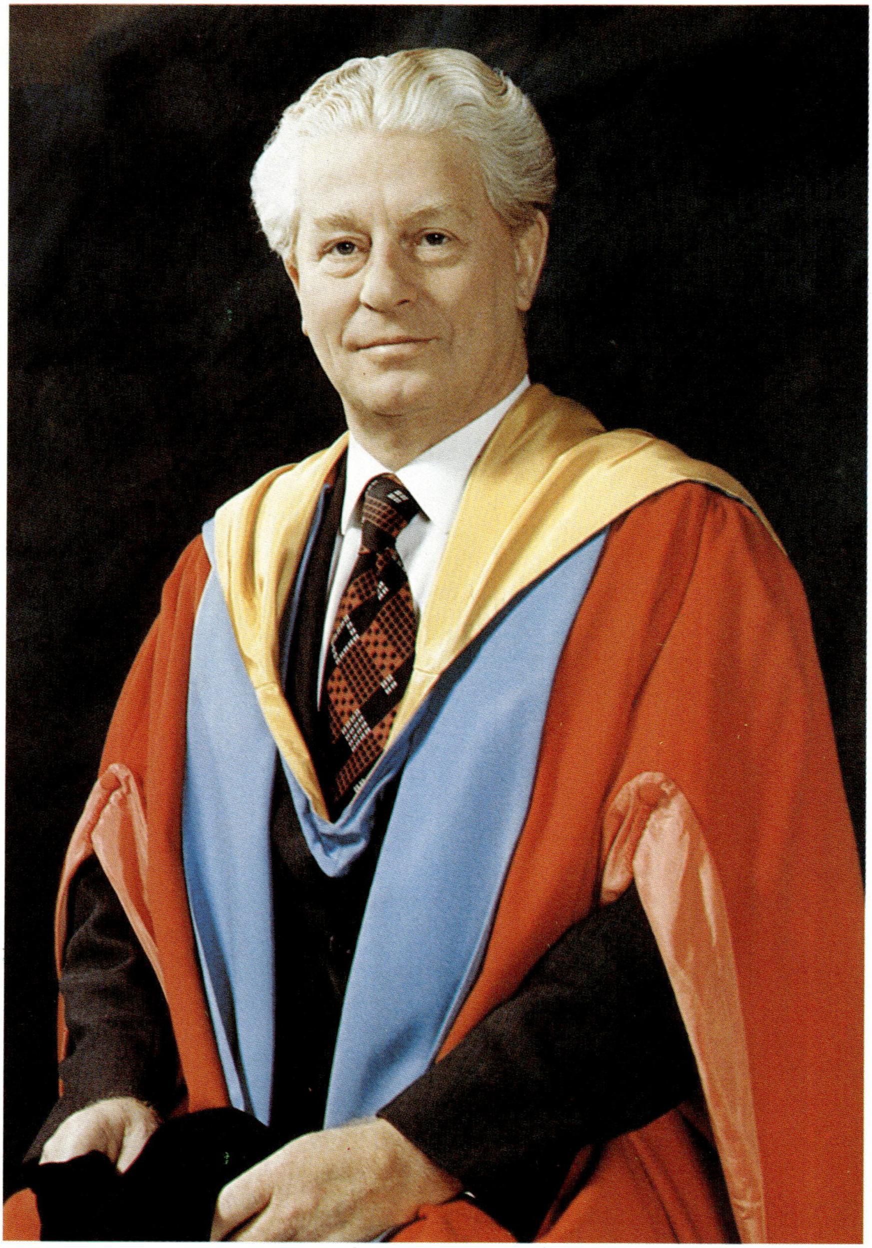

TOM GIBSON (1915- )
*President, 1976 to 1978.*
*Portrait by Elliot Robertson, 1977.*

# THOMAS GIBSON

DSc, MB, FRCSGlasg, FRCSEdin,
FRACS(Hon), FRSE
(1915- )

*The portrait/photograph was commissioned from Elliot Robertson by Strathclyde University in 1977 for the Wolfson Centre of Bioengineering and it is for this reason that the DSc gown of Strathclyde University is worn. It was this portrait which inspired Council to record similarly the surviving Past Presidents of the College and if possible continue the practice with future Presidents.*

Tom Gibson had his schooling in Kilbarchan School and Paisley Grammar School, proceeded to Glasgow University and graduated MB,ChB in 1938. He became a Fellow of the Royal College of Surgeons of Edinburgh in 1941. From 1942 to 1944 he was assistant surgeon to the Medical Research Council in their Unit in the Burns Wards of Glasgow Royal Infirmary. In 1944 he joined the RAMC as a surgical specialist in maxillofacial surgery and served first with No. 5 Maxillofacial Surgical Unit in North Europe and latterly as OC No.1 Indian Maxillofacial Unit. After demobilisation he was appointed Consultant Plastic Surgeon to the West of Scotland Plastic and Oral Surgery Service and was its Director from 1970 to 1980 when he retired.

He became associated with Dr (later Professor) R. M. Kenedi of Strathclyde University's Engineering Department in the early 1960s and from this collaboration there developed the present Bioengineering Centre. He was appointed in 1970 as their Visiting Professor and continues to serve in this capacity. Strathclyde University awarded him their honorary DSc in 1972.

For some years he was a member of Council of the British Association of Plastic Surgeons, became their President in 1970 and was the Editor of their official organ, the *British Journal of Plastic Surgery*, from 1969 to 1979.

His publications are on tissue immunology, burns, bioengineering and various aspects of plastic surgery including its history.

He became a Fellow of the Royal Faculty of Physicians and Surgeons of Glasgow in 1955, the Honorary Librarian and a member of Council from 1964 to 1974 and is now the Honorary Curator of the Art Collection. As the College's representative at the Jubilee celebrations of the Royal Australasian College of Surgeons, he was awarded their Honorary Fellowship.

Tom Gibson was President of the Royal College of Physicians and Surgeons of Glasgow from 1976 to 1978.

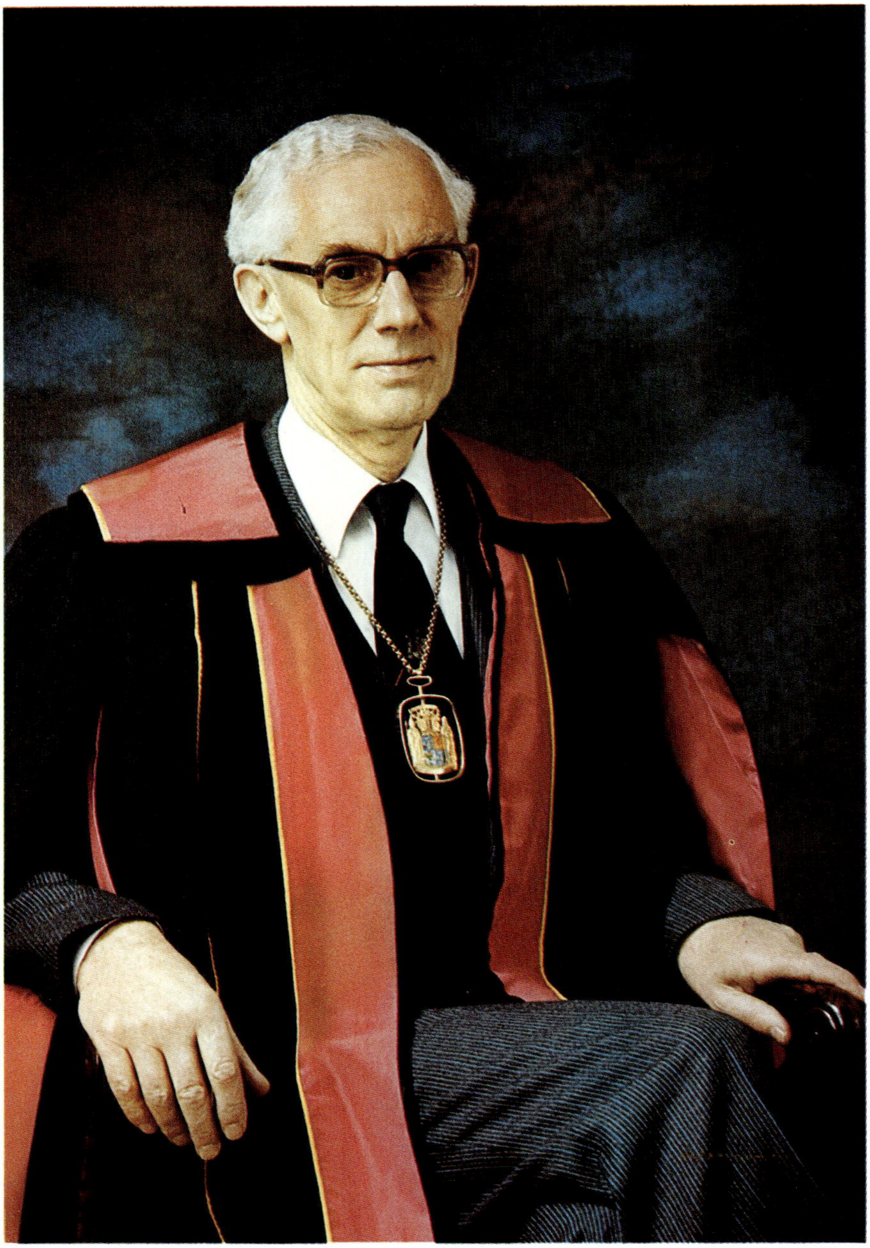

GAVIN B. SHAW (1919- )
*President, 1978 to 1980.*
*Portrait by Elliot Robertson, 1981.*

# GAVIN (BROWN) SHAW

CBE, BSc, MB,ChB, FRCPGlasg, FRCPLond, FRCPEdin, FRCPIrel(Hon), FACP(Hon), FRCPsych(Hon), FRCGP(Hon)
(1919- )

*The portrait/photograph was made by Elliot Robertson in 1978.*

Gavin Shaw received his education in Glasgow Academy and Glasgow University where he graduated BSc in 1939 and MB,ChB in 1942. He served in the Royal Naval Volunteer Reserve from 1943 to 1946 and in the last year was a Specialist in Laboratory Medicine. On his return to civilian life he was Clinical Tutor in Medicine to the Regius Professor at Glasgow University, Sir John McNee, until 1948 when he became Senior Registrar in Medicine in the Southern General Hospital. Appointed Consultant Physician with duties in cardiology in 1956, he was further promoted to Consultant Physician and Cardiologist in Charge of Wards in the Southern General Hospital in 1963, a post which he still holds.

He is a Fellow of all the Royal Colleges of Physicians of the UK, an Honorary Fellow of the American College of Physicians (1979) and of the Royal College of Physicians of Ireland (1979). In 1980, he was awarded the Honorary FRCPsych and the Honorary FRCGP.

His main clinical interests have been in the field of cardiology including coronary care and the use of pacemakers, and his many scientific papers reflect these. He has been deeply involved in undergraduate and postgraduate education, as a member and chairman of a number of committees set up to promote such teaching, and to organise courses, closed and open circuit television programmes, symposia and examinations. He has been an examiner in the MB,ChB Final Examination of Glasgow University since 1968 and examines in cardiology and internal medicine for the MRCP in Glasgow, Edinburgh and London. He is a member of the National Medical Consultative Committee, its Executive, and its sub-committees for Medicine. He was awarded the CBE in 1980.

His long association in office in the Royal College of Physicians and Surgeons started when he was a Member of Council from 1953 to 1957 when he became Honorary Secretary until 1965. He returned to the Council for a second four-year period from 1970 to 1974 and continued to serve on College committees until he was elected Visitor in 1976 and subsequently President from 1978 to 1980.

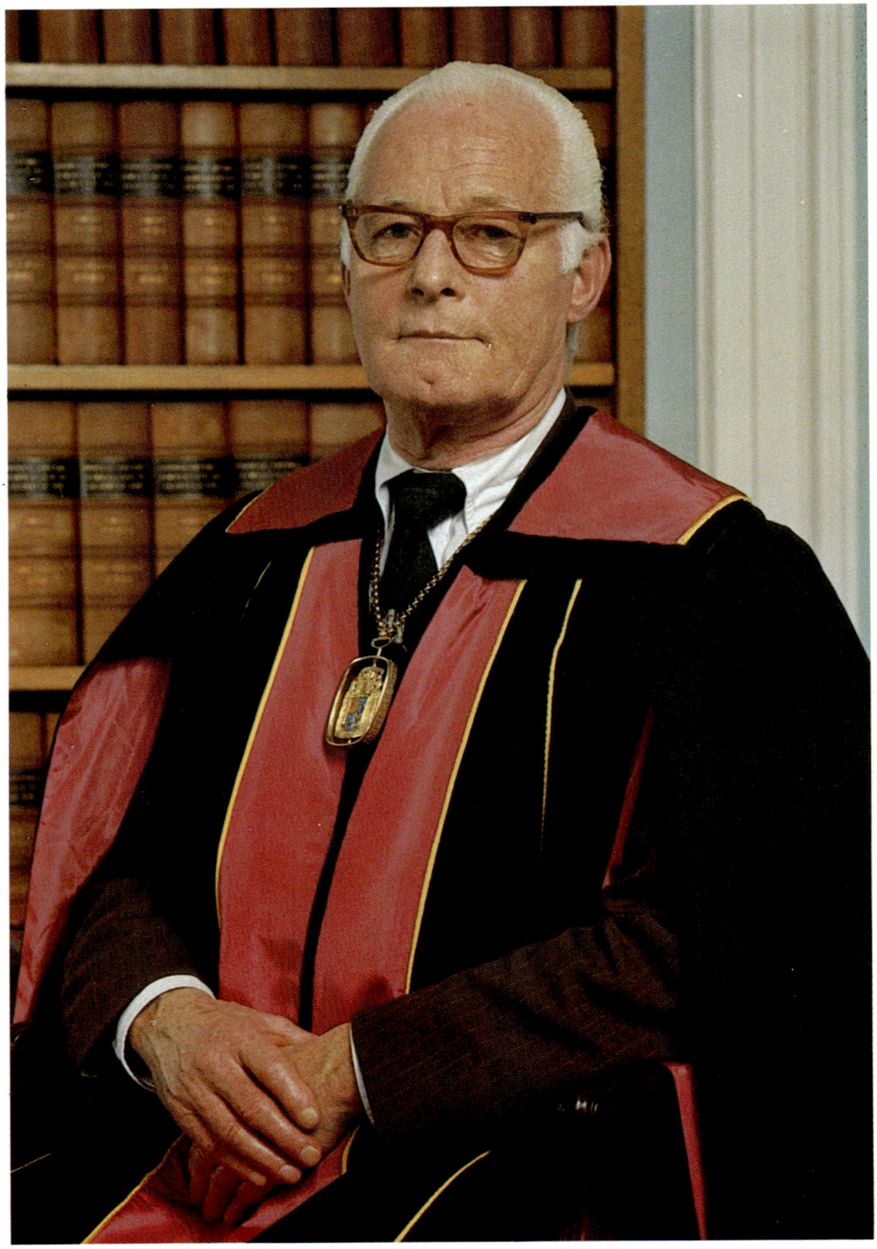

DOUGLAS H. CLARK (1917- )
*President, 1980 to 1982.*
*Portrait by Elliot Robertson, 1982.*

# DOUGLAS (HENDERSON) CLARK

MD, ChM, FRCSEd, FRCSGlasg, FRCSEng(Hon), FRCSIrel(Hon), FCS SA(Hon), FRCPEd
(1917- )

*The portrait/photograph by Elliot Robertson was made in 1982.*

Douglas Clark was born in Ayrshire and after his schooling at Ayr Academy, and with the aid of bursaries from the Rainy Foundation and the Miners Welfare, took the medical course at Glasgow University and graduated there MB,ChB in 1940. A residency post with the recently appointed Professor of Surgery in Glasgow University, Charles (later Sir) Illingworth, was followed by a period of almost six years army service in Britain, India, Burma and Malaysia. After demobilisation he rejoined the surgical professional unit in the Western Infirmary in 1948 as a Senior Registrar, having acquired the Fellowship of the Royal College of Surgeons of Edinburgh and that of the Royal Faculty of Physicians and Surgeons of Glasgow. His researches into peptic ulceration led to a ChM in 1950 and MD with Honours in 1957. He became a consultant surgeon to the Western Infirmary in 1953 and remained so for the rest of his professional life.

In 1952 he was appointed the 'William Stewart Halsted Fellow' to the Johns Hopkins Hospital in Baltimore. Here he made many international friends including Dr 'Tommy' Johns of Richmond, Virginia, whom the College created an Honorary Fellow in 1975, and with whom he exchanged surgical trainees for many years.

Douglas Clark has travelled much: as guest lecturer and visiting professor in Richmond, Virginia; Duke University, North Carolina; UCLA; Queensland University; Stellenbosch University, South Africa; Vanderbilt University, Nashville, USA; Johns Hopkins University, Baltimore; and as President of the Royal College roving around South Africa, Hong Kong, Malaysia and Australia.

He is widely acknowledged as an excellent under- and post-graduate surgical teacher. Recently, many of his younger colleagues and assistants subscribed to have his portrait painted by Alexander Goudie and he is or has been an external examiner in surgery in Sheffield, Leeds, Aberdeen, Edinburgh, Manchester, Belfast and Liverpool.

In addition to being awarded Honorary Fellowships from the Surgical Colleges of England, Ireland and South Africa, he is also a Fellow of the Royal College of Physicians of Edinburgh and a Member of the Academy of Medicine of Singapore. He is now Director of that most prestigious surgical travelling club 'The James IV Association of Surgeons'.

His extensive writings have been mainly on gastro-enterology and thyroid disease.

Douglas Clark was President from 1980 to 1982.

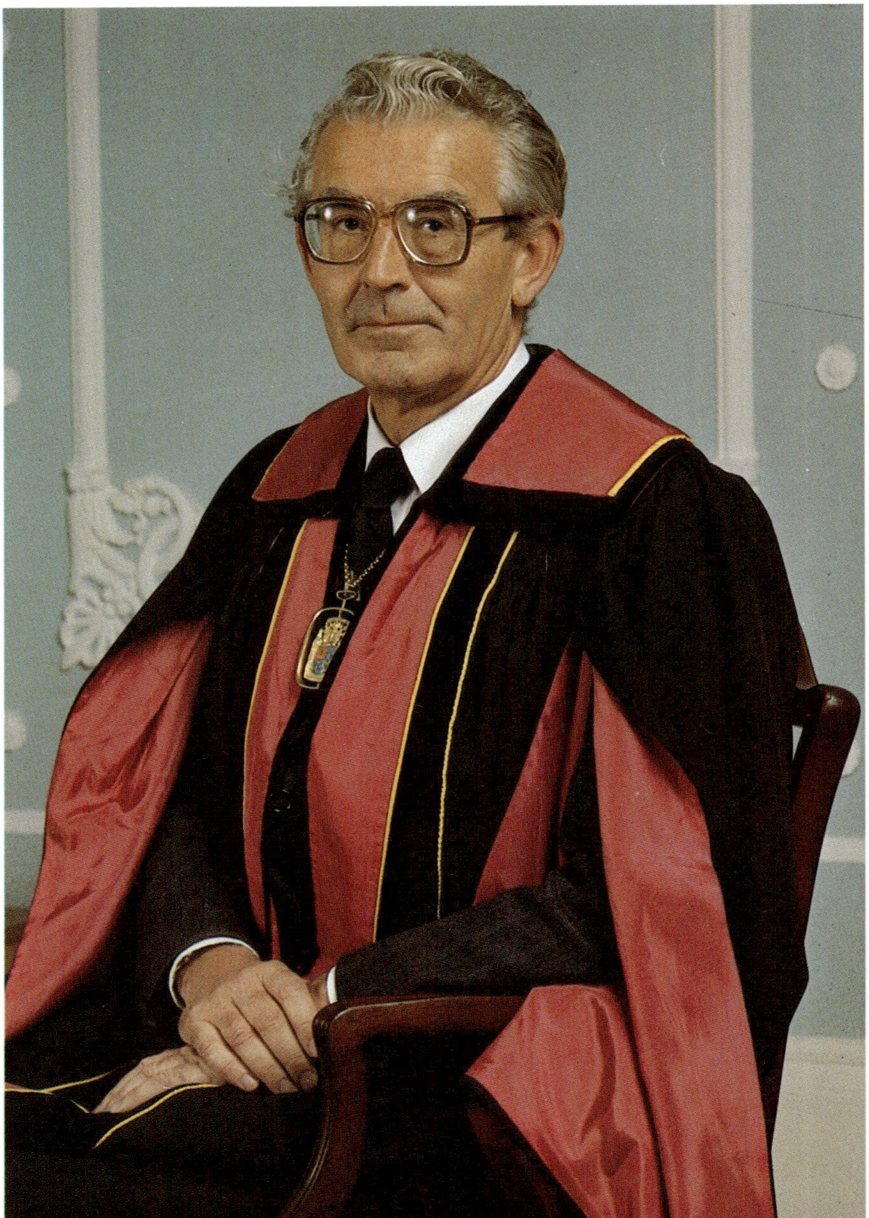

THOMAS J. THOMSON
*President, 1982*
*Portrait by Elliot Robertson, 1982.*

# THOMAS (JAMES) THOMSON

OBE, FRFPSGlasg 1949, FRCPGlasg 1964,
FRCPLond 1969, FRCPEdin 1981

*The portrait/photograph by Elliot Robertson was made in 1982.*

Thomas Thomson was born in Airdrie in 1923 and was educated in Airdrie Academy and later in Glasgow University where he graduated MB,ChB in 1945. His main interest has always been the practice and teaching of clinical medicine and he has held posts in clinical medicine in teaching hospitals continuously since 1948. In 1953 he became a Lecturer in the Department of Materia Medica of Glasgow University until 1961 when he was created Honorary Lecturer. He is now Consultant Physician and Consultant Gastroenterologist to Stobhill General Hospital in Glasgow.

In addition to teaching undergraduates in clinical medicine and materia medica, he has been intensely interested in postgraduate training and was Postgraduate Clinical Tutor to the Glasgow Northern Hospitals from 1961 to 1981. The same interest led to his appointment as Honorary Secretary of the Royal College of Physicians and Surgeons of Glasgow from 1965 to 1973 when he was deeply involved in the organisation of the College's postgraduate activities.

His administrative abilities have been widely recognised and he was Secretary of the Specialist Advisory Committee for General Internal Medicine for the United Kingdom from 1970 to 1974, and Chairman of the Medico-Pharmaceutical Forum from 1978 to 1980. At present he is Chairman of both the Conference of Royal Colleges and Faculties in Scotland and the National Medical Consultative Committee of Scotland. In addition he takes an active part in postgraduate medical educational committees, locally, nationally and internationally.

His many publications have been mainly concerned with materia medica, clinical pharmacology and gastroenterology and he has contributed to and/or acted as joint editor to several well known textbooks of medical treatment and gastroenterology. He was awarded the OBE in 1978.

He became President of the Royal College of Physicians and Surgeons of Glasgow in 1982.

# INDEX

The subjects of the portraits are in capitals. The reproduction of the portrait faces the first page of each biographical sketch. References to other illustrations or their captions are given by the page number.